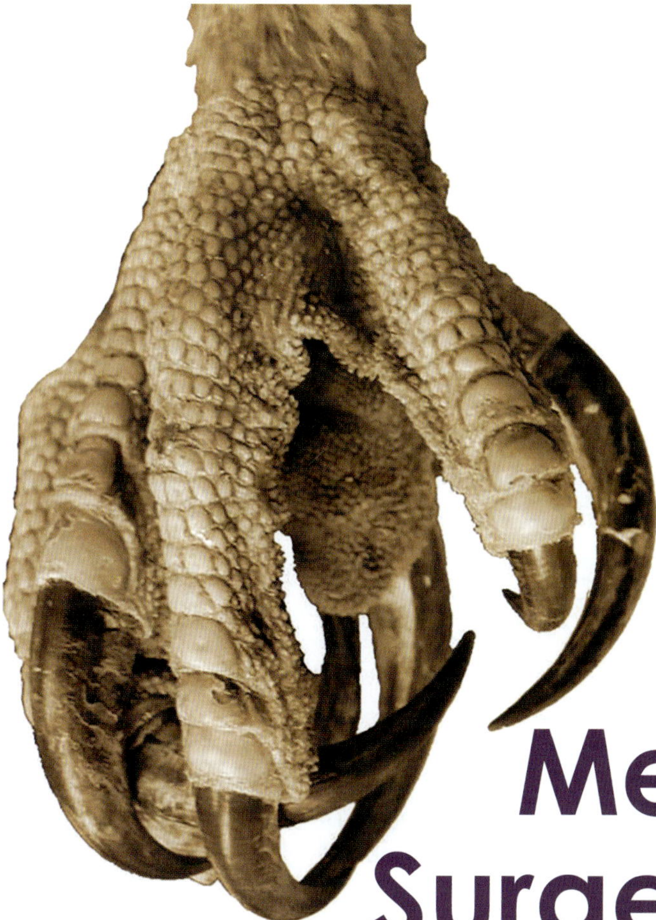

Raptor Medicine, Surgery, and Rehabilitation

3rd Edition

Raptor Medicine, Surgery, and Rehabilitation

3rd Edition

David E. Scott, DVM

Staff Veterinarian, Carolina Raptor Center, Charlotte, North Carolina, USA

CABI

CABI is a trading name of CAB International

CABI
Nosworthy Way
Wallingford
Oxfordshire OX10 8DE
UK

Tel: +44 (0)1491 832111
Fax: +44 (0)1491 833508
E-mail: info@cabi.org
Website: www.cabi.org

CABI
WeWork
One Lincoln St
24th Floor
Boston, MA 02111
USA

Tel: +1 (617)682-9015
E-mail: cabi-nao@cabi.org

A catalogue record for this book is available from the British Library, London, UK.

Library of Congress Cataloging-in-Publication Data

Names: Scott, David E., 1966- author.
Title: Raptor medicine, surgery, and rehabilitation / David E. Scott, DVM, Staff Veterinarian, Carolina Raptor Center, Charlotte, North Carolina, USA.
Description: Third edition. | Wallingford, Oxfordshire ; Boston, MA : CAB International, [2020] | Includes bibliographical references and index. | Summary: "Comprehensive and extensively illustrated, this book accumulates years of practical knowledge when dealing with injured birds of prey. It outlines everything from handling and the intake examination through to practical procedures and the treatment of a range of conditions and injuries, as well as advice on housing, rehabilitation and release"-- Provided by publisher.
Identifiers: LCCN 2020023974 (print) | LCCN 2020023975 (ebook) | ISBN 9781789246100 (hardback) | ISBN 9781789246117 (ebook) | ISBN 9781789246124 (epub)
Subjects: LCSH: Birds of prey--Diseases. | Birds of prey--Surgery.
Classification: LCC SF994.5 .S36 2020 (print) | LCC SF994.5 (ebook) | DDC 639.97/89--dc23
LC record available at https://lccn.loc.gov/2020023974
LC ebook record available at https://lccn.loc.gov/2020023975

References to Internet websites (URLs) were accurate at the time of writing.

ISBN-13: 9781789246100 (hardback)
9781789246117 (ePDF)
9781789246124 (ePub)

Commissioning Editor: Alex Lainsbury
Editorial Assistant: Lauren Davies/Emma McCann
Production Editor: Shankari Wilford

Typeset by SPi, Pondicherry, India
Printed and bound in the UK by Bell & Bain Ltd, Glasgow

Contents

About the Author

David Scott is the staff veterinarian at the Carolina Raptor Center in Charlotte, North Carolina, USA.

He received his BS Electrical Engineering from the University of Illinois in 1988 and DVM from the University of Illinois in 1997, and has worked with many wildlife rehabilitation groups since then.

He is also a software engineer and has developed the RaptorMed™ medical records software (www.raptormed.com) specifically designed for the medical management and husbandry of all types of animals. It is used at rehabilitation centers, in aquariums, and for permanent collections all over the world.

Foreword

This book is not intended to be a complete reference for avian practice or for the rehabilitation of birds of prey. Instead, it has been written by a practicing veterinarian as a helpful and concise, day-to-day, clinical handbook. The intended audience is anyone new to raptor rehabilitation as well as the seasoned veterinarian, technician, or rehabilitator who needs a refresher or a quick reference.

There are many great references listed in this book. I used many of them extensively when researching this book and I continue to use them regularly in my practice.

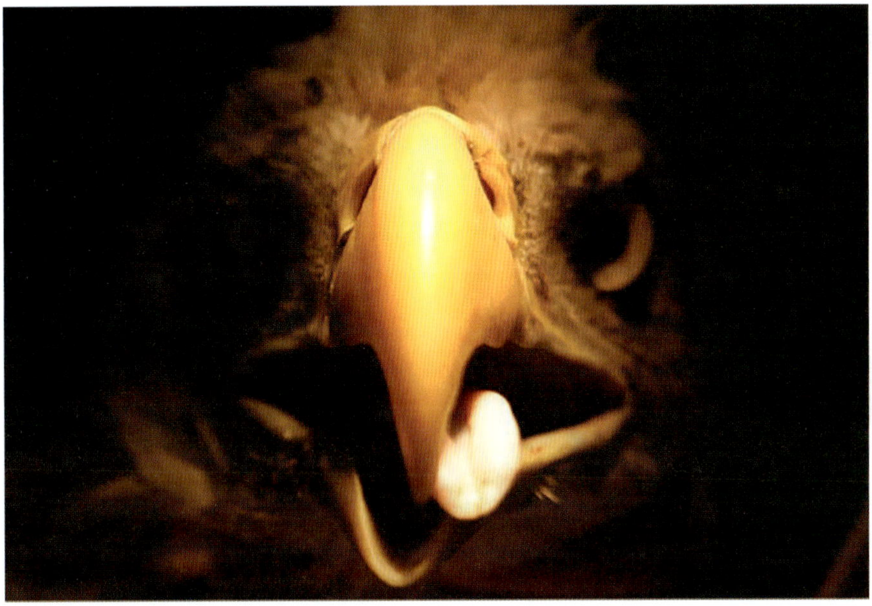

rap•tor | raptər |
noun
a bird of prey, e.g. an eagle, hawk, falcon, or owl.
ORIGIN late Middle English: from Latin, literally "plunderer", from ***rapt- "seized"***, from the verb ***rapere***.[1]

[1]Dictionary, Mac OSX version 2.2.1 (accessed February 2016).

Acknowledgments

To Carolina Raptor Center and the many volunteers—for providing me with an incredible place to work and learn.

To Dr Michelle Hawkins (Veterinary Ophthalmology Service, University of California, Davis, CA) and Dr Ralph Hamor (Comparative Ophthalmology Service, University of Illinois, Urbana, IL)—for supplying some great images of retinas.

To Carly Smith, Katie Kissel, and Ashley Whitesell, DVM—for assisting in the laborious research that went into producing the Species Overview in Chapter 3.

To Mathias and Carly—the most amazing, caring, and hard-working people I have ever met. This book would not have been possible without your daily support and friendship.

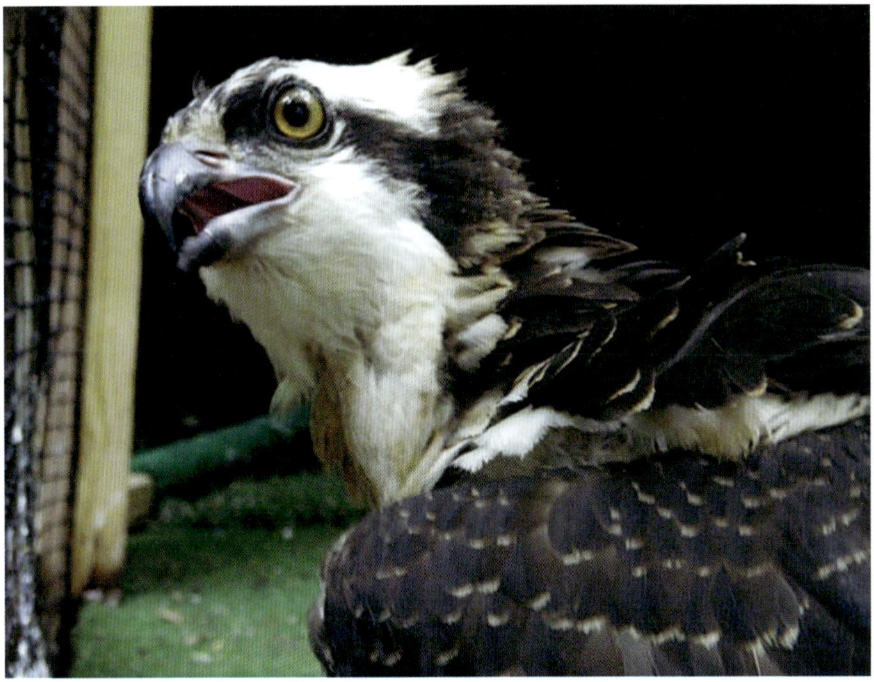

Abbreviations

BAR	bright, alert, and responsive
BID	twice daily, q12h
BW	body weight
CBC	complete blood count
D5W	dextrose in 5% water
E3D	every third day
EOD	every other day
EPH	protein electrophoresis
ESF	external skeletal fixator
ET	endotracheal
GI	gastrointestinal
IC	intracardiac
IM	intramedullary
IM	intramuscular
IO	intraosseous
IT	intratracheal
IV	intravenous
LRS	lactated Ringer's solution
NPO	nothing per os
NSAID	non-steroidal anti-inflammatory drug
PCR	polymerase chain reaction
PCV	packed cell volume
PLR	pupillary light reflex
PO	per os (given orally)
PRN	as needed
PT	physical therapy
QAR	quiet, alert, and responsive
QID	four times daily, q6h
q3d	every third day
qxd	every x days
q4h	every 4 h
qxh	every x hours

RBC	red blood cell
ROM	range of motion
SC	subcutaneous
SID	once daily, q24h
SQ	subcutaneous
TID	three times daily, q8h
TP	total protein
TS	total solids
URT	upper respiratory tract
VI	virus isolation
WBC	white blood cell

1 Handling and Physical Examination

Birds of prey are actually quite easy to work with if you have the proper training and a little experience. On the other hand, they can be incredibly dangerous if handled improperly. As with all wild animals, it is important to work fast and to minimize stress whenever working with birds of prey. Proper handling techniques and being prepared can go a long way to help create a safe and stress-free interaction.

Learning Objectives

1. Proper handling techniques.
2. Performing a physical exam.
3. Intake protocols for common problems.

Handling and Restraint

Proper restraint is important for the patient's well-being and for staff safety. Always remember that the talons are in most cases the most dangerous part of the bird and, as such, should be restrained at all times.

Appropriately sized leather gloves should always be worn. They must be thick enough to protect the wearer but not too thick as they can make handling cumbersome.

The legs should be held with the index finger between them. This is more comfortable for the bird (the legs will not rub) and the grip is much more secure (see arrowhead in Fig. 1.1).

The legs should always be grabbed as close to the body as is possible (i.e. above the stifle joints) to avoid iatrogenic fractures. This is especially important in birds with long, thin legs such as Cooper's hawks. Once the bird is adequately restrained, the grip should be moved closer to the feet for better control of the talons.

When transporting a bird, secure the legs with an underhanded grip, cover the bird's head with a towel and place the bird's back to your chest (Fig. 1.1). With your other hand, gently place the towel across the chest (be careful not to interfere with respiration) and hold the beak up. This protects the bird's face from its talons and also restrains both wings.

The eyes and head should be covered with a light towel whenever possible since this will have a calming effect on birds of prey.

Remember to protect your face with one hand when grabbing a bird from a kennel.

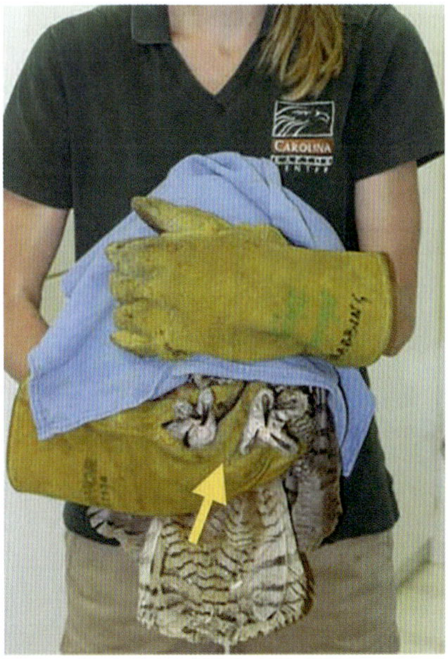

Fig. 1.1. Proper handling for transport.

To decrease stress, consider using isoflurane anesthesia when doing examinations or treatments.

Vultures use their beak for defense so their head must be gently restrained at all times. This can be done by covering the head with a towel and loosely encircling the neck with your fingers just under the mandible.

Young birds should be handled with extreme caution. In most cases these birds should be handled as little as possible, should not be manipulated onto their back unless absolutely necessary and should be transported in a box, rather than hand-carried. *Young birds/hatchlings should never be grabbed by the legs.* Always use a body grab from behind with the wings carefully folded up against the body (see Chapter 12).

Long-handled nets are very useful when capturing birds, but they need to be constructed and used properly to avoid injury. The actual net should be made from solid, lightweight cloth and not from fenestrated net material since the strands can cause serious damage to the feathers. The rim of the net should be padded with foam. Plumbing pipe insulation foam works very well.

Different-sized nets are needed to safely capture all the common species. Nets should range in size from an 18″ (45 cm) net with a 2′ (0.6 m) handle to a 36″ (90 cm) net with a 5′ (1.5 m) handle.

Birds in flight should be netted "cleanly" without allowing their wings to touch the hoop. This can take some practice but is easy once you become accustomed to using the net.

Never swing a net at a bird to capture as this will almost certainly result in injury. Instead, place the net in the bird's path and let it fly into the net.

Physical Examination

Most of the physical exam can be achieved with the bird restrained on its back and a complete exam can be done in less than 10 min. Most procedures involving birds of prey, including examinations, require two people. This allows you to be most efficient, keep staff safe and, most importantly, minimize stress to the patient.

Have all supplies and expected treatments ready before beginning the exam or treatment. Be as quiet as possible. This is a general rule that applies whenever working with wildlife, especially for birds of prey. Give butorphanol or midazolam, if needed, *at the beginning of your exam* for analgesia and as a mild sedative (see Appendix B, Formulary, for dosage). Have a physical exam checklist available to refer to (see Table 1.1).

Try to collect a minimum database as quickly as possible but never try to do too much if the bird is stressed or severely compromised. In many cases it is safer to simply stabilize your patient on admission and stage your workup. Your minimum database may include blood work and/or radiographs.

> **Raptor Tip**
>
> Don't forget to roll the bird over on its sternum to examine the spine and dorsal pelvis.

Although a detailed history is rarely available with wildlife, try to collect as much information regarding where and how the bird was found. If it was transferred from another facility, ask about previous treatments and medications received.

Always record a keel score with the weight (measured in grams) (Fig. 1.2). The keel score, or body condition score, is a measure of the amount of pectoral muscle mass present and is a good indication of the general health status. Keel scores range from 1 to 5. A healthy bird has a score of 3–4. The determination of a keel score requires palpation and a visual assessment. Using alcohol to clear the feathers from the pectoral muscle helps to determine an accurate score.

With a score of 1 or 2, the muscle mass is clearly concave (or non-existent) and the keel bone is extremely prominent. This is an emaciated bird.

With a score of 3, the muscle mass bulges ventrally and is convex.

With a score of 4, the muscle mass comes out almost horizontally from the keel bone.

Table 1.1. Physical examination checklist.

Region/area	Findings	Comments
Weight		
Age	plumage—eye color	
Sex	brood patch—egg—plumage—wing chord	
Behavior	BAR—QAR—lethargic—comatose—neurologic—seizures—habituated—imprinted—unable to stand	
Head	"reading"—tilt—hanging low—wounds—eyes closed	
Mouth (tongue, glottis, choana)	pale—bloody—parasite—cheesy exudate/lesions	
Nares	discharge—bloody—clogged	
Cere	swollen—wound—color	
Beak/jaw	fractured—worn—dirty—cracked—scissor-beak	
Ears	parasites—bloody	
Right eye		
Lids	swollen—wounds—irritated—bruised	
Nicitans	swollen—wounds—irritated—bruised	
Cornea	cloudy—ulcerated—collapsed—perforated	
Anterior chamber	cloudy—fibrinous material—blood clot—synechia	
Lens	cataract—synechia—luxated	
Posterior chamber	blood clot—fibrinous material—chorioretinitis—detachment—craters	
PLR/menace	positive or negative	
Left eye		
Lids	swollen—wounds—irritated—bruised	
Nicitans	swollen—wounds—irritated—bruised	
Cornea	cloudy—ulcerated—collapsed—perforated	
Anterior chamber	cloudy—fibrinous material—blood clot—synechia	
Lens	cataract—synechia—luxated	
Posterior chamber	blood clot—fibrinous material—chorioretinitis—detachment—craters	
PLR/menace	positive or negative	
Body		
Crop	full—empty—sour	
Neck	bruised—wounds	
Keel	bruised—wounds	
Keel score	1 2 3 4 5	
Keel fat	yes or no	
Furcular fat	yes or no	
Abdominal fat	yes or no	

Continued

Table 1.1. Continued.

Region/area	Findings	Comments
Back/spine	bruised—wounds	
Pelvis	bruised—wounds	
Vent	soiled—bloody—flaccid	
Right wing	drooped	
Coracoid/ scapula/clavicle	fracture (open, closed)—wounds—subcutaneous air—swelling—bruised	
Humerus	fracture (open, closed)—wounds—subcutaneous air—swelling—bruised	
Elbow	swollen—wounds—dislocated—poor ROM	
Ulna/radius	fracture (open, closed)—wounds—swelling—bruised	
Wrist	swollen—wounds—dislocated—poor ROM	
Metacarpals	fracture (open, closed)—wounds—swelling—bruised	
Feathers	soiled—frayed—tipped—broken—in blood	
Left wing	drooped	
Coracoid/ scapula/clavicle	fracture (open, closed)—wounds—subcutaneous air—swelling—bruised	
Humerus	fracture (open, closed)—wounds—subcutaneous air—swelling—bruised	
Elbow	swollen—wounds—dislocated—poor ROM	
Ulna/radius	fracture (open, closed)—wounds—swelling—bruised	
Wrist	swollen—wounds—dislocated—poor ROM	
Metacarpals	fracture (open, closed)—wounds—swelling—bruised	
Feathers	soiled—frayed—tipped—broken—in blood	
Right leg	flaccid—not weight bearing	
Femur	fracture (open, closed)—wounds—subcutaneous air—swelling—bruised	
Stifle	swollen—wounds—dislocated—poor ROM	
Tibiotarsus	fracture (open, closed)—wounds—swelling—bruised	
Hock	swollen—wounds—dislocated—poor ROM	
Tarsometatarsus	fracture (open, closed)—wounds—swelling—bruised	
"Ankle"	swollen—wounds—dislocated	
Digits/talons	fracture (open, closed)—wounds—swelling—bruised—worn/smooth pad—bumblefoot—broken talon	
Left leg	flaccid—not weight bearing	
Femur	fracture (open, closed)—wounds—subcutaneous air—swelling—bruised	
Stifle	swollen—wounds—dislocated—poor ROM	
Tibiotarsus	fracture (open, closed)—wounds—swelling—bruised	

Continued

Table 1.1. Continued.

Region/area	Findings	Comments
Hock	swollen—wounds—dislocated—poor ROM	
Tarsometatarsus	fracture (open, closed)—wounds—swelling—bruised	
"Ankle"	swollen—wounds—dislocated	
Digits/talons	fracture (open, closed)—wounds—swelling—bruised—worn/smooth pad—bumblefoot—broken talon	
Other		
Ectoparasites	lice—flat flies—maggots	
Mutes	gritty—runny—bloody—odor—color	
Feathers	soiled—oiled—broken—frayed	

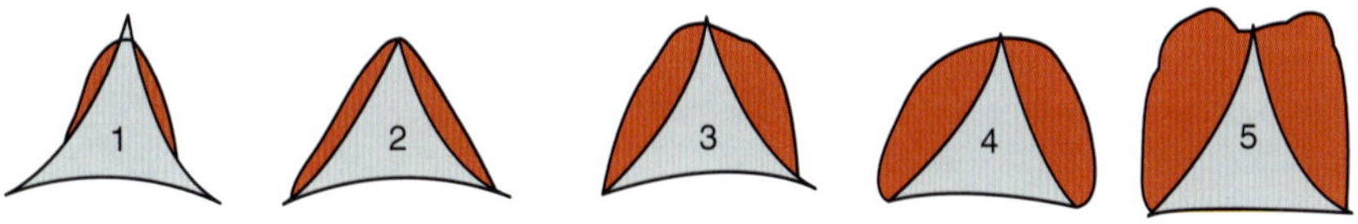

Fig. 1.2. Keel scores.

With a score of 5, the muscle mass rises above the edge of the keel bone.

Note that the keel score measures muscle mass and is relatively independent of the fat that overlies the pectoral muscle. For this reason, it is important to assess the pectoral muscle mass as well as the amount of fat, especially in an overweight bird.

Fat is deposited externally in several places in a bird. Three sites that are easy to check are: over the pectoral muscle/sternum, on the abdomen, and in the furcular hollow formed by the clavicle bones. All three areas should be evaluated.

It is important to realize that the edge of the keel bone will be visible and palpable in all but the most obese birds.

> **Raptor Tip**
>
> Intranasal midazolam can provide mild sedation for exams and procedures.

Do not forget to examine the eyes carefully. Both anterior and posterior chamber damage is quite common. In a recent study, 40% of admitted wild raptors had significant damage in at least one posterior chamber (Scott, 2015). It takes practice to become proficient at fundic exams, and recognizing a normal retina is the first step to being able to properly evaluate a traumatized retina. Euthanasia should be considered in any bird that has serious injury to one or both eyes (see Chapter 5).

Blood in the mouth or ears is usually associated with head trauma.

Apply a small amount of alcohol along the ventral side of the wing including the elbows and wrists. This helps clear feathers away and makes visualization of bruises much easier. Make sure there are no open wounds first since the application of alcohol is very painful.

Avian bruises can be quite alarming in both color and extent. As will be discussed later, biliverdin is an important pigment in birds and their bruises will, after a few days, turn green. Do not worry; this is normal (Fig. 1.3).

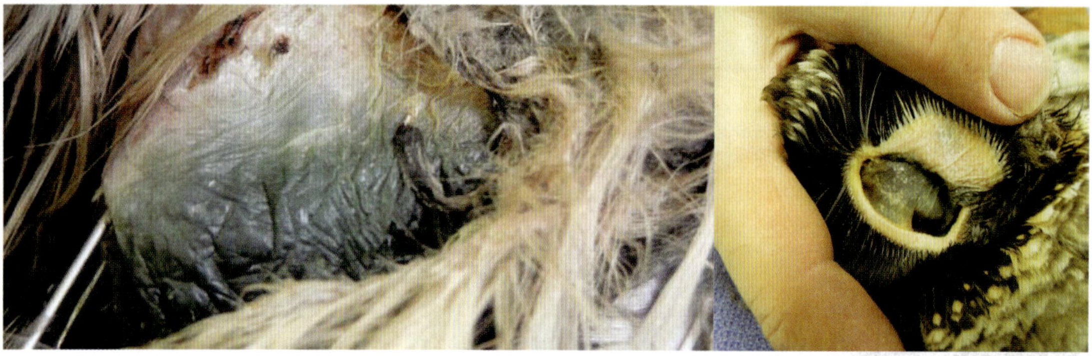

Fig. 1.3. Avian bruises can be very bright green. The right image shows a bruise in the ear of a barred owl (*Strix varia*).

Physical Exam Checklist

The checklist in Table 1.1 serves as a reminder so that important parts of the examination are not easily forgotten. In addition, always doing your examination in the same order will help ensure that important areas are not forgotten. This checklist can be laminated and used with an erasable marker. Findings can be quickly circled or written in while the exam is being completed.

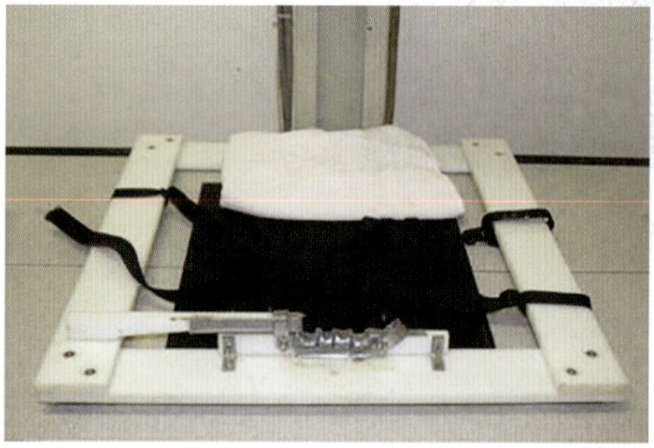

Fig. 1.4. Radiographic restraint device.

Radiographic Restraint and Positioning

Both lateral and ventral–dorsal (VD) views are helpful. However, a VD view may be adequate for many cases. General anesthesia is recommended but VD radiographs can oftentimes be done with just simple restraint. The exceptions are very large or powerful birds such as vultures and eagles for which general anesthesia is typically required. The head should be covered with a light towel to decrease stress.

Manual restraint can be achieved with a simple device as shown in Figs 1.4 and 1.5. It uses a frame that allows the tarsometatarsi to be restrained under a padded sliding bar and the abdomen and thorax to be secured by nylon strips. The wings can then be secured with masking tape.

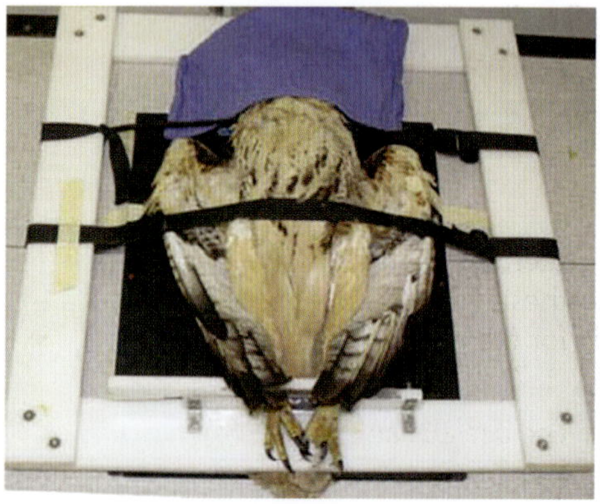

Fig. 1.5. Hawk positioned for radiograph.

To get a good VD radiograph (Fig. 1.6):

- The keel must overlie the spine.
- The legs are pulled down symmetrically.

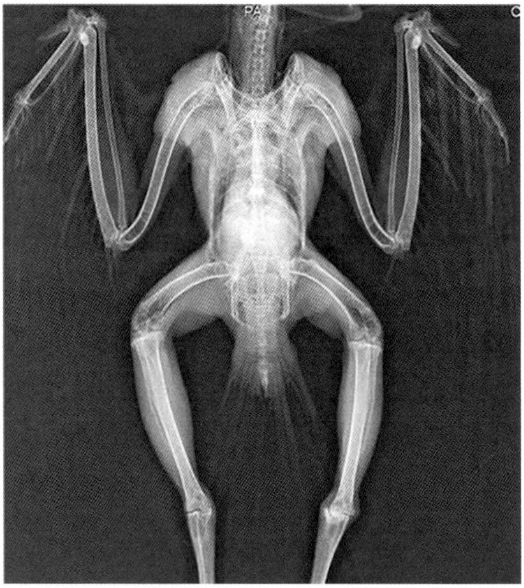

Fig. 1.6. A good ventral–dorsal (VD) radiograph.

- The wings are pulled out symmetrically.
- The elbows and stifles should not overlap.

Raptor Tip

On the VD radiograph, make sure the keel and spine are overlapped.

Lateral radiographs almost always require anesthesia as the positioning is very uncomfortable for the bird. To get a good lateral radiograph (Fig. 1.7):

- The acetabulae should overlap.
- The coracoids should overlap.
- The wings should be extended dorsally.
- The legs should be pulled back caudally if you are interested in the abdomen. They should be spread if you are interested in the actual femur bones themselves.

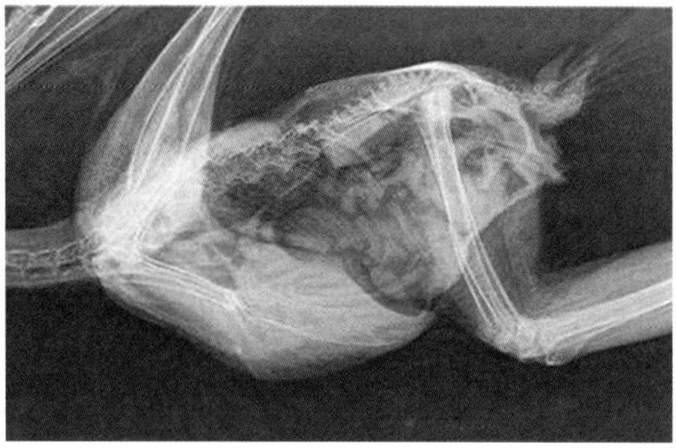

Fig. 1.7. A good lateral radiograph.

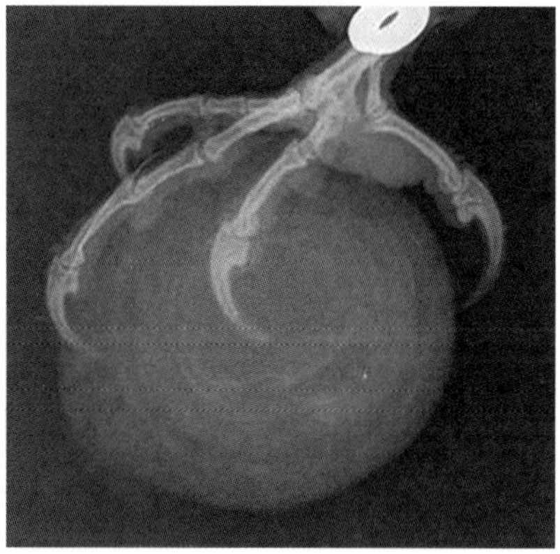

Fig. 1.8. Use of a gauze ball to assist in taking radiographs of the foot.

A gauze ball wrapped in elastic bandage material can be useful when taking radiographs of the feet since it helps spread the digits and eliminates superposition problems (Fig. 1.8). Anesthesia is usually required to get good results.

Intake Protocols

Table 1.2 is a quick-reference guide for treating some commonly seen problems. Refer to the Formulary for dosages.

Table 1.2. Intake protocols.

Problem	Treatment
Blood in oral cavity	Swab oral cavity Start broad-spectrum antibiotic and meloxicam Butorphanol 2 mg/kg BID/TID Treat as with head trauma (see below)
Caught in chimney	Rehydrate Flush and stain eyes to check for corneal ulcers Check wrists, beak, and talons for trauma Wipe down feathers with damp cloth Watch for possible respiratory trouble secondary to inhalation of soot Plan to bathe as soon as possible if necessary Treat for emaciation if present
Chorioretinitis	Give one injection of dexamethasone 2 mg/kg IM if less than 24 h Meloxicam
Corneal abrasion	Fluorescein stain to confirm Apply triple-antibiotic ointment with sterile applicator Do not use topical corticosteroids
Dehydration	Rehydrate Assume 5 or 10%. Replace deficit over 48 h Maintenance is 50 ml/kg/day Any appropriate route based on clinical condition. SQ usually works well in most cases See Chapters 4 and 7 for more details
Emaciation	Rehydrate for 18 h before feeding. Assume 10% dehydration and calculate for 2 × maintenance. LRS is usually the best choice Add Vitamin-B complex to fluids. Use enough to tinge the fluids a light yellow color (approximately 0.5 ml per 30 ml) Iron dextran 0.1 ml/kg IM Fenbendazole 25 mg/kg PO Begin antifungals in most species (terbinafine, itraconazole, or voriconazole) Place in warm incubator After 18 h, begin feeding furless/boneless meat at 20 g per kg BW TID. Tube-feeding with formula is also an option. Slowly increase the food amount over the next 2–3 days
External parasites (feather lice and flat flies)	Apply topical insecticidal spray. Products with permethrin, pyrethrins, and piperonyl butoxide (e.g. Bronco Equine Spray®, Farnum, Phoenix, AZ, USA) are safe and seem to work well. Use with caution since many insecticides are toxic to birds
Fracture	Butorphanol 2 mg/kg BID/TID Stabilize (fluids, etc.) Get radiograph if possible. Use general anesthesia via mask Flush wounds Cover/protect exposed bone with hydrogel bandage (e.g. Duoderm® extra thin, ConvaTec, Mulgrave, VIC, Australia). Close wound with sutures if possible Immobilize joint above and below fracture Start enrofloxacin and clindamycin if bone is exposed Start meloxicam Plan surgical repair within 24 h if possible

Continued

Table 1.2. Continued.

Problem	Treatment
Head trauma	Give one injection of dexamethasone 2 mg/kg IM. Note that this treatment is controversial but seems to be beneficial for acute retinal injury which is also common in these cases If trauma occurred within 24 h, give mannitol at 500 mg/kg IV/IO slowly TID × 3 followed by crystalloids for diuresis Butorphanol 2 mg/kg BID/TID Use midazolam as necessary Place in oxygen cage Do not apply heat (i.e. in a warm incubator)
Maggots and fly eggs	Physically remove eggs and maggots Apply nitenpyram (Capstar®, Novartis, Greensboro, NC, USA) topically on wounds (mix with water and spray on wounds). See Formulary for recipe Wait a few minutes and remove dead maggots Flush and clean wounds Give nitenpyram ½ tablet orally Check BID for recurrence Manage wounds as necessary with antibiotics and debridement
Oiled	Give activated charcoal 10–30 ml/kg PO if risk of aspiration is low Stabilize (fluids, etc.) Once stabilized, bathe bird under general anesthesia with warm water and Dawn dish soap® (Procter & Gamble, Cincinnati, OH, USA) (see Chapter 7)
Open-mouthed breathing	Administer oxygen via mask (intubate if necessary) Place air sac tube if no improvement (see Chapter 4 for more details)
Poisoning (suspected)	If organophosphorus toxicity: atropine 0.4 ml/kg IM. Repeat q4h as needed If lead toxicity: run blood lead test as soon as possible. Begin chelation therapy Give activated charcoal 10–30 ml/kg PO if risk of aspiration is low Give Vitamin-B complex 0.1 ml/kg IM Supportive care (fluids, etc.) Keep NPO
Seizures	Midazolam 1 mg/kg IM, repeat as needed Keep NPO Provide supportive care (oxygen, fluids, etc.) Run blood lead test as soon as possible
Shock	Administer oxygen via mask (intubate if necessary) Place 20- or 22-gauge IO catheter Begin fluid therapy immediately (see Chapter 4 for more details)
Soft tissue wounds/ tendon or bone exposure	Butorphanol 2 mg/kg BID/TID Stabilize (fluids, etc.) Start broad-spectrum antibiotic and meloxicam Flush wounds Cover/protect exposed tissue with silver sulfadiazine cream and hydrogel bandage (e.g. Duoderm® extra thin). Close wound with temporary sutures if possible Immobilize wound Plan surgical debridement and closure as soon as possible if tendon or bone is exposed

Continued

Table 1.2. Continued.

Problem	Treatment
Subcutaneous air	Aspirate with 18-gauge needle. Make small nick with needle as you are withdrawing to make a larger hole Repeat as necessary Do not give SQ fluids Determine cause as soon as possible
Unable to stand/ spinal trauma	Give one injection of dexamethasone 2 mg/kg IM. Note that this treatment may or may not be beneficial and is controversial Supportive care (fluids, etc.) Clean and evacuate vent/cloaca BID Keep on thick padding Provide nutritional support Run blood lead test if no evidence of trauma Meloxicam Trimethoprim–sulfamethoxazole: aids in controlling intestinal bacterial overgrowth but be certain to maintain adequate hydration Place a tail wrap
Uveitis	Rule out corneal ulcer with fluorescein stain Use prednisone drops if stain negative Can also use topical NSAID drops Meloxicam
Wing droop	Radiograph to check for fractures. Many of these cases can have a coracoid fracture Apply figure-8 bandage ± body wrap as needed Meloxicam Tramadol or another analgesic

Bibliography

Chitty, L. (2008) *BSAVA Manual of Raptors, Pigeons and Passerine Birds*. BSAVA, Gloucester, UK.

Redig, P. (1993) *Medical Management of Birds of Prey*, 3rd edn. The Raptor Center, St. Paul, MN, USA.

Scott, D. (2015) *RaptorMed™ clinical database at Carolina Raptor Center*, Charlotte, NC, USA.

2 Anatomy and Physiology

In order to treat birds effectively, it is important to know about some of the unique features of avian anatomy and physiology. This chapter provides a quick overview of some of the more clinically relevant features.

Learning Objectives

1. Skeletal anatomy.
2. Soft tissue anatomy.
3. Avian physiology of clinical importance.

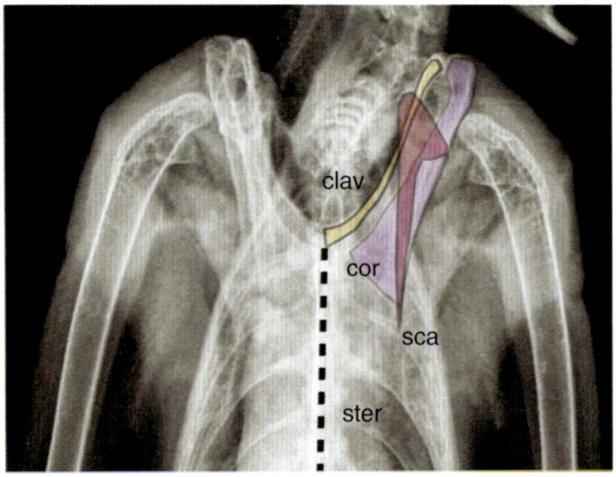

Fig. 2.1. The shoulder joint: coracoid (cor), clavicle (clav), scapula (sca), sternum/keel (ster).

Shoulder

The shoulder is a complex joint formed by the head of the humerus, the scapula, the clavicle (furcula), and the coracoid (Fig. 2.1). The coracoid is a fan-shaped bone that forms a strut between the shoulder and a synovial joint attachment to the sternum. This bone is commonly fractured as a result of blunt trauma.

Thoracic Limb

The humerus is a pneumatic bone and is connected to the thoracic air sacs (Fig. 2.2). This is important and clinically relevant because:

- When repairing humeral fractures, it is important not to flush into the proximal humerus as this can lead to flooding of the air sacs.
- Infections can be transmitted between the humerus and thorax via the air sacs.

Ulna

The ulna is much larger than the radius and, despite its larger size, ulna fractures are more common than fractures of the radius. The olecranon articulates with the ventral humeral condyle and the head of the radius articulates with the dorsal humeral condyle.

Wrist/Carpal Joint

The wrist/carpal joint is composed of several small bones including the radial carpal bone, the ulnar carpal bone, and the major/minor metacarpal bones. The alular metacarpal bone is fused to the major metacarpal bone.

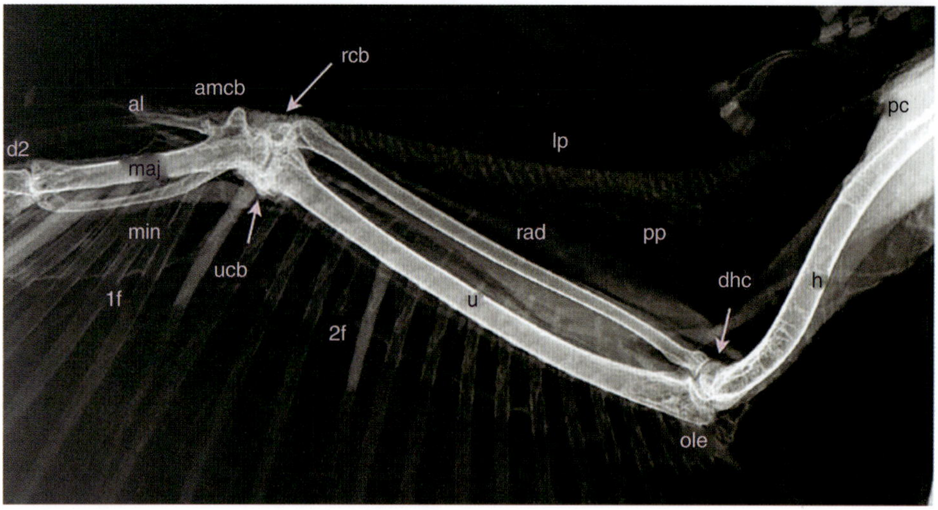

Fig. 2.2. The thoracic limb: alula (al), alular metacarpal bone (amcb), radial carpal bone (rcb), ulnar carpal bone (ucb), major metacarpal bone (maj), minor metacarpal bone (min), second digit (d2), primary feathers (1f), secondary feathers (2f), radius (rad), ulna (u), ligamentum propatagialis pars longus (lp), propatagium (pp), dorsal humeral condyle (dhc), olecranon (ole), humerus (h), pectoral crest (pc).

Propatagium or Wing Web

The propatagium or wing web is bordered cranially by the ligamentum propatagialis pars longus, a fibro-elastic length of connective tissue that stretches from the shoulder to the carpal joint. This structure forms the leading edge of the wing and is important in maintaining an effective airfoil. The ligamentum propatagialis pars brevis is a similar structure that runs from the shoulder to the proximal ulna/radius.

Spine, Sternum, and Pelvis

The vertebral column is separated into several sections (Fig. 2.3). The actual number of vertebrae in each section is dependent on species.

Cervical vertebrae

These comprise a variable number of highly mobile vertebrae.

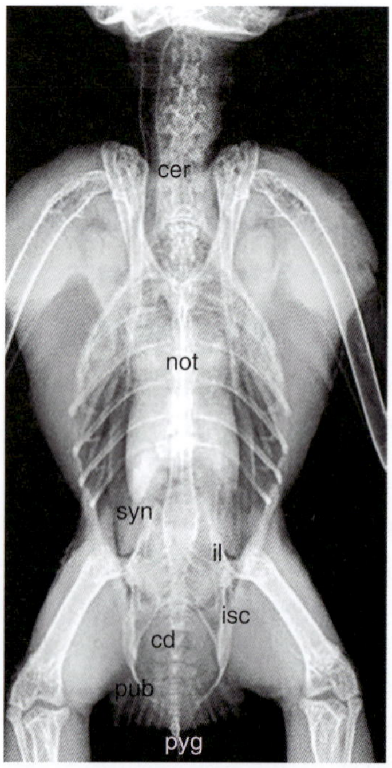

Fig. 2.3. The spine and pelvis: cervical vertebrae (cer), notarium (not), synsacrum (syn), ilium (il), ischium (isc), caudal vertebrae (cd), pubis (pub), pygostyle (pyg).

Notarium

Each thoracic vertebra has a rib attached to it and they are fused to form the notarium. Uncinate processes project caudally from the ribs, except on the last rib. There are also sternal ribs that originate on the sternum and join with the vertebral ribs.

Synsacrum

The lumbar, sacral, and caudal vertebrae are fused to form the synsacrum. The synsacrum is fused to the ilium portion of the pelvis.

Free caudal vertebrae

Some birds have a few free caudal vertebrae.

Pygostyle

This is formed from the fusion of the caudal-most vertebrae.

Sternum (or keel bone)

The sternum is a broad but thin bone that provides the attachments for the main flight muscles as well as protecting the coelomic cavity.

Pelvis

The pelvis is composed of the ilium, ischium, and pubis bones and it is fused to the synsacrum via the ilium bone. The pubic bones are not fused ventrally in raptors and most birds. The acetabulum is deep and is formed by the fusion of the ilium cranially and ischium caudally.

Legs

As with the humerus, the femur is also a pneumatic bone that communicates with the air sac system. Various fusions have occurred in the avian leg so that the bird has a tibiotarsus bone (not a tibia) distal to the stifle joint and a tarsometatarsus bone distal to the hock joint (Fig. 2.4).

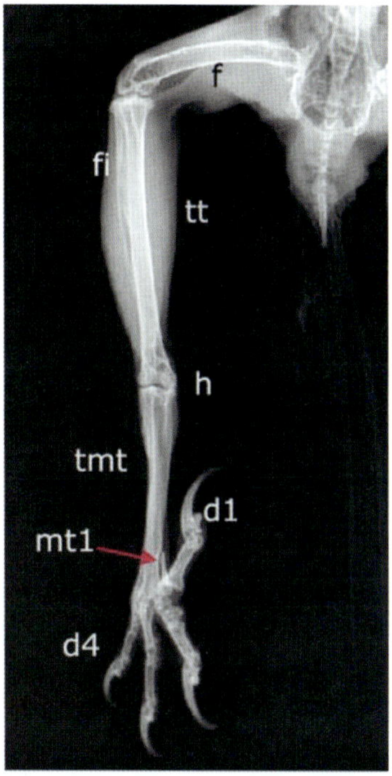

Fig. 2.4. The leg: femur (f), fibula (fi), tibiotarsus (tt), hock joint (h), tarsometatarsus (tmt), metatarsal 1 (mt1), digit 1 (d1), digit 4 (d4).

All raptors have four digits. The hallux is the caudal-most digit and is assigned number 1. The remaining digits are numbered medially to laterally. Digits 1 and 2 are generally considered the most important and their function is considered crucial for releasability in most species. In accipiters, digit 3 is much longer than the others and is especially important for hunting while in flight.

Hawks, eagles, and falcons have anisodactyl feet with digits 2, 3, and 4 directed cranially. Owls and ospreys have zygodactyl feet in which digit 4 can rotate forward or backward. Interestingly, the number of phalanges in each digit is equal to the digit number plus one. So, for example, digit 2 has three phalanges (Fig. 2.5).

It is important to note that the talon consists of a complete bone core extending almost to the tip. Therefore, talon fractures and injuries must be treated seriously because complications such as osteomyelitis may result. In addition, talon

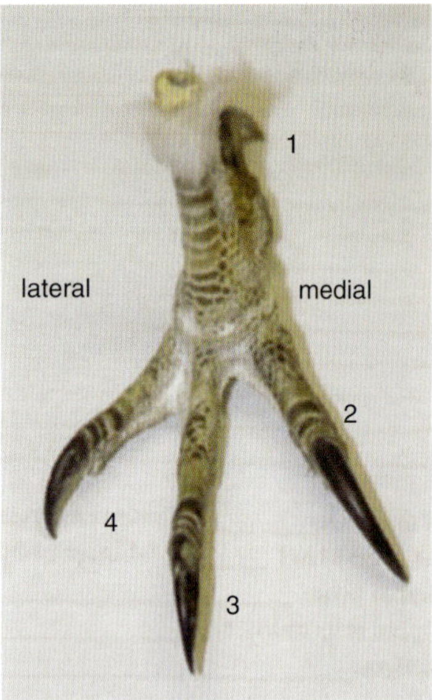

Fig. 2.5. Digit numbering.

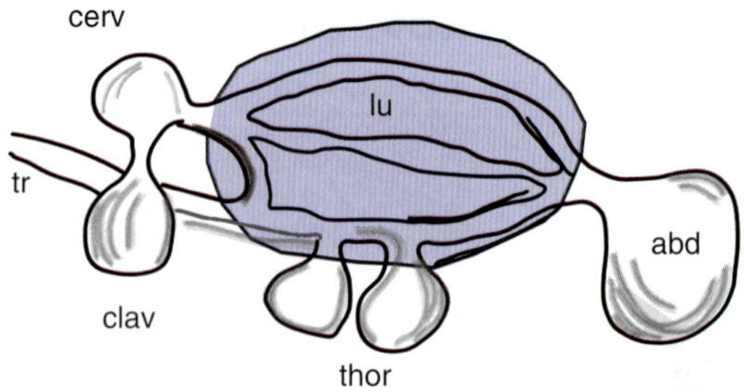

Fig. 2.6. Schematic of the avian air sacs. Trachea (tr), cervicocephalic (cerv), clavicular (clav), cranial and caudal thoracic (thor), abdominal (abd). The lungs (lu) are highlighted.

trimming can be dangerous and painful if done too aggressively.

Respiratory System

The glottis is located at the base of the tongue and is easily accessible for intubation. However, the small diameter of the glottis in species such as the eastern screech owl and American kestrel can make intubation tricky. The trachea is formed by complete cartilaginous rings and, therefore, cannot expand. This is important because inflatable ET tubes can cause serious mucosal necrosis and should never be used.

The trachea narrows and bifurcates into the two main-stem bronchi at the syrinx. The syrinx is the source of the avian voice and is also a common location for obstruction, either due to a foreign body or from a neoplastic or granulomatous mass. Loss of voice, change in voice, or dyspnea should always indicate careful (i.e. endoscopic) evaluation of the syrinx.

Avian lungs lie dorsally, are attached to the thoracic ribs and vertebrae, and fill the intercostal spaces. They are best seen on lateral radiographs.

The avian respiratory system also includes a series of air sacs (Figs 2.6 and 2.7). The typical bird has four pairs of air sacs (cervical, cranial thoracic, caudal thoracic, and abdominal). There is also a fused clavicular air sac. In addition, there is a cervicocephalic air sac that is not connected to the other air sacs. The cervicocephalic air sac does, however, connect to the infraorbital sinus located below the eyes. This sinus has many diverticuli and may be involved in cases of sinusitis which can present as swellings under the eyes. The air sacs are best seen on the VD view and should be dark (i.e. air density).

The air sacs are not involved in oxygen exchange. They act as bellows and serve entirely to direct air flow into and through the lungs. They penetrate and fill the medullary cavities of the humerus, femur, as well as several other bones. This is clinically relevant for reasons stated above.

Birds do not have a diaphragm separating the abdominal and thoracic cavity. Breathing is achieved by muscles which move the ribs and sternum. Negative pressure is created by increasing the volume of the coelomic cavity and involves the movement of the keel bone both cranially and ventrally. Because of this, it is critically important that birds not be restrained too tightly across the chest.

The avian respiratory cycle is complicated but also very efficient. It takes two cycles for air to move completely through the respiratory tract, but this process ensures fresh air is moving through the lungs both on inspiration and exhalation. During inhalation of the first cycle, half the air volume is drawn into the lungs and half into the caudal air sacs. Air already in the lungs moves

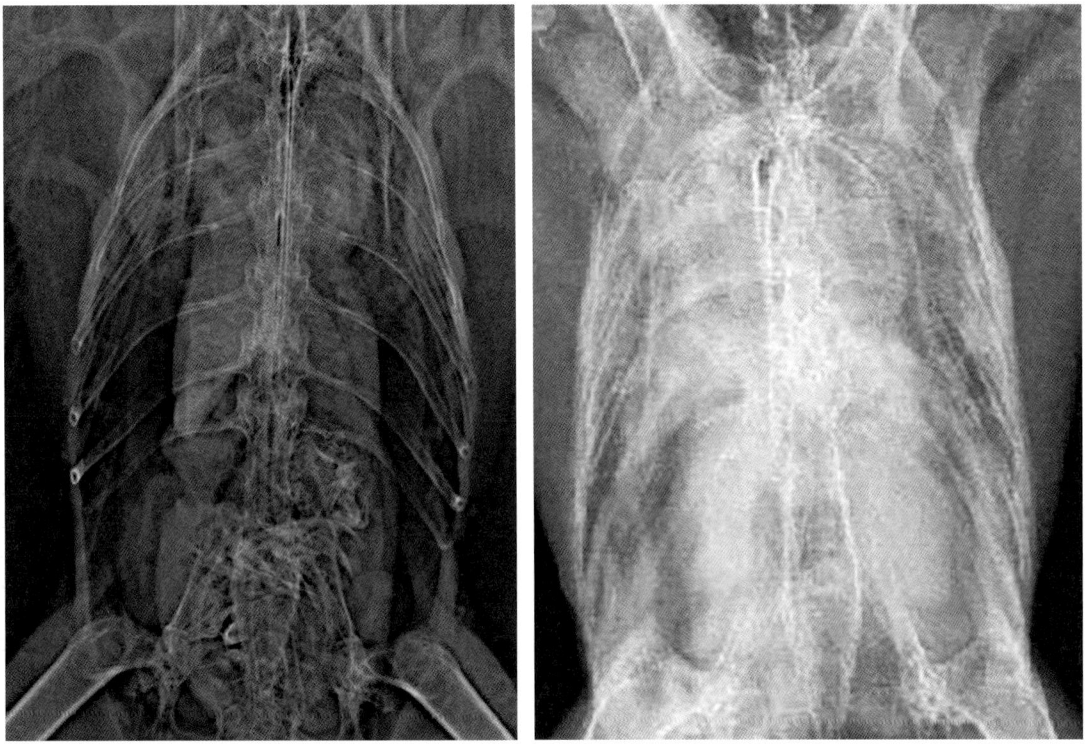

Fig. 2.7. Healthy air sacs (left) appear dark. There may be (as in this radiograph) an hourglass appearance formed by the heart and liver, but this is not always present. Compare to the radiograph on the right from a bird with severe air sacculitis due to Aspergillosis.

into the cranial air sacs. On exhalation, air in the caudal air sacs moves into the lungs and air in the cranial air sacs exits through the trachea. This repeats during the second cycle so all the air inspired during the first cycle has now passed through the lungs and has been exhaled. Refer to Altman *et al*. (1997) for a good description.

Gastrointestinal System

The crop is on the right side of the neck. It is a widening or out-pouching of the esophagus and the actual shape of the crop depends upon the species (Fig. 2.8). The crop is clinically important as it can be the site of infection and/or injury. Note that owls do not have a crop.

The avian stomach is composed of two parts. The proventriculus is the gastric or glandular part and the ventriculus (gizzard) is responsible for mechanical breakdown of food. In raptors, the glandular portion (proventriculus) is well developed but the wall of the ventriculus is relatively thin when compared to granivorous species that require extensive grinding of coarse food material.

Raptors will form a pellet of undigestible material in the stomach and expel or "cast" them orally before the next meal. This is normal in a healthy bird and should be noted in daily records. Owl pellets will contain bones. Other types of raptors have a lower gastric pH which dissolves the bones, so their pellets rarely contain bones.

Liver

The avian liver is composed of two main lobes. Not all birds have a gall bladder, but when one is present, it is usually associated with the right liver lobe. The combination of the heart and liver typically forms an hourglass shape when seen on a VD radiograph.

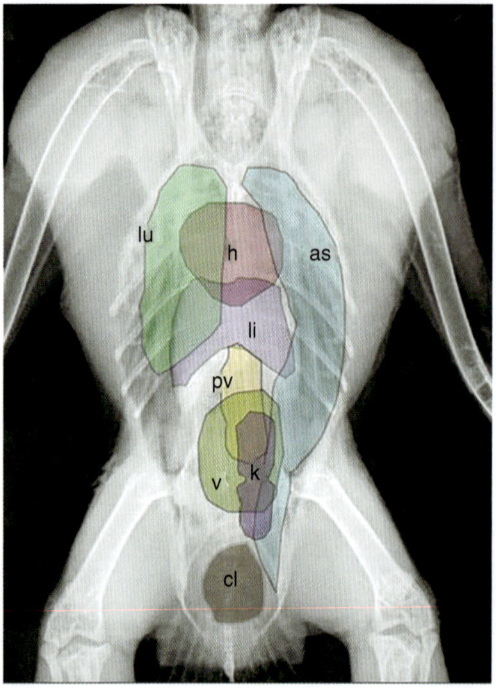

Fig. 2.8. Soft tissue structures seen on VD view: heart (h), lung (lu), air sacs (as), liver (li), proventriculus (pv), ventriculus (v), kidney (k) cloaca (cl).

Biliverdin versus bilirubin

Birds lack biliverdin reductase, so the end-product of hemoglobin catabolism is biliverdin, not bilirubin as in mammals (Fig. 2.9). Biliverdin is normally excreted by the liver into the bile and this gives birds' feces the characteristic green coloration. In a healthy animal, most of the bile is reabsorbed. With liver disease, bile is not reabsorbed, biliverdin accumulates, and is eliminated in the feces and excreted by the kidneys, resulting in green urates. Note that biliverdinuria and green urates can also result when a healthy liver is overwhelmed in cases of hemolysis such as malaria. Jaundice and icterus are not normally seen in birds.

> **Raptor Tip**
>
> Green urates may indicate liver disease.

Nitrogenous Wastes

Uric acid (UA) crystals are synthesized in the liver as the main waste product of protein metabolism. These white crystals are excreted by the kidney as the urate portion of bird droppings. Elevated levels of UA can be the result of:

- A transient postprandial elevation.
- Kidney damage.
- Dehydration.

Clinical Pathology

Of the commonly measured enzymes, only aspartate aminotransferase (AST) is useful for evaluating the avian liver. It is sensitive but not specific for detecting liver necrosis. However, as it is also produced in muscle tissue, AST levels should always be evaluated in conjunction with creatine kinase (CK).

As in mammals, bile acid (BA) levels are a sensitive measurement of liver function and should always be checked when liver disease is suspected. Note that normal levels for BA may vary considerably with species.

Spleen

The spleen is oval in shape. It is attached dorsally at the isthmus between the proventriculus and ventriculus. It functions in erythrophagocytosis, lymphopoiesis, and the production of antibodies. The spleen does not serve as a reserve pool for RBC as it does in mammals. It is best seen on the lateral radiograph (Fig. 2.10). Enlargement can be seen secondary to systemic infection.

> **Raptor Tip**
>
> Birds do not have lymph nodes.

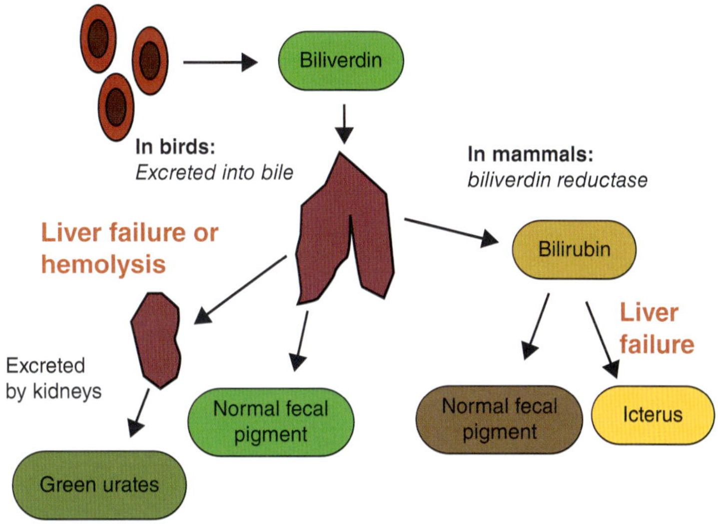

Fig. 2.9. Metabolism of biliverdin.

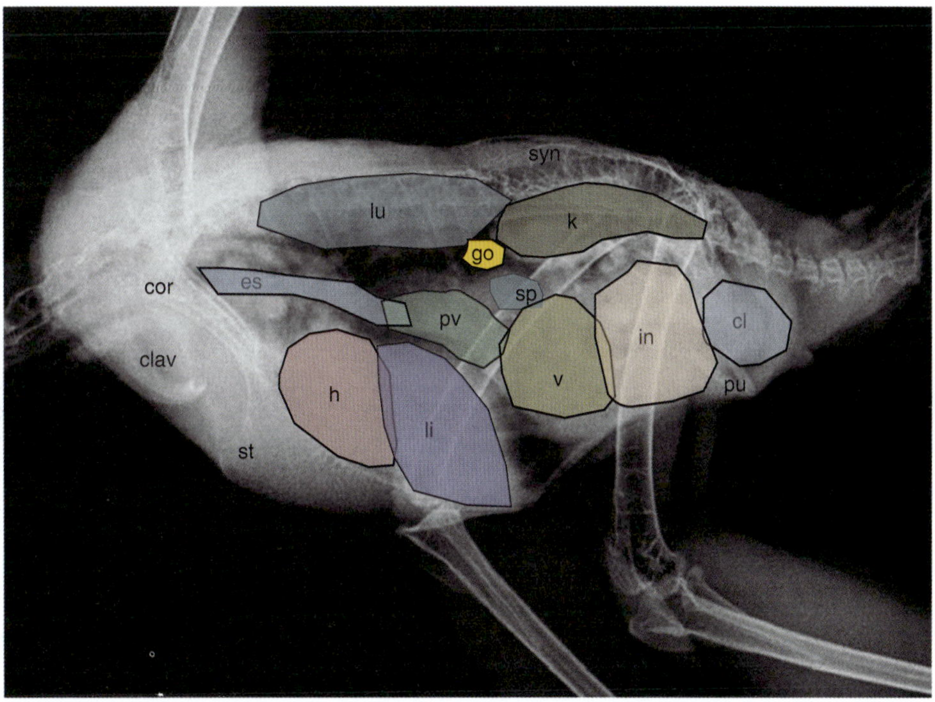

Fig. 2.10. Structures seen on lateral view: clavicle (clav), coracoid (cor), sternum (st), heart (h), liver (li), esophagus (es), proventriculus (pv), spleen (sp), ventriculus (v), lung (lu), kidney (k), gonad (go), intestines (in), pubis (pu), cloaca (cl), synsacrum (syn).

Urogenital System

Kidneys

The kidneys in birds are firmly attached in depressions ventral to the synsacrum. In most species each kidney is divided into cranial, middle, and caudal lobes. Large nerves from the lumbosacral plexus run adjacent to or through the parenchyma of the kidneys so that any mass or inflammation in the area (e.g. renal tumor) can result in leg lameness on the affected side.

There are no distinct cortical and medullary regions in the avian kidney. The functions are mixed side-by-side and are carried out by two types of nephrons.

The cortical or reptilian nephron is the most common type and produces the urate portion of the dropping. Urates contain UA, a relatively inert and less toxic (when compared to urea or ammonia) form of processed nitrogenous waste. Because this is the primary mechanism of excretion, assessment of UA is the best measurement of renal function. Measurement of blood urea nitrogen (BUN) and creatinine is generally of little diagnostic value.

The medullary or mammalian nephron produces urine.

It is important to realize that avian droppings contain three parts: a brown or green fecal portion, a white, pasty urate portion, as well as a clear liquid urine portion.

Raptor Tip

Birds have a renal portal system so injections in the thighs are generally not a good idea.

Birds have a renal portal system that allows blood to be shunted from the caudal half of the body directly to the kidneys. This is clinically relevant because potentially nephrotoxic drugs can be dangerous and renally excreted drugs may be eliminated before being systemically available. Because of this, injections should be given in the pectoral muscles rather than in the muscles of the leg or thigh.

Reproductive Tract

The female reproductive tract normally develops only on the left side; however, a report in psittacines indicates that partial development of a right oviduct is not uncommon (Nemetz, 2010), especially in younger birds. The oviduct consists of the magnum, infundibulum, isthmus, and shell gland (from cranial to caudal) and each portion plays a different role in the production of an egg. The oviduct can be very thin and difficult to locate in immature birds; but it is usually easily identified as it runs over the surface of the left kidney in a more mature bird. The ovary is located medially near the cranial pole of the left kidney (Fig. 2.11).

The paired testes lie medial to the cranial extent of the kidneys and are adjacent to the adrenal glands. The size and color vary depending on species, season, and age. They are typically smooth and elongated in shape but can vary greatly in size, and the color can range from pale tan to almost black.

The Cloaca

The cloaca is the common collection point for the GI and urogenital tracts. The cloaca has three chambers.

The coprodeum receives the rectum and in many birds is just a widening of the distal colon.

The urodeum receives the ureters and oviduct/ductus deferens via openings in the dorsal wall. It is separated from the other chambers by two mucosal folds.

The proctodeum is the last chamber and is held closed by the vent sphincter muscle. The cloacal bursa (the bursa of Fabricius) is in the dorsal wall of the proctodeum. The bursa is the site of B lymphocyte maturation in the young bird and it regresses so that it is not grossly visible by the time most birds have fledged (Fig. 2.12).

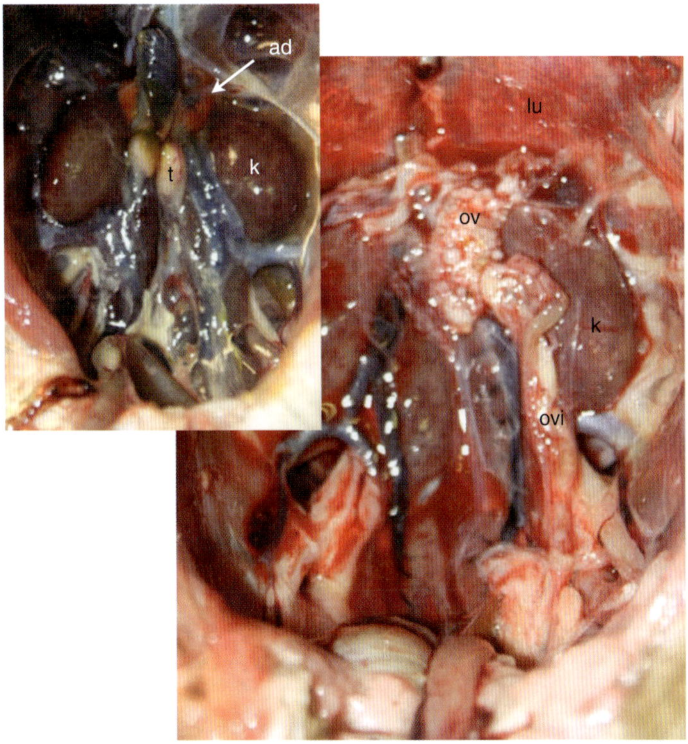

Fig. 2.11. Reproductive tract: ovary with follicles (ov), oviduct (ovi), testes (t), adrenal gland (ad), kidney (k), lung (lu).

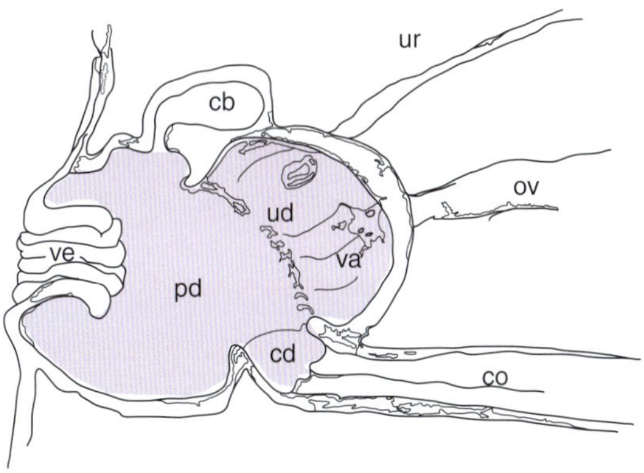

Fig. 2.12. Cloaca anatomy: cloacal bursa (cb), ureter (ur), oviduct (ov), colon (co), coprodeum (cd), proctodeum (pd), vagina (va), urodeum (ud), vent (ve).

Bibliography

Altman, R.B., Clubb, S.L., Dorrestein, G.M. and Quesenberry, K. (1997) *Avian Medicine and Surgery*. W.B. Saunders Company, Philadelphia, PA, USA.

Nemetz, L. (2010) Clinical pathology of a persistent right oviduct in psittacine birds. *Proceedings of the 31st Conference of the Association of Avian Veterinarians, San Diego, CA, USA*. Association of Avian Veterinarians, Teaneck, NJ, USA, pp. 73–77.

Orosz, S. (1999) The avian respiratory system. *Compendium of Small Animal/Exotic Medicine* 21(19), 935–943.

Ritchie, B.W., Harrison, G.J. and Harrison, L.R. (1994) *Avian Medicine: Principles and Application*. Wingers Publishing, Inc., Lake Worth, FL, USA.

Samour, J. (2008) *Avian Medicine*, 2nd edn. Mosby-Elsevier, Philadelphia, PA, USA.

3 Species Overview

A short species summary is presented including the common name, scientific name, abbreviation, the normal weight range, the typical diet, and habitat, as well as reproductive details. The species are arranged by continent, but it is very common for a species to be present in many parts of the world. These data were compiled from multiple sources listed below but many species are not well documented.

The weights are provided in as much detail as current research allows. Note that the weight ranges can vary significantly based on geographic location and latitude. Ranges are printed separately for each sex, if available, or combined if not. In some cases, multiple sources are listed if a discrepancy existed in the published literature. In rare cases, only a few individual weights are provided.

Africa

Name	Abbrev.	Weight range	Diet	Habitat
African barred owlet (*Glaucidium capense*)		Male: 83–132 g Female: 93–139 g	Insects, small rodents, and birds	Woodland and forests, and on forest edges, more open savannah, and along rivers
Reproduction: Uses natural cavities or pre-existing nests. 2–3 eggs. Incubation period unknown. Fledges at 30–33 days Note: Sexually dimorphic				
African cuckoo-hawk (*Aviceda cuculoides*)		220–296 g	Preys on small vertebrates, including hairy caterpillars, which make up a large percentage of the diet	Occurs in moist forests, along forest edges, clearings, and in riparian and suburban habitats
Reproduction: Stick nests in tree forks. 2 eggs. Incubation for 32–33 days. Fledges at 5–6 weeks				
African fish eagle (*Haliaeetus vocifer*)		Male: 2000–2500 g Female: 3200–3600 g	Feeds mainly on fish but also on small prey and termites. Occasionally feeds on carrion	Near bodies of water. Immatures sometimes found far from water
Reproduction: Large stick nest, usually high in trees. 1–4 eggs (usually 2). Incubation for 42–45 days by both parents. Fledges at 70–75 days Note: Sexually dimorphic. Siblicide does not normally occur				

Continued

<table>
<tr><th>Name</th><th>Abbrev.</th><th>Weight range</th><th>Diet</th><th>Habitat</th></tr>
<tr><td>African goshawk
(Accipiter tachiro)</td><td></td><td>220–360 g</td><td>Preys on a wide variety of small invertebrates but mainly small birds</td><td>Moist dense forests and woodlands</td></tr>
<tr><td colspan="5">Reproduction: Small stick nest. 2–3 eggs. Incubation for 30 days. Fledges at 35 days</td></tr>
<tr><td>African harrier-hawk
(Polyboroides typus)</td><td></td><td>635–950 g</td><td>Opportunistic feeder. Small mammals, frogs, lizards, insects, fruit, and carrion</td><td>Wide variety of open and forested habitat from semi-desert to rainforest</td></tr>
<tr><td colspan="5">Reproduction: Builds stick nest lined with green leaves. 2 eggs. Incubation for 36 days by both parents. Fledges at 52 days
Note: This species has a reversible intertarsal ("knee") joint which can bend backward, as well as forward, enabling the bird to reach into deep holes to extract the contents</td></tr>
<tr><td>African hawk-eagle
(Aquila spilogaster)</td><td></td><td>Male: 1150–1300 g
Female: 1440–1640 g</td><td>Small mammals up to the size of a hare and gamebirds</td><td>Semi-arid open woodland, savannah, and dry riparian forest</td></tr>
<tr><td colspan="5">Reproduction: Large stick nest. 2 eggs. Incubation for 43–44 days by both parents. Fledges at 73 days</td></tr>
<tr><td>African hobby
(Falco cuvierii)</td><td></td><td>Male: 125–178 g
Female: 186–224 g</td><td>Small birds, bats, and insects</td><td>Open, moist woodland, damp wooded savannah, forest edges, and large clearings</td></tr>
<tr><td colspan="5">Reproduction: Takes over nests of other species. 2–3 eggs. Incubation for 30–32 days. Fledges around 30 days</td></tr>
<tr><td>African marsh harrier
(Circus ranivorus)</td><td></td><td>382–590 g</td><td>Feeds mainly on small rodents (70% of diet), occasionally birds as large as ducks, frogs, carrion, and insects</td><td>Confined mainly to wetlands</td></tr>
<tr><td colspan="5">Reproduction: Platform nest of vegetation usually placed in a reed bed above water level. 2–5 eggs. Incubation for 32–34 days. Fledges at 38–40 days</td></tr>
<tr><td>African scops owl
(Otus senegalensis)</td><td></td><td>45–120 g</td><td>Feeds mainly on insects but occasionally takes small vertebrates</td><td>Well-wooded savannahs, sometimes mangroves and gardens</td></tr>
<tr><td colspan="5">Reproduction: Tree or fence cavities, natural holes. 4–6 eggs. Incubation for 25–27 days. Fledges at 1 month</td></tr>
<tr><td>African wood owl
(Strix woodfordii)</td><td></td><td>240–350 g</td><td>Mostly insects, but will eat reptiles, small birds, and rodents</td><td>Forest, from the edge of primary forest to dense woodland</td></tr>
<tr><td colspan="5">Reproduction: Usually ground nests at base of tree trunk. 1–3 eggs. Incubation for 31 days. Will start leaving nest at 23–27 days but are not fully fledged until 46 days</td></tr>
<tr><td>Amur falcon
(Falco amurensis)</td><td></td><td>Male: 97–155 g
Female: 110–188 g</td><td>Insects, voles, small birds, amphibians</td><td>Open areas, woodland edge, wooded steppe, and moist grasslands</td></tr>
<tr><td colspan="5">Reproduction: Often uses old Corvidae nests or tree holes. 2–6 eggs. Incubation for 28–30 days. Fledges at 30–31 days
Note: This species undertakes the longest regular overwater migration of any raptor, crossing over the Indian Ocean between India and East Africa. This is a journey of more than 4000 km, which also includes nocturnal flight</td></tr>
</table>

Continued

Name	Abbrev.	Weight range	Diet	Habitat
Augur buzzard (*Buteo augur*)		1100–1300 g	Reptiles, but also on hares, hyraxes, gamebirds, and insects	Hilly and mountainous country at all elevations, and forest or open woodlands for nesting
Reproduction: Nest built in tree usually on a cliff ledge. 1–3 eggs. Incubation for 39–40 days. Fledges at 48–60 days. Usually only 1 chick survives due to siblicide				
Ayres's hawk-eagle (*Aquila ayresii*)		685–1050 g	Mostly smaller birds, tree-dwelling rodents, and bats	Evergreen forests, forest edges, clearings, and woodlands
Reproduction: Usually unstable stick/twig nest. 1 egg. Incubation for 43–45 days. Fledges at 73–75 days				
Barn owl	See North America			
Bat owl (*Macheiramphus alcinus*)		600–650 g	Primarily insectivorous bats, but also insects and birds	Clear spaces in moist wooded and forest edge habitats
Reproduction: Large stick nest on tree branch. 1–2 eggs. Incubation for 42 days. Fledges at 67 days				
Bateleur (*Terathopius ecaudatus*)		1800–2900 g	Carrion and live animals such as young hares, rodents, and reptiles. May eat fish and ground birds	Bushy savannahs, open woodlands, coastal plains, and semi-deserts
Reproduction: High tree nests. 1 egg. Incubation for 52–59 days. Fledges at 110 days				
Bearded vulture (*Gypaetus barbatus*)		4.5–7.0 kg	Mainly on bones and marrow, but it may take carrion, some small rodents, or birds and reptiles. The only living bird species that specializes in feeding on marrow	Mainly mountains and surrounding plains with rocky areas for nesting and breaking bones
Reproduction: Stick nests built on cliffs, ledges, or in caves. 1–2 eggs laid at 4–5-day interval. Incubation for 53–60 days. Fledges at 110–130 days. Will commonly depend on parents for 2 years, forcing them to nest every other year Note: Main threats to this species are poison baits				
Beaudouin's snake eagle (*Circaetus beaudouini*)		1500–2500 g	Both venomous and non-venomous snakes (up to 2.8 m long), lizards, birds, insects, and rodents.	Arid, open, and dense woodland up to 2500 m above sea level.
Reproduction: Green leaf-lined stick nest. 1 egg. Incubation for 48–53 days. Fledges at 96–113 days				
Black harrier (*Circus maurus*)		400–600 g	Small mammals (rodents), small birds, reptiles, amphibians, and insects	Fynbos scrub and bushlands, with marshes
Reproduction: Platform of reed stems usually built in reed bed on ground or in moist vegetation. 3–4 eggs. Incubation for 34 days. Fledges at 36 days				

Continued

Name	Abbrev.	Weight range	Diet	Habitat
Black kite	See Australia			
Black sparrowhawk (*Accipiter melanoleucus*)		Male: 450–650 g Female: 750–1020 g	Preys mostly on mid-sized birds	Forests of all types, riparian woodland, and tree plantations
Reproduction: Stick nests in trees. 2–4 eggs. Incubation for 34–38 days. Fledges at 37–50 days Note: Known to attempt multiple brooding on occasions. This behavior is exceedingly rare in birds of prey. The second brood may be raised in the same nest, or in a second nest nearby				
Black-breasted snake eagle (*Circaetus pectoralis*)		1200–2300 g	Snakes and other reptiles, rodents, amphibians, insects, small birds, bats, and fish	Light woodland, savannah, plains, and other open country
Reproduction: Small stick nest in small tree or other vegetation. 1 egg. Incubation for 51 days. Fledges at 90 days				
Black-winged kite	See Australia			
Bonelli's eagle (*Aquila fasciata*)		1600–2600 g	Mid-sized birds, lizards, and small mammals. They rarely eat carrion	Mostly dry, open, and semi-open habitat, mountainous regions
Reproduction: Usually nests on cliffs, electricity towers, rarely trees. 1–3 eggs. Incubation for 37–40 days. Fledges at 55–65 days Note: Electrocution is a major threat to this species				
Booted eagle (*Hieraaetus pennatus*)		Male: 710 g Female: 975 g	Small and medium-sized birds, small mammals, reptiles, and large insects	Mountainous areas with forests and open lands
Reproduction: Stick nests on cliff faces, in small trees. 1–3 eggs at 2–3-day intervals. Incubation for 36–40 days. Fledges at 50–55 days. All chicks usually survive				
Brown snake eagle (*Circaetus cinereus*)		1500–2500 g	Snakes up to 3 m long, but it also consumes lizards, gamebirds, and sometimes mammals	Savannahs, woodlands, and dry wooded countries with tall trees
Reproduction: Stick nest in trees. 1 egg. Incubation for 47–53 days. Fledges at 96–113 days Note: They hunt by swooping down from a perch and catching their prey on the ground. Unlike other snake eagles, they rarely or never eat in flight				
Cape eagle owl (*Bubo carpensis*)		900–1800 g	Mostly medium-sized mammals and birds but also eats reptiles, crabs, and large insects	Mountainous regions, rocky areas, wooded gullies. Also hunts in open savannah
Reproduction: Often reuses nests of larger birds. 1–3 eggs. Incubation for 34–38 days. Fledges at 45 days				
Cape vulture (*Gyps coprotheres*)		7–11 kg	Scavenger. Carrion	Mountains, in open grassland, arid savannahs, and steppes

Continued

Name	Abbrev.	Weight range	Diet	Habitat
Reproduction: Cliff platform nests. 1 egg. Incubation for 55 days. Fledges at 140 days Note: The 2 prominent bare skin patches at the base of the neck are thought to be temperature sensors and used for detecting the presence of thermals Note: The Cape vulture is a rare species. These vultures suffer from poisoning, electrocution from powerlines, persecution, and are killed for traditional medicine				
Cassin's hawk-eagle (*Aquila africana*)		900–1200 g	Birds and squirrels	Primary lowland rainforest
Reproduction: Leaf-lined stick nest in trees. 1–2 eggs. Incubation period and fledging age unknown				
Chestnut-flanked sparrowhawk (*Accipiter castanilius*)		135–200 g	Small mammals, reptiles, and amphibians, as well as birds	Occupies moist lowland rainforest habitats
Reproduction: Unknown				
Cinereous vulture (*Aegypius monachus*)	CIVU	Male: 6.3–11.5 kg Female: 7.5 –14.0 kg	Carrion-feeder, occasionally attacks live prey, including birds, reptiles, calves, and lambs	Arid hilly and montane habitat, including wooded areas, and semi-desert
Reproduction: Large (2 m across and 3 m deep) nests in trees along cliffs. 1 egg. Incubation for 50–62 days. Fledges at 100–120 days				
Common buzzard (*Buteo buteo*)		Male: 525–1180 g Female: 625–1365 g	Small and medium-sized mammals, reptiles, amphibians, and insects	All types of forests but always close to open area
Reproduction: 2–4 eggs. Incubation for 28–30 days. Fledges at 50–60 days Note: This species probably has the keenest vision of all the raptors				
Common kestrel (*Falco tinnunculus*)	COKE	Male: 135–250 g Female: 155–315 g	Small mammals, passerines, lizards, and insects	Numerous kinds of open or slightly wooded areas with tall grass and low shrubs
Reproduction: Nests in tree cavities, holes, crevices. 3–6 eggs. Incubation for 27–30 days. Fledges at 27–35 days				
Congo serpent eagle (*Dryotriorchis spectabilis*)			Snakes, lizards, and amphibians, and possibly small mammals	Lowland and medium-altitude primary rainforests
Reproduction: Unknown				
Crowned hawk-eagle (*Stephanoaetus coronatus*)		Male: 2700–4100 g Female: 3100–4700 g	Primarily feeds on mammals, sometimes on lizards or large snakes	Lowland and evergreen forest, dense woodland, ravines and gorges in open savannahs
Reproduction: Bulky stick platform nests in large trees. 1–2 eggs. Incubation for 49–50 days. Fledges at 103–115 days Note: Most of its prey is killed on the ground, except the monkeys caught in tree-tops				

Continued

Name	Abbrev.	Weight range	Diet	Habitat
Dark chanting goshawk (*Melierax metabates*)		Male: 645–695 g Female: 841–852 g	Reptiles, birds, insects, and small rodents	Savannahs and open woodlands
Reproduction: Small nest in main fork of tree. 1–2 eggs. Incubation for 36 days. Fledges at 50 days				
Dickinson's kestrel (*Falco dickinsoni*)		167–246 g	Mainly large insects, but also rodents, lizards, small birds, frogs, and crustaceans	Savannah and open woodland, particularly swampy areas near water
Reproduction: Usually nests in holes in baobab trees, or crowns of dead palms. 2–4 eggs. Incubation for 30 days. Fledges at 33–35 days				
Eastern chanting goshawk (*Melierax poliopterus*)		514–802 g	Small birds, rodents, lizards, and insects, hunting mainly on the ground	Savannah, steppe, semi-arid, and arid regions
Reproduction: Small twig platform usually in a tree canopy. 1–2 eggs. Incubation for 35 days. Fledges at 49–56 days				
Eastern imperial eagle (*Aquila heliaca*)		2.4–4.5 kg	Small mammals, but also takes waterfowl and feeds on carrion. Rarely eats fish	Open woodlands mixed with open areas and low-elevation mountainous areas
Reproduction: Tree-top stick nests. 1–4 eggs. Incubation for 43–52 days. Fledges at 63–77 days. Siblicide is common Note: They are a lowland species, but due to habitat loss and hunting they have been pushed to higher elevations in some parts of the world				
Egyptian vulture (*Neophron percnopterus*)	EGVU	1.6–2.2 kg	Mostly carrion but also small mammals, birds, eggs, and reptiles	Arid woodlands and semi-arid bush country, especially canyons and rocky areas
Reproduction: Stick nest in canyons and rocky areas. Lined with masses of wool and hair. 1–3 eggs. Incubation for 42–47 days. Fledges at 70–90 days Note: The species demonstrates the use of tools by using a pebble as a hammer to crack eggs, also by using twigs to roll up wool for use in their nest				
Eleonora's falcon (*Falco eleonorae*)		Male: 350 g Female: 390 g	Large flying insects and small passerines. It may also hunt small mammals and lizards	Cliffs, tops of rocky islets near water. Also in rainforest and sparsely wooded terrain
Reproduction: Nests in cliff ledges, crevices, under vegetation. 2–3 eggs. Incubation for 28–30 days. Fledges at 37 days				
Eurasian hobby	See Europe			
Eurasian sparrowhawk	See Europe			
European honey buzzard	See Europe			

Continued

Name	Abbrev.	Weight range	Diet	Habitat
European scops owl	See Europe			
Forest buzzard (*Buteo trizonatus*)		700 g	Small mammals, reptiles, amphibians, and insects	Evergreen woodlands, including introduced eucalyptus and pines
Reproduction: Stick platform nest. 2 eggs. Incubation unknown. Fledges at 50 days				
Fox kestrel (*Falco alopex*)		250–300 g	Large insects, lizards, small mammals, and birds	Semi-desert, rocky hills, cliffs, and outcrops along open savannah
Reproduction: Nests on rock ledges. 2–3 eggs. Incubation and fledging unknown				
Fraser's eagle owl (*Bubo poensis*)		Male: 575–770 g Female: 685–1052 g	Small mammals, birds, frogs, reptiles, as well as insects and other arthropods	Lowland primary evergreen rainforest, forest edges, and clearings
Reproduction: Nests on ground or in tree-hollows				
Gabar goshawk (*Micronisus gabar*)		Male: 90–173 g Female: 167–240 g	Small mammals, birds, reptiles, and insects	Savannahs, open woodland, thorn bush, and steppe habitats
Reproduction: Stick nests on bushes. 2–4 eggs. Incubation for 32–35 days. Fledges at 35 days				
Grasshopper buzzard (*Butastur rufipennis*)		Male: 310–340 g Female: 300–380 g	Insects (particularly grasshoppers). It can also take small birds, rodents, and reptiles	Woodland, forest edges, and arid thorny savannahs
Reproduction: Nests in tree fork. 1–3 eggs. Incubation for 30 days. Fledges at 36 days				
Grayish eagle owl (*Bubo cinerascens*)		500 g	Insects, invertebrates, small mammals	Dry rocky deserts and open savannah, as well as lowland forests
Reproduction: 1–3 eggs. Incubation and fledging unknown				
Greater kestrel (*Falco rupicoloides*)		178–334 g	Small birds, mammals, insects, mainly caught on the ground	Open grasslands and semi-arid steppes
Reproduction: Usually uses abandoned nests in trees. 3–5 eggs. Incubation for 32 days. Fledges at 30–34 days				
Greater spotted eagle (*Clanga clanga*)		Male: 1700–1900 g Female: 1800–2500 g	Small mammals, reptiles, amphibians, fish, insects, and carrion	Lowland forest and forest edges near a variety of wet areas
Reproduction: Nests in trees, on rocks, or ground. 1–3 eggs. Incubation for 42–44 days. Fledges at 60–67 days				
Grey kestrel (*Falco ardosiaceus*)		Male: 205–255 g Female: 240–300 g	Grasshoppers and small reptiles. It may take small birds, rodents, and bats	Savannah with large trees or palms, and open woodland
Reproduction: Nests in tree cavities. 2–5 eggs. Incubation for 26–31 days. Fledges at 30 days				

Continued

Name	Abbrev.	Weight range	Diet	Habitat
Griffon vulture (*Gyps fulvus*)		6–11 kg	Feeds almost exclusively on carrion of medium-sized and large domestic and wild animals	Mountains, plateaus, grassland, scrubland, and semi-desert
Reproduction: Nests on cliff face or ledge. 1 egg. Incubation for 52–60 days. Fledges at 110 days				
Hen harrier (*Circus cyaneus*)		Male: 290–400 g Female: 370–708 g	Small mammals and birds, reptiles, amphibians, insects, sometimes carrion	Open habitats from tundra and taiga to desert
Reproduction: Ground nest in vegetation. 3–6 eggs. Incubation for 29–31 days. Fledges at 29–42 days				
Hooded vulture (*Necrosyrtes monachus*)		1500–2600 g	Carrion, including dead fish, small mammals, bird eggs, trash, excreta, and insects	Wide range of open, cultivated, and urban habitats
Reproduction: Reuses nest yearly. 1 egg. Incubation for 48–54 days. Fledges at 3–4 months Note: Endangered				
Jackal buzzard (*Buteo rufofuscus*)		865–1080 g	Insects, small reptiles, mammals, birds, and carrion	Mainly hilly and mountainous habitats
Reproduction: Nests on cliff ledges, base of bushes, or in trees. 1–3 eggs. Incubation for 39–40 days by both parents. Fledges at 50–53 days				
Lanner falcon (*Falco biarmicus*)	LAFA	Male: 500–600 g Female: 700–900 g	Small mammals, insects, reptiles, and occasionally carrion	Extreme desert to wet forested mountains. Needs rocky crags and cliffs nearby for nesting
Reproduction: Nests on rock ledges on high cliffs. 2–5 eggs. Incubation for 30–35 days by both sexes. Fledges at 35–47 days				
Lappet-faced vulture (*Torgos tracheliotus*)		4400–9400 g	Mainly a scavenger, but also takes small mammals and live domestic stock	Prefers open, semi-arid, or arid habitat
Reproduction: Large stick platform nest in trees. 1 egg. Incubation for 7–8 weeks. Fledges at 125–135 days				
Lesser kestrel (*Falco naumanni*)	LEKE	Male: 90–172 g Female: 138–208 g	Primarily insects, both aerial and terrestrial, and other invertebrates	Dry, warm, semi-desert areas, and steppes. Prefers open habitat including farm fields
Reproduction: Nests in a variety of natural and man-made cavities. 3–6 eggs. Incubation for 26–28 days. Fledges at 36 days				
Lesser spotted eagle (*Lophaetus pomarinus, Aquila pomarina*)		1.2–2.6 kg	Small mammals, medium-sized birds, frogs, lizards, snakes, and insects	Lowland forest close to wetlands, dry upland forest, forest steppe
Reproduction: Reuses stick nests usually in trees. 2 eggs. Incubation for 43–45 days. Fledges at 58 days. Siblicide is common				

Continued

Name	Abbrev.	Weight range	Diet	Habitat
Levant sparrowhawk (*Accipiter brevipes*)		Male: 140–275 g Female: 180–290 g	Small birds and mammals. Young are fed insects and small reptiles	Wooded plains, particularly within river basins, foothills, and mountain slopes
Reproduction: Stick-and-twig nests in trees. 3–5 eggs. Incubation for 29–35 days mostly by female. Fledges at 29–31/40–45 days Note: Migrates in small flocks				
Little owl (*Athene noctua*)		105–260 g	Insects, small reptiles, small mammals, and birds	Variety of semi-open habitats
Reproduction: Nests in hollow branches, holes, and natural cavities. 3–6 eggs at 2-day intervals. Incubation for 22–28 days. Fledges at 35 days				
Little sparrowhawk (*Accipiter minullus*)		Male: 74–85 g Female: 68–105 g	Mostly small birds on the fly, some bats, lizards, and insects	Patches of forest and forest edges, riparian habitat, woodlands, and dense bush
Reproduction: Small stick nest in tree fork. 1–3 eggs. Incubation for 31–32 days. Fledges at 25–27 days				
Lizard buzzard (*Kaupifalco monogrammicus*)		Male: 220–275 g Female: 248–410 g	Small reptiles, large insects, birds, frogs, and rodents	Mature broadleaved woodland is the typical habitat, but this species will occur in other areas with good tree cover
Reproduction: Nests in fork of tree. 1–3 eggs. Incubation for 33 days. Fledges at 40 days				
Long-crested eagle (*Lophaetus occipitalis*)		Male: 912–1300 g Female: 1300–1500 g	Mostly rodents. Also small birds, lizards, arthropods, and fish	Wooded areas, in the vicinity of marshes, wetlands, and rivers
Reproduction: Green leaf-lined stick nest in tree. 1–2 eggs. Incubation for 42 days. Fledges at 53–58 days				
Long-eared owl	See North America			
Long-legged buzzard (*Buteo rufinus*)		Male: 1100 g Female: 1300 g	Small mammals, reptiles, and insects	Arid steppe or semi-desert, as well as in mountainous regions
Reproduction: Nests on rock or cliff ledges and trees. 3–5 eggs. Incubation for 33–35 days. Fledges at 43–45 days				
Long-tailed hawk (*Urotriorchis macrourus*)		492 g	Small mammals (mainly squirrels) and birds	Lowland tropical evergreen forest, rarely in open
Reproduction: Nest in high trees				
Madagascar long-eared owl (*Asio madagascariensis*)			Small mammals, birds, reptiles, and insects.	Drier western forests but appears to be quite adaptable
Reproduction: Mostly unknown. Thought to lay its eggs in stick nests created by other animals				
Madagascar red owl (*Tyto soumagnei*)		323–435 g	Small rodents and insects	Humid forest areas, but hunts in adjacent open country

Continued

Name	Abbrev.	Weight range	Diet	Habitat
Reproduction: Nests in tree cavities. Probably 2 eggs. Incubation unknown. Fledges at 10 weeks				
Madagascar scops owl (*Otus rutilus*)		Male: 85–107 g Female: 112–116 g	Insects, especially moths and beetles. May also take small vertebrates	Rainforest and humid bushy country
Reproduction: Nests in natural tree holes. 4–5 eggs. Incubation and fledging unknown				
Marsh owl (*Asio carpensis*)		225–485 g	Small mammals, such as rodents, birds, amphibians, reptiles, and large insects	Multitude of habitats, ranging from estuaries, mangroves, grasslands, and open savannah
Reproduction: Ground nest in tall grass. 2–6 eggs. Incubation for 27–28 days. Fledges at 29–35 days				
Martial eagle (*Polemaetus bellicosus*)		3000–4700 g	Mammals as large as small antelopes. It may also eat snakes, large lizards, and birds	Grassland, wooded savannah, and riparian forests
Reproduction: Nests in tree or cliff. 1–2 eggs. Incubation for 45–53 days. Fledges at 90–190 days				
Merlin	See North America			
Montagu's harrier (*Circus pygargus*)		Male: 227–305 g Female: 320–445 g	Small rodents, birds, snakes, lizards, and large insects	Open country, steppe, lightly forested areas, grasslands, and marshlands
Reproduction: Nests on ground in tall vegetation. 3–5 eggs. Incubation for 28–29 days by female. Fledges at 30–40 days Note: Migratory—winters in sub-Saharan Africa				
Mountain buzzard (*Buteo oreophilus*)		700 g	Small mammals, reptiles, and insects	Patches of hilly and montane forests, including exotic plantations
Reproduction: Nests in fork of high tree. 2 eggs. Incubation unknown. Fledges at 7 weeks				
Northern goshawk	See North America			
Northern white-faced owl (*Ptilopsis leucotis*)		185–220 g	Invertebrates and small vertebrates such as reptiles, birds, and mammals	Savannahs, open and riverine woodlands, and thornveld with acacias
Reproduction: Nests in natural hollows or crevices, or old nests of other birds. 2–4 eggs. Incubation for 30 days. Fledges at 30–32 days				
Osprey	See North America			
Ovambo sparrowhawk (*Accipiter ovampensis*)		Male: 105–190 g Female: 180–305 g	Mainly on small birds up to the size of doves. Some flying insects may also be taken	Forest, woodland, and exotic tree plantations
Reproduction: Stick-and-leaf nest in crown of tree. 1–5 eggs. Incubation for 33–36 days. Fledges at 33 days				
Pale chanting goshawk (*Melierax canorus*)		Male: 410–750 g Female: 750–1000 g	Hares, rodents, birds, snakes, lizards, and insects	Savannahs, arid steppes, and dry, open semi-desert

Continued

Name	Abbrev.	Weight range	Diet	Habitat
Reproduction: Nest in thorn acacias. 1–2 eggs. Incubation for 37 days. Fledges at 7–8 weeks				
Pallid harrier (*Circus macrourus*)		Male: 315 g Female: 445 g	Small mammals, birds, and large insects	Open country, mainly steppes and grasslands
Reproduction: Grass nests on ground under vegetation. 3–6 eggs. Incubation for 30 days. Fledges at 35–40 days				
Pallid scops owl (*Otus brucei*)		100–110 g	Mostly insects, but also lizards, spiders, and small mammals	A wide variety of semi-open, cultivated, and arid areas
Reproduction: Nests in tree cavities. 4–6 eggs. Incubation for 26–28 days. Fledges at 30 days				
Palm-nut vulture (*Gypohierax angolensis*)		1360–1700 g	Mainly fruit of the oil palm, though it also feeds on crabs, mollusks, locusts, and fish	Tropical forest edges, lakes, estuaries, large rivers, and seashores
Reproduction: Bulky tree nests. 1 egg. Incubation for 6–7 weeks. Fledges at 3 months				
Pearl-spotted owlet (*Glaucidium perlatum*)		Male: 36–86 g Female: 61–147 g	Mainly arthropods, but also bats, birds, rodents, and lizards	Lightly wooded areas, forest, open woodland, and grassland
Reproduction: Natural cavity nests. 2–4 eggs. Incubation for 30 days. Fledges at 31 days				
Pel's fishing owl (*Scotopelia peli*)		2000–2300 g	Fish	Forest or woodland along the edges of rivers, swamps, lakes, and estuaries
Reproduction: Nests in shady trees close to the water. 2 eggs (only 1 chick is raised). Incubation for 32–33 days. Fledges at 68–70 days				
Peregrine falcon	See North America			
Pharaoh eagle owl (*Bubo ascalaphus*)		1900–2300 g	Small vertebrates (mammals, birds, and reptiles), larger insects	Arid habitats, including open desert plains, rocky outcrops, mountain cliffs, and wadis
Reproduction: Nests in shallow scrapes in rocks. 2 eggs. Incubation for 31–36 days. Starts fledging at 20–35 days, but not fully fledged for another month				
Pygmy falcon (*Polihierax semitorquatus*)		54–67 g	Small lizards and large insects. It also takes some rodents and birds	Arid and semi-arid steppes with sparse vegetation and some large trees or plants
Reproduction: Nests in a large weaver nest. 3 eggs. Incubation for 28–30 days. Fledges at 27–40 days				
Red kite	See Europe			
Red-breasted goshawk (*Accipiter toussenelii*)		Male: 150–235 g Female: 170–265 g	Main foods are frogs and freshwater crabs, also small mammals, lizards, large insects, and birds	Low-altitude forests, especially rainforests and dense second growth, often near wetlands
Reproduction: Leaf-lined stick nests. 2–3 eggs. Incubation for 4–5 weeks. Fledges at 32–36 days				

Continued

Name	Abbrev.	Weight range	Diet	Habitat
Red-footed falcon (*Falco vespertinus*)		130–197 g	Variety of insects, amphibians, reptiles, mammals, and birds.	Variety of open habitats with some tree cover.
Reproduction: Colonial breeder, reusing the old nests of corvids. 3–4 eggs. Incubation for 27–28 days. Fledges at 27–30 days				
Red-necked buzzard (*Buteo auguralis*)		Male: 525–620 g Female: 580–890 g	Small animals, including insects, reptiles, and mammals	Prefers forest edges and clearings
Reproduction: Stick nest in large tree. 1–2 eggs. Incubation unknown				
Red-necked falcon (*Falco chicquera*)		Male: 139–178 g Female: 190–305 g	Primarily small birds, such as larks and sparrows, but will occasionally take larger prey	Semi-desert, open grasslands with large trees, watercourses, flood and coastal plains
Reproduction: Reuses old nests of other raptors or corvids. 2–5 eggs. Incubation for 32–35 days. Fledges at 35–40 days				
Red-thighed sparrowhawk (*Accipiter erythropus*)		Male: 78–94 g Female: 132–170 g	Small birds up to the size of pigeons, lizards, amphibians, and insects	Lowland primary and older secondary forest and forest edges
Reproduction: 2 eggs. Incubation and fledging unknown				
Rock kestrel (*Falco rupicolus*)		136–314 g	Small mammals (rodents), insects, small birds, and reptiles including snakes	Wide range of habitats. Seems to favor mountainous, hilly, and rocky areas
Reproduction: Usually nests in rocky cliffs. 1–6 eggs. Incubation for 27–31 days. Fledges at 30–36 days				
Rufous-breasted sparrowhawk (*Accipiter rufiventris*)		180–210 g	Almost exclusively small birds, but will go to the ground to hunt insects, reptiles, and small mammals	Open habitats such as savannah, grassland
Reproduction: New platform nest built yearly. 2–4 eggs. Incubation for 34 days. Fledges at 4–5 weeks				
Rüppell's vulture or **Ruepell's griffon** (*Gyps rueppellii*)		6800–9000 g	Feeds solely on carrion	Open savannah, mountains, and semi-arid country
Reproduction: Roosts and nests on cliffs in colonies. 1 egg. Incubation for 55 days. Fledges at 150 days. Note: Critically endangered				
Saker falcon	See Europe			
Sandy scops owl or **Cinnamon scops owl** (*Otus icterorhynchus*)		Male: 69–80 g Female: 61–80 g	Crickets and grasshoppers	Humid lowland forest
Reproduction: Unknown				

Continued

Name	Abbrev.	Weight range	Diet	Habitat
Scissor-tailed kite (*Chelictinia riocourii*)		110 g	Mainly insects and arachnids. Will take more lizards and rodents in breeding season	Arid sub-Saharan steppe and scrub savannah
Reproduction: Nests in thorny bushes. 4 eggs.				
Secretarybird (*Sagittarius serpentarius*)		2200–4300 g	Large insects, reptiles, and small mammals, which it often stamps on before swallowing whole	Open country, mostly savannahs, scrub, and grasslands
Reproduction: Nests in acacia trees. 1–3 eggs. Incubation for 42–46 days. Fledges at 65–106 days Note: Although it can fly, this species is largely terrestrial and can cover 30 km/day Note: This species is both taller and longer than any other species of raptor				
Seychelles scops owl (*Otus insularis*)		130–159 g	Lizards, insects, and possibly tree frogs	Forests, slopes, and valleys usually close to a water source
Reproduction: Nests in trees. 1 egg. Incubation for 25–30 days. Fledges at 4–6 weeks				
Shelley's eagle owl (*Bubo shelleyi*)		1257 g	Medium-sized mammals and large birds	Lowland primary rainforest and forest edge
Reproduction: 3 eggs. Incubation for 34 days				
Shikra	See Europe			
Short-eared owl	See North America			
Short-toed snake eagle (*Circaetus gallicus*)		Male: 1200–2000 g Female: 1300–2300 g	Snakes make up majority of their diet. They can be over 150 cm long and are usually eaten whole	Lowland forest, wetlands, grassland, and desert
Reproduction: Usually tree nest of sticks. 1 egg. Incubation for 47 days. Fledges at 70–80 days				
Sokoke scops owl (*Otus ireneae*)		45–55 g	Mainly on insects such as crickets and beetles	In tropical coastal forests where *Cynometra* and *Brachylaena* are growing
Reproduction: Nests in natural cavities				
Sooty falcon (*Falco concolor*)		350 g	Small birds, bats, and insects. Hunts on the wing	During summer breeding season it occupies hot, arid areas. Winter near water sources
Reproduction: Nests on cliff ledges. 2–4 eggs. Incubation for 27–30 days. Fledges at 32–38 days				
Southern banded snake eagle (*Circaetus fasciolatus*)		950–1110 g	Snakes, lizards, chameleons, frogs, and insects. Some small mammals	Coastal and subcoastal forest close to rivers, marshes, or flood plains

Continued

Name	Abbrev.	Weight range	Diet	Habitat
Reproduction: Nest in tree fork. 1 egg. Incubation for 49–51 days. Fledges at 10–15 weeks Note: The chicks are fed by both parents with a diet of shredded snake flesh				
Southern white-faced owl (*Ptilopsis granti*)		Male: 185–240 g Female: 225–275 g	Large insects, spiders, small birds, reptiles, and small mammals	Savannah, dry open woods, wooded areas along rivers, forest edges, and clearings
Reproduction: Nests in natural holes or platform nests of other larger birds. 2–3 eggs. Incubation for 30 days. Fledges at 30–32 days				
Spotted eagle owl (*Bubo africanus*)		Male: 487–620 g Female: 640–850 g	Invertebrates, small mammals, birds, and reptiles	Open woodlands, rocky hills, and ravines, savannahs, semi-deserts, and grasslands
Reproduction: Nests in many natural cavities, large abandoned nests, and in bushes on the ground. 2–4 eggs. Incubation for 32 days. Fledges at 7 weeks				
Spotted owlet (*Athene brama*)		110–115 g	Mainly insects, but also lizards, mice, and small birds	Open or semi-open country, including semi-desert
Reproduction: Nests in cavities in cliff-sides or ravines. 3–5 eggs				
Steppe eagle	See Europe			
Taita falcon (*Falco fasciinucha*)		Male: 212–233 g Female: 297–346 g	Mainly small birds caught in flight but also insects and bats	Large cliffs, gorges, or rocky out-cropping frequently in areas of Mopane woodland
Reproduction: Nests normally on bare rock. 2–4 eggs. Incubation for 31–33 days. Fledges at 42 days				
Tawny eagle	See Europe			
Torotoroka scops owl (*Otus madagascariensis*)		108 g	Insects and small vertebrates	Moist and drier forests, thickets, humid bush country, and parks
Reproduction: Nests in natural tree cavities. 2–5 eggs				
Vermiculated fishing owl (*Scotopelia bouvieri*)		637 g	Small fish, frogs, crustaceans, fiddler crabs, and small birds and mammals	Gallery forest along rivers and pools in primary forest. Flooded forest
Reproduction: Unknown				
Verreaux's eagle (*Aquila verreauxii*)		Male: 3.1–4.1 kg Female: 3.1–5.8 kg	Mainly rock hyraxes, but also francolins, guinea fowl, herons, egrets, reptiles, hares, monkeys	Rocky areas, cliffs, mountains, savannah, woodland, and sub-desert habitats
Reproduction: Stick nest usually on cliff ledges. 1–3 eggs. Incubation for 43–47 days. Fledges at 84–99 days Note: Cooperative hunting is utilized for hunting hyraxes, where one eagle flies above to distract the hyrax colony and the other eagle attacks. They are also reported to push hyraxes off cliffs				
Verreaux's owl (*Bubo lacteus*)		Male: 1615–1960 g Female: 2475–3115 g	Birds, insects, mammals such as hedgehogs, hares, mongooses, small rodents	Arid semi-desert, to moist, tall woodlands

Continued

Name	Abbrev.	Weight range	Diet	Habitat
Reproduction: Usually uses old stick nests of other birds. 2 eggs. Incubation for 38 days. Only 1 chick will survive beyond 2 weeks as the adults preferentially only feed one. Fledges at 9 weeks				
Wahlberg's eagle (*Aquila wahlbergi*)		Male: 437–845 g Female: 670–1400 g	Mainly reptiles, mammals, and birds	Woodland, wooded savannah, grassland, often close to rivers
Reproduction: Nest in tall trees. 1–2 eggs. Incubation for 44–46 days. Fledges at 62–80 days.				
Western banded snake eagle (*Circaetus cinerascens*)		1125 g	Snakes and amphibians, but also small mammals, fish, and insects	Woodland, forest edges, and wooded savannah, often close to rivers
Reproduction: Stick nest in well-concealed vegetation. 1 egg. Incubation for 35–55 days. Fledges at 10–15 weeks				
Western marsh harrier (*Circus aeruginosus*)		405–670 g	Frogs, small mammals, snakes, lizards, and insects. Easy prey such as bird eggs and chicks, injured or sick birds	Freshwater wetlands, fishponds, and marshes
Reproduction: Nests in reeds. 3–8 eggs. Incubation for 33–38 days. Fledges at 35–40 days Note: This species flies at about 50 km/h, being the fastest harrier despite its larger size				
White-backed vulture (*Gyps africanus*)		4150–7200 g	Scavenger. Carrion	Open savannah and wooded country
Reproduction: Platform nest in large tree. 1 egg. Incubation for 56–58 days. Fledges at 120–130 days Note: Critically endangered				
White-browed hawk owl (*Ninox superciliaris*)			Mainly insects and spiders, small vertebrates such as rodents and birds. Perch-hunter	Open terrain with few trees, semi-arid thorn scrub, savannah, and deciduous dry forest
Reproduction: Nests in open tree cavity or in depression in ground. 3–5 eggs				
White-headed vulture (*Trigonoceps occipitalis*)		3300–5300 g	Feeds mainly on carrion, but also consumes freshly killed prey such as flamingos and small antelope	Dry regions, in open areas such as plains and desert, savannah and thorn bush
Reproduction: Platform stick nest in tall trees. 1 egg. Incubation for 43–54 days. Fledges at 115 days Note: This vulture prefers freshly killed prey, unlike other vulture species				
Yellow-billed kite (*Milvus parasitus*)		Male: 630–930 g Female: 750–940 g	Wide range of small vertebrates and insects, much of which is scavenged	Found in almost all habitats, including parks in suburban areas
Reproduction: Small stick nest in tree. 2–3 eggs. Incubation for 30 days. Fledges at 48 days				

Asia

Name	Abbrev.	Weight range	Diet	Habitat
African scops owl	See Africa			
Amur falcon	See Africa			
Andaman hawk owl (*Ninox affinis*)		Unknown	Mainly insects	Mainly lowland forest
Reproduction: Unknown Note: Endemic to the Andaman Islands				
Andaman scops owl (*Otus balli*)		Unknown	Primarily insects	Trees in semi-open areas, settlements, and cultivated areas and gardens
Reproduction: Unknown				
Andaman serpent eagle (*Spilornis elgini*)		790–1000 g	Birds, frogs, lizards, snakes, and rats	Rainforests of the interior of the island
Reproduction: Unknown				
Asian barred owlet (*Glaucidium cuculoides*)		150–240 g	Beetles, grasshoppers, cicadas, and other large insects. Lizards, mice, and small birds	Open sub-montane or montane forest of pine, oak, and rhododendron. Also inhabits subtropical and tropical evergreen jungle at lower elevations
Reproduction: Nests in cavities. 4 eggs. Incubation unknown Note: Generally a diurnal bird				
Australasian grass owl (*Tyto longimembris*)		250–582 g	Mainly rodents	Tall grasslands and swampy country
Reproduction: Nests on the ground in dense tussocks of grass or sedges, usually well away from trees. It is enveloped in grasses and is approached by a series of at least 3 tunnels. 3–8 eggs. Incubation for 42 days. Fledges at 2 months Note: Also called the Eastern grass owl				
Barn owl	See North America			
Barred eagle owl (*Bubo sumatranus*)		Unknown	Very broad, opportunistic diet	Evergreen forest with ponds and streams, gardens with large, densely foliaged trees, groves in cultivated country, sometimes not far from habitation
Reproduction: Unknown				
Bat hawk	See Australia			
Bawean serpent eagle (*Spilornis baweanus*)		Unknown	Mostly snakes and lizards	The only diurnal raptor that lives on the island of Bawean in the Java Sea
Reproduction: Unknown Note: Critically endangered species with only 65–70 individuals reported				

Continued

Name	Abbrev.	Weight range	Diet	Habitat
Bearded vulture	See Europe			
Besra (*Accipiter virgatus*)		80–210 g	Large insects, small birds, mammals, reptiles, and frogs	Deciduous and evergreen forests, dense forests, savannah, and cultivated lands
Reproduction: Nests in trees. 2–5 eggs				
Black baza (*Aviceda leuphotes*)		168–224 g	Primarily large insects, but will eat lizards and small mammals	Open deciduous or evergreen tropical forest, often around clearings, near streams or rivers
Reproduction: Both sexes build a small, compact nest with twigs and thin sticks in a large tree in the forest, often near water. 2–3 eggs				
Black kite	See Australia			
Black-thighed falconet (*Microhierax fringillarius*)		28–55 g	Mainly feeds on insects, including moths, butterflies, dragonflies, termites, and cicadas; occasionally small birds and lizards	Forest, forest edge, and wooded open area
Reproduction: Nests in old nest holes of barbets, or occasionally old woodpecker holes. 2–5 eggs. Incubation and fledging times unknown Note: Smallest bird of prey				
Black-winged kite	See Australia			
Blakiston's fish owl (*Ketupa blakistoni*)		2.25–4.6 kg	Mainly fish and small vertebrates	Riverine forest and coniferous forest
Reproduction: Nests in large tree-hollows. 1–3 eggs. Incubation for 35 days. Fledges at 35–40 days				
Blyth's hawk-eagle (*Nisaetus alboniger*)		830 g	Small mammals, birds, lizards, and bats	Tropical areas where there is montane and hilly forest
Reproduction: The nest is deep, cup-shaped, and usually set in a tree higher than the rest of the canopy. Clutch size is unknown, but all observed nests have had 1 egg. Incubation and fledging length unknown				
Bonelli's eagle	See Africa			
Booted eagle	See Africa			
Boreal owl	See North America			
Brahminy kite	See Australia			
Brown fish owl (*Ketupa zeylonensis*)		1105–1308 g	Fish, frogs, and crabs, but will also take rodents, birds, reptiles, and large beetles	Thick lowland forest and open but well-wooded country. Always near water
Reproduction: Typically nests in cavities. They will also use abandoned stick nests of large birds, or a rock ledge, or ruins of an old building. 1–2 eggs. Incubation for 34–38 days. Fledges at about 50 days				

Continued

Name	Abbrev.	Weight range	Diet	Habitat
Brown hawk owl (*Ninox scutulata*)		170–230 g	Large insects such as beetles and grasshoppers, but also frogs, lizards, small birds, mice, and occasionally small insectivorous bats or crabs	In northern regions, inhabits forest and woodland. In South-east Asia, occurs exclusively in primary lowland rainforest, far from human habitation
Reproduction: Nests in cavities. 2–5 eggs. Incubation for around 25 days. Fledges at 24–27 days Note: Also known as the Brown boobook				
Brown wood owl (*Strix leptogrammica*)		800–1100 g	Small mammals, small birds, and reptiles. Fish have been reported	Heavy tropical forest along the sea coast, in lowlands, and in lower hills
Reproduction: Nests in cavities. 2 eggs. Incubation and fledging length unknown				
Buffy fish owl (*Ketupa ketupu*)		1028–2100 g	Mainly fish, as well as crustaceans, reptiles, frogs, toads, and insects	Unknown
Reproduction: Often nests on tip of bird's-nest ferns, or in fork of a thick branch covered by ferns, moss, and orchids. Will also nest in tree-hollows or other raptors' nests, and sometimes may resort to caves in rocky sites. 1–2 eggs. Incubation for 28–29 days. Fledges at 6 weeks. Typically only 1 chick survives				
Central Nicobar serpent eagle (*Spilornis minimus*)		Unknown	Unknown. Possibly lizards, domestic chicken, and crab	Found in forest near rivers, but not frequenting the shore or clearings. Occurs mostly below 100 m
Reproduction: Unknown Note: A subspecies of the widespread Crested serpent eagle				
Chestnut-backed owlet (*Glaucidium castanonotum*)			Mainly insects such as beetles, but also consumes mice, lizards, and small birds	Wet dense forests, and can be seen from lowlands up to 2000 m in elevation
Reproduction: Nests in cavities. Typically 2 eggs. Reproduction details unknown				
Chinese goshawk (*Accipiter soloensis*)			Frogs, lizards, large insects, and caterpillars	Frequents forest edge, selectively logged forest, open woodland, open country with trees, lightly wooded cultivation, and rice fields
Reproduction: The nest is a flat saucer of sticks, lined with green leaves and placed in fork or on lateral branch of a tree, often near a wetland. 2–5 eggs Note: Complete long-distance, trans-equatorial migrant. Migrates in large soaring flocks				
Chocolate boobook (*Ninox randi*)		200–220 g	Insects (moths and dragonflies)	Lowland mangroves and rainforests
Reproduction: Unknown				

Continued

Name	Abbrev.	Weight range	Diet	Habitat
Cinereous vulture	See Africa			
Cinnabar hawk owl (*Ninox ios*)			Feeds predominantly upon flying insects	Forests
Reproduction: Unknown Note: Discovered in 1999				
Collared falconet (*Microhierax caerulescens*)		30–50 g	Mainly insects, especially butterflies, but also dragonflies, lantern flies, grasshoppers, beetles, and cicadas; also takes small forest and open habitat birds and lizards	Deciduous to moist-deciduous and evergreen forest-dwelling species
Reproduction: Nests in cavities in trees, often in holes positioned on the underside of a bare branch; nest holes are half-filled with a bed-like layer of dried leaves and insect parts. 4 eggs				
Collared owlet (*Glaucidium brodiei*)		52–63 g	Mainly small birds, but will also take mice, lizards, cicadas, grasshoppers, beetles, and other large insects	Usually sub-montane and montane forests with open spaces, clearing, and forest edges. Woodland with scrub
Reproduction: Unknown Note: This bird is both diurnal and crepuscular				
Collared scops owl (*Otus lettia*)		100–170 g	Mainly beetles, grasshoppers, and other insects, but will also take lizards, mice, and small birds	Forest, scrub, second growth; also groves of trees and bamboo stands around habitations, open country and towns
Reproduction: Nests in cavities				
Common buzzard	See Africa			
Common kestrel	See Africa			
Crested goshawk (*Accipiter trivirgatus*)		224–450 g	Squirrels, rodents, bats, and birds	Occurs in broadleaved and coniferous forest, urban parkland, and marshes
Reproduction: Stick nest placed in fork near the top of a tree. 2–3 eggs				
Crested hawk-eagle (*Nisaetus cirrhatus*)		1.3–1.9 kg	Birds (up to the size of domestic chickens), medium-sized mammals, snakes, and lizards	Dry deciduous to semi-evergreen forest, including late second-growth logged forest with clearings, and cultivated areas
Reproduction: Stick nest placed high in a main branch fork of a large tree. 1 egg. Incubation for 35–44 days. Fledges at 65–70 days Note: The most widespread and common Asiatic hawk-eagle species				

Continued

Name	Abbrev.	Weight range	Diet	Habitat
Crested honey buzzard (*Pernis ptilorhyncus*)		750–1490 g	A specialist feeder, living mainly on the larvae of social bees and wasps, also eating bits of comb and honey. It will take other small insect prey such as cicadas	Lowland and montane deciduous broadleaved or mixed broadleaved/coniferous forests with river valleys
Reproduction: Stick nest placed in a tall tree. 1–2 eggs. Incubation for 28–35 days by both parents. Fledges at 35–45 days Note: Also called the Oriental honey buzzard				
Crested serpent eagle (*Spilornis cheela*)		420–1800 g	Mainly snakes, but they also catch lizards, frogs, toads, large insects, and small birds	Wide range of habitats, including rainforest, open savannah, mangrove swamps, plantations, ravines, evergreen and deciduous forest, and tidal creeks
Reproduction: Nest made of sticks and lined with leaves in trees often close to water. 1 egg. Incubation by female for 35 days. Fledges at 60 days Note: There are at least 15 subspecies of this bird				
Dusky eagle owl (*Bubo coromandus*)			Small mammals, birds, reptiles, fish, and large insects	Forest and forest edge, plantation. Prefers watered and well-wooded areas. Mango tree groves, and old tamarind and other densely foliaged trees
Reproduction: Nest made of sticks in the fork of the trunk of a large tree preferably near water and often in the vicinity of human habitation. 1–3 eggs				
Eastern buzzard (*Buteo japonicus*)			Small and medium-sized mammals, birds, reptiles, amphibians, and insects	All types of forests, but always close to open area
Reproduction: Unknown Note: Considered a subspecies of the widespread Common buzzard				
Eastern imperial eagle	See Africa			
Eastern marsh harrier (*Circus spilonotus*)		350–800 g	Small mammals, birds, frogs, and reptiles	Open country including marshland, paddy fields, and grassland
Reproduction: Nest made of sticks on the ground, usually in a reed bed. 4–7 eggs. Incubation for 33–48 days. Fledges at 35–40 days Note: Mostly migratory				
Egyptian vulture	See Africa			
Enggano scops owl (*Otus enganensis*)			Mainly on insects, spiders, and other arthropods	It is thought to occupy forest and wooded areas

Continued

Name	Abbrev.	Weight range	Diet	Habitat
Reproduction: Unknown Note: Endemic to Enggano Island				
Eurasian eagle owl	See Europe			
Eurasian hobby	See Europe			
Eurasian pygmy owl	See Europe			
Eurasian sparrowhawk	See Europe			
European honey buzzard	See Europe			
European scops owl	See Europe			
Flores hawk-eagle (*Nisaetus floris*)			Small mammals, birds, and lizards	Lowland rainforest
Reproduction: Unknown Note: Considered a critically endangered species Note: Formerly classified as a subspecies of *Nisaetus cirrhatus* (Crested hawk-eagle)				
Forest owlet (*Athene blewitti*)			Reptiles, insects, rodents, birds, frogs, and invertebrates	Riparian jungle, mangrove groves, and open deciduous forests
Reproduction: Unknown Note: Believed extinct until rediscovered in 1997. Critically endangered				
Golden eagle	See North America			
Great gray owl	See North America			
Great Nicobar serpent eagle (*Spilornis klossi*)			Reptiles, rodents, and birds	Primary forest, often within the canopy
Reproduction: Unknown Note: Considered a subspecies of *Spilornis cheela* (Crested serpent eagle)				
Greater spotted eagle	See Africa			
Grey-faced buzzard (*Butastur indicus*)			Frogs, snakes, lizards, insects, and small rodents	Varied habitats. Woodlands, paddy fields, streams, and grasslands. In its breeding range: coniferous and mixed evergreen forests in mountains, at forest edges, fields, meadows, marshes, and around agricultural lands
Reproduction: Small stick nest in a tree. 3–4 eggs. Incubation about 1 month. Fledges at around 35–39 days Note: Complete, long-distance, trans-equatorial migrant. This is one of the species that dominates the "East Asian Continental Flyway"				
Grey-headed fish eagle (*Ichthyophaga ichthyaetus*)		1600–2700 g	Fish, small birds, mammals, and dead fish	Lowland forests close to fresh water, streams, large ponds, rivers, and marshes. Also along sea coasts and near estuaries
Reproduction: Large stick nest in tall tree. 1–2 eggs. Incubation by both parents for 45–50 days. Fledges at around 70 days				

Continued

Name	Abbrev.	Weight range	Diet	Habitat
Griffon vulture	See Africa			
Gyrfalcon	See North America			
Hen harrier	See Africa			
Himalayan vulture (*Gyps himalayensis*)		8–12 kg	Only carrion	Mountains between 1500 and 4000 m in elevation
Reproduction: May be solitary nester or form small, loose colonies of about 5–6 pairs, usually well above the treeline. Large stick nest. 1 egg. Incubation by both parents for 54–58 days. Chick stays with parents 6–7 months				
Hume's owl (*Strix butleri*)		162–225 g	Small mammals, birds, reptiles, insects, and scorpions	Semi-deserts and rocky ravines with water
Reproduction: Unknown Note: Unusual for owls, this species is mostly independent of forests				
Indian black eagle (*Ictinaetus malayensis*)		1.0–1.6 kg	Small mammals such as bats, rats, squirrels, and flying squirrels. Reptiles, frogs, insects, and some birds	Lowland, evergreen, and montane forests, up to 4000 m above sea level. They prefer slopes and mountainous country and areas where there is forest cover
Reproduction: Large stick nest/platform usually set in fork of a tree with a dense canopy above. 1–2 eggs. Incubation for 35–40 days. Fledges at 60 days				
Indian scops owl (*Otus bakkamoena*)		125–152 g	Mainly insects including beetles and grasshoppers. Occasionally small vertebrates	Forest and secondary woodland, desert vegetation and groups of densely foliaged trees in gardens, mango orchards, and other fruit trees around villages and cultivations
Reproduction: Nests in cavities. 3–4 eggs. Incubation for 27–28 days. Fledges at 4–5 weeks				
Indian spotted eagle (*Clanga hastata*)			Mammals, frogs, and birds	Wetlands, open forest, forest clearings, and cultivated areas
Reproduction: The nest is a flat platform placed in fork of a tree. 1–2 eggs. Incubation by both sexes for 31 days. Fledges at around 71 days				
Indian vulture (*Gyps indicus*)		5.5–6.3 kg	Carrion	Hilly crags in India. Can be found in cities near cultivated areas or around garbage dumps and slaughterhouses
Reproduction: Nests mainly on cliffs but has also been known to nest in trees. 1 egg. Incubation by both sexes for 50 days Note: Serious declines in population due to poisoning by diclofenac use in cattle				
Japanese scops owl (*Otus semitorques*)		130 g	Mainly large insects, but also feeds on spiders, small mammals, frogs, and birds	Forest and wooded gardens, often near villages and suburbs
Reproduction: Nests in cavities. 4–5 eggs				

Continued

Name	Abbrev.	Weight range	Diet	Habitat
Japanese sparrowhawk (*Accipiter gularis*)		85–193 g	Small- to medium-sized birds	Breeds mainly in deciduous forests and also in urban parks. Avoids closed-canopy forest and plantation monocultures
Reproduction: Stick nest usually near trunk of a tree. 2–5 eggs. Incubation for 25–28 days. Fledges at about 1 month				
Javan hawk-eagle (*Nisaetus bartelsi*)			Small mammals, birds, snakes, and lizards	Primary forest, secondary forest, tree plantations, and semi-deciduous forest
Reproduction: Stick nest lined with green leaves in a large tree in undisturbed forest. 1 egg. Incubation for 47–48 days. Fledges at 68–72 days. Pairs breed every 2 years if nesting is successful, since juveniles may remain close to the nest for 1 year after they fledge Note: Endangered. Endemic to the island of Java in Indonesia				
Javan owlet (*Glaucidium castanopterum*)			Mainly insects but also spiders, scorpions, lizards, small mammals, birds, and sometimes snakes	Dense primary lowland rainforests and thick bamboo jungle
Reproduction: Unknown Note: Endemic to Java and Bali				
Javan scops owl (*Otus angelinae*)		75–91 g	Prefers larger insects	Humid primary forests with thick undergrowth
Reproduction: Unknown Note: Rare owl that lives in the mountains of Java				
Jerdon's baza (*Aviceda jerdoni*)		Around 350 g	Snakes, lizards, frogs, and insects	Primary forest and freshwater swamp forest in lowlands and foothills. Also at forest edges and in partially cleared areas
Reproduction: The nest is a bulky structure with a fairly deep cup placed in a tree. 2–3 eggs				
Jungle owlet (*Glaucidium radiatum*)		88–114 g	Grasshoppers, locusts, cicadas, and other large insects	Himalayan foothills, sub-montane moist deciduous forest, and secondary jungle with bamboos. Also in dry to moist deciduous forests
Reproduction: Nests are in natural tree-hollows, or abandoned woodpecker or barbet holes. 2–3 eggs Note: Generally crepuscular				
Kinabalu serpent eagle (*Spilornis kinabaluensis*)			Snakes and lizards	Restricted to montane forest, from 750 to 2900 m above sea level
Reproduction: Unknown				
Laggar falcon (*Falco jugger*)		525–850 g	Primarily birds	Dry open woodland and other open habitats with scattered trees

Continued

Name	Abbrev.	Weight range	Diet	Habitat
Reproduction: Generally uses the old nest of vultures, kites, or crows placed in a tree, cliff, or building. 3–4 eggs. Incubation for 30 days. Fledges at 42–49 days Note: It is slower than other falcons, but can use its surroundings effectively to hunt, often flying with the sun behind it which makes it very difficult for prey to see the hunter				
Lanner falcon	See Africa			
Lappet-faced vulture	See Africa			
Legge's hawk-eagle (*Nisaetus kelaarti*)			Small mammals, birds, and reptiles	Primary evergreen forest and forest patches
Reproduction: Unknown				
Lesser fish eagle (*Ichthyophaga humilis*)		780–785 g	Primarily fish	Forested rivers, lakes, and wetlands. Sometimes found around open bodies of water
Reproduction: Stick nest lined with green leaves in a tree close to water. 2–4 eggs Note: Unlike the related Grey-headed fish eagle, which prefers standing and sluggish wetlands, Lesser fish eagles occur more often along hill streams, fast-flowing rivers, and other moving water				
Lesser kestrel	See Africa			
Lesser spotted eagle	See Africa			
Levant sparrowhawk	See Africa			
Little owl	See Africa			
Long-legged buzzard	See Africa			
Luzon scops owl (*Otus longicornis*)			Little known, but mainly insects	Humid, closed-canopy forests in foothills and pine forests on mountains up to 2200 m
Reproduction: Unknown Note: Endemic to Luzon				
Mantanani scops owl (*Otus mantananensis*)		106–110 g	Mainly insects and arthropods, occasionally small vertebrates	Wooded areas and forests. Also coconut groves and casuarina plantations
Reproduction: Nests in cavities Note: Found on small islands between Borneo and the Philippines				
Mentawai scops owl (*Otus mentawi*)			Mainly insects	Lowland rainforest but also found in secondary growth and in villages near human habitation
Reproduction: Unknown Note: Endemic to larger islands of Mentawai, off west Sumatra, Indonesia. Locally common but little studied				
Mentawai serpent eagle (*Spilornis sipora*)			Tree snakes and other reptiles	Forest on Mentawai Islands, below 450 m from sea level

Continued

Name	Abbrev.	Weight range	Diet	Habitat
Reproduction: No data Note: Non-migratory				
Merlin	See North America			
Minahassa owl (*Tyto inexspectata*)			Small mammals	Tropical rainforest as well as drier, degraded forests on Minahassa Peninsula in northern Sulawesi
Reproduction: Likely nests in hollow trees in early April. Fledged juveniles observed being fed in early to mid-September Note: Non-migratory				
Mindanao eagle owl (*Mimizuku gurneyi*)			Small mammals and birds, and large insects	Grassland, lowland rainforest, and secondary growth in southern Philippines
Reproduction: Unknown Note: Non-migratory				
Mindanao scops owl (*Otus mirus*)			Insects	High-elevation mountain rainforest on the island of Mindanao
Reproduction: No data Note: Non-migratory				
Mindoro scops owl (*Otus mindorensis*)			Insects	Montane forest above 870 m in Mindoro
Reproduction: No data Note: Non-migratory				
Moluccan scops owl (*Otus magicus*)		114–165 g	Insects and small vertebrates	Primary forests and coastal swamp forests
Reproduction: No data Note: Non-migratory				
Montagu's harrier (*Circus pygargus*)		230–440 g	Small mammals and ground birds, reptiles, and invertebrates	Variable but mainly lowland river valleys and plains
Reproduction: 4–5 eggs. Incubation for 40 days. Fledges at 42 days Note: Elaborate mating ritual. Breeding pairs formed at 2–3 years of age may be lifelong				
Morepork (*Ninox novaeseelandiae*)		150–216 g	Huge variety of large invertebrates and insects	Trees ranging from tropical forests to isolated strands. Most common in temperate woodland in New Zealand
Reproduction: 2–3 eggs. Incubation for 30 days. Fledges at 35 days but remains with adult for another 3 months				
Mottled wood owl (*Strix ocellata*)			Palm squirrels, mice, and other small mammals	Lightly wooded plains, open woodland, and groves of mature trees on outskirts of cultivated land
Reproduction: 2–3 eggs. Breeding season: February to April				

Continued

Name	Abbrev.	Weight range	Diet	Habitat
Mountain hawk-eagle (*Nisaetus nipalensis*)			Small mammals, especially hares, and terrestrial birds	Inhabits subtropical and broadleaved forests and fir forest at higher elevations
Reproduction: 1–2 eggs				
Mountain scops owl (*Otus spilocephalus*)		53–112 g	Insects (beetles and moths)	Humid forest including temperate and subtropical or tropical rainforest, both lowland and montane
Reproduction: 2–5 eggs. Incubation by female only				
Natuna serpent eagle (*Spilornis natunensis*)			Snakes, lizards.	Wooded hills, lowland, semi-open country
Reproduction: Unknown				
Nias serpent eagle (*Spilornis asturinus*)		420–565 g	Snakes, lizards	Forested slopes on the island of Nias
Reproduction: Unknown Note: Adults non-migratory				
Nicobar scops owl (*Otus alius*)			Insects, small lizards	Coastal forest on Nicobar Island
Reproduction: Unknown Note: Non-migratory				
Nicobar sparrowhawk (*Accipiter butleri*)			Lizards, insects	Forest
Reproduction: Unknown Note: Non-migratory				
Northern boobook (*Ninox japonica*)		167–168 g	Invertebrates (beetles and moths)	Lowland deciduous forests with tall trees, wooded parks, and gardens
Reproduction: 3–4 eggs. Incubation for 25–31 days by female only. Fledges at 25–28 days				
Northern goshawk	See North America			
Northern hawk owl (*Surnia ulula*)		215–392 g	Small mammals, birds, frogs, and fish	Open boreal coniferous forest
Reproduction: 5–13 eggs. Incubation for 23–30 days by female only. Fledges at 23–30 days				
Northern long-eared owl	See North America (Long-eared owl)			
Northern Philippine hawk-eagle (*Nisaetus philippensis*)		1.1–1.2 kg	Most likely birds and small mammals	Primary dipterocarp forest and second-growth forest
Reproduction: Unknown Note: Adults non-migratory				

Continued

Name	Abbrev.	Weight range	Diet	Habitat
Ochre-bellied hawk owl (*Ninox ochracea*)			Mainly insects	Primary and tall secondary lowland forest and riverine forest
Reproduction: Unknown				
Oriental bay owl (*Phodilus badius*)		255–308 g	Small rodents, bats, birds, lizards, frogs, and large insects	Woodland, plantation, and mangrove swamps
Reproduction: 3–5 eggs. Incubation by female alone				
Oriental hobby (*Falco severus*)		168–249 g	Feeds on small birds, bats, and insects	Forest edges, clearings, secondary growth, mangroves, and native gardens
Reproduction: 2–4 eggs				
Oriental scops owl (*Otus sunia*)		75–95 g	Insects and spiders, small rodents, and small birds	Deciduous and mixed forest, also in open evergreen forest
Reproduction: Unknown				
Osprey	See North America			
Palawan scops owl (*Otus fuliginosus*)			Insects most likely	Lowland forest on the island of Palawan
Reproduction: Unknown				
Pallas's fish eagle (*Haliaeetus leucoryphus*)		2.0–3.7 kg	Mostly fish. Some birds and nestlings, mammals, reptiles, and carrion	Near freshwater systems up to 5000 m in elevation
Reproduction: 2–4 eggs. Incubation for 40–45 days. Fledges at 70–105 days. Chicks depend on parents for an additional 30 days				
Pallid harrier	See Africa			
Pallid scops owl	See Africa			
Pere David's owl (*Strix davidi*)			Unknown	Coniferous and mixed forest with adjacent open areas
Reproduction: Unknown				
Peregrine falcon	See North America			
Pharaoh eagle owl	See Africa			
Philippine eagle (*Pithecophaga jefferyi*)		4.7–8.0 kg	Large mammals including flying lemurs and squirrels, macaques, pigs, dogs, fruit bats, and small deer. Also birds, cobras, and monitor lizards	Primary dipterocarp forest, mid-montane forests, primarily along mountainsides
Reproduction: 1–2 eggs. Incubation for 58–68 days. Fledges at 4–5 months and dependent on parents for 17 more months Note: Some of the largest eagles in the world and most endangered. Captive birds have lived to be over 40 years old. Philippine national bird				

Continued

Name	Abbrev.	Weight range	Diet	Habitat
Philippine eagle owl (*Bubo philippensis*)			Presumed small mammals, birds, and possibly fish	Lowland forest, often near lakes and rivers
Reproduction: Unknown Note: One of the largest owls in the world				
Philippine hawk owl (*Ninox philippensis*)		125 g	Insects, small birds, frogs, and lizards.	Primary and second-growth rainforest
Reproduction: Unknown				
Philippine scops owl (*Otus megalotis*)		200–310 g	Insects	Tropical forest, secondary woodland, and forest edge
Reproduction: 1–2 eggs				
Philippine serpent eagle (*Spilornis holospilus*)		603–1600 g	Snakes and lizards	Large range including riparian forest, foothills, and open country
Reproduction: Unknown				
Pied falconet (*Microhierax melanoleucus*)		55–75 g	Large insects, and small to medium birds	Evergreen and deciduous woodland
Reproduction: Nests in woodpecker or barbet holes. 3–4 eggs				
Pied harrier (*Circus melanoleucus*)		254–455 g	Small rodents (voles), frogs, small birds, and nestlings	Open ground, including grasslands, steppe, and the edges of wet meadows
Reproduction: Nests on the ground, in tall grass or bushes. 3–6 eggs				
Rajah scops owl (*Otus brookii*)			Insects (moths)	Montane rainforest
Reproduction: Unknown				
Reddish scops owl (*Otus rufescens*)		70–83 g	Insects (grasshoppers, crickets) and crabs	Lowland forest
Reproduction: Unknown				
Red-footed falcon	See Africa			
Red-headed vulture (*Sarcogyps calvus*)		3.6–5.4 kg	Carrion (ungulates, birds, turtles, and fish)	Wide range including open countryside, semi-desert, cultivated areas, and savannah
Reproduction: 1 egg. Incubation for 45 days				
Red-necked falcon (*Falco chicquera*)		139–305 g	Small birds	Arid, lightly wooded, open savannah and grassland
Reproduction: 2–5 eggs. Incubation for 32–35 days. Fledges at 35–40 days				
Rock eagle owl (*Bubo bengalensis*)		1100 g	Rats, mice, birds, reptiles, frogs, crabs, and large insects	Rocky hills and wooded country
Reproduction: 2–4 eggs. Incubation for 35 days				
Rough-legged hawk	See North America			

Continued

Name	Abbrev.	Weight range	Diet	Habitat
Rufous-bellied eagle (*Lophotriorchis kienerii*)		732–800 g	Small mammals, birds, and reptiles	Evergreen, deciduous, mixed, and disturbed forest
Reproduction: 1 egg				
Rufous-winged buzzard (*Butastur liventer*)		336–340 g	Small mammals, reptiles, frogs, and large insects	Open, lightly wooded, cultivated areas and forest edge
Reproduction: Unknown				
Ryukyu scops owl (*Otus elegans*)		100–107 g	Insects (beetles, grasshoppers, crickets, moths), spiders, and small vertebrates	Subtropical evergreen forest
Reproduction: 2–5 eggs. Incubation for 30 days. Fledges at 32 days				
Ryukyu serpent eagle (*Spilornis perplexus*)			Snakes and frogs	Subtropical evergreen forest and coastal lowlands and farmlands
Reproduction: Unknown				
Saker falcon	See Europe			
Sangihe scops owl (*Otus collari*)		76 g	Probably insects	Forest, mixed plantations, secondary growth in lowlands
Reproduction: Unknown Note: Found on Sangihe Island				
Serendib scops owl (*Otus thilohoffmanni*)			Probably large insects and small vertebrates	Rainforest in Sri Lanka
Reproduction: Unknown Note: Endangered				
Shikra	See Europe			
Short-eared owl	See North America			
Short-toed snake eagle (*Circaetus gallicus*)		1.2–2.3 kg	Snakes, lizards, frogs, and some small mammals	Wide range including dense forest, open woodland, arid grassland, and semi-desert
Reproduction: 1 egg. Incubation for 42–47 days. Fledges at 60–80 days				
Simeulue scops owl (*Otus umbra*)		90–100 g	Insects, arthropods	Forest edge, remnant forest, and steep slopes in coastal forests
Reproduction: Unknown Note: Endemic to the island of Simeulue off north-west coast of Sumatra				
Simeulue serpent eagle (*Spilornis abbotti*)				Lowland forests
Reproduction: Unknown Note: Endemic to the island of Simeulue off the north-west coast of Sumatra				

Continued

Name	Abbrev.	Weight range	Diet	Habitat
Slender-billed vulture (*Gyps tenuirostris*)			Carrion (cattle, deer, and pigs)	Lowland, open, and partly wooded land
Reproduction: Unknown Note: Critically endangered				
Snowy owl	See North America			
Socotra buzzard (*Buteo socotraensis*)		500–1000 g	Reptiles and invertebrates	Foothills and plateau, mostly where deep ravines exist
Reproduction: Nests on cliffs or crevices. 1–3 eggs Note: Endemic to Socotra Island, Yemen				
Sooty falcon (*Falco concolor*)	See Africa			
Southern Philippine hawk-eagle (*Nisaetus pinskeri*)		1200 g	Birds	Mature forest in lowlands and low mountains
Reproduction: Unknown				
Speckled hawk owl (*Ninox punctulata*)		151 g (n = 1)	Unknown	Lowland and hilly forest
Reproduction: Unknown				
Spot-bellied eagle owl (*Bubo nipalensis*)		1300–1500 g	Mostly birds. Also snakes, lizards, and fish	Wide range including dense evergreen and moist deciduous forest, and dense riparian forest
Reproduction: 1 egg				
Spotted eagle owl (*Bubo africanus*)		550–850 g	Large insects, arthropods, small mammals, birds, and reptiles	Wide range including rocky desert outcrops, woodland, and savannah
Reproduction: 2–4 eggs. Incubation for 30–32 days. Fledges at 42 days				
Spotted owlet (*Athene brama*)		110–114 g	Insects (beetles, moths), earthworms, lizards, and mice	Open or semi-open country including farmland, near human settlements. Semi-desert. Avoids thick forest
Reproduction: Nests in cavity in tree or building. 3–5 eggs. Fledges at 20–28 days				
Spotted wood owl (*Strix seloputo*)		Male: 1010 g Females: larger	Mostly small rodents, small birds, and large insects	Wide variety of habitats
Reproduction: Nests in tree-hollow or sometimes in platform-like epiphytic fern in tree. 2–3 eggs				
Steller's sea eagle (*Haliaeetus pelagicus*)		Male: 5–6 kg Female: 7–9 kg	Large fish, especially salmon, birds, hares, young seals, and carrion	Near water in coastal habitats, or along large river valleys
Reproduction: Reuses massive stick nests in trees. 1–3 eggs. Incubation for 38–45 days. Fledges at 70 days Note: This eagle is protected by law, and is designated a National Treasure in Japan				
Steppe eagle	See Europe			

Continued

Name	Abbrev.	Weight range	Diet	Habitat
Sulawesi goshawk (*Accipiter griseiceps*)		Male: 212 g Female: 299 g	Small mammals, birds, lizards, and large insects	Primary lowland, hilly, or montane forest. Mangroves
Reproduction: Unknown				
Sulawesi hawk-eagle (*Nisaetus lanceolatus*)			Small and medium-sized birds, small mammals, snakes, and lizards	Primary and old secondary forest
Reproduction: Stick nest on large horizontal branch in large tree. 1 egg. Incubation presumed for 40–50 days. Fledges at several weeks				
Sulawesi masked owl (*Tyto rosenbergii*)			Mainly rats and other small rodents and bats	Cultivated areas with scattered trees, grasslands, and open country with dead trees. Rainforest and forest edge
Reproduction: Nests in cavities. Probably 2–3 eggs. Incubation for 35–42 days. Fledges at 49–56 days				
Sulawesi scops owl (*Otus manadensis*)		83–93 g	Nocturnal insects and other invertebrates. Also small vertebrates and probably geckos	Humid primary forest, second-growth forest, forest clearings and edges
Reproduction: Typically nests in tree cavities. 2–7 eggs. Incubation for 25–35 days				
Sulawesi serpent eagle (*Spilornis rufipectus*)			Lizards, small snakes, and occasionally small mammals	Lowland, hill, and montane forest
Reproduction: Unknown				
Sunda scops owl (*Otus lempiji*)		100–170 g	Mainly insects. Also rodents, lizards, and small birds	Second-growth evergreen and deciduous forest. Forest edge, open areas with scattered trees
Reproduction: Nests in tree-hollows. 2–3 eggs				
Tawny eagle	See Europe			
Tawny fish owl (*Ketupa flavipes*)			Mostly fish. Also crayfish, crabs, rodents, lizards, large beetles, and large birds	Evergreen-forested streams or rivers at lower elevations, and freshwater swamp forest
Reproduction: Usually uses abandoned large raptor nests in tall trees near water but may also use a hollow in a ravine or riverbank. 1–2 eggs				
Tawny owl	See Europe			
Togian hawk owl (*Ninox burhani*)		100 g	Most likely insects	Disturbed lowland and hill forest, mixed gardens, and sago swamp
Reproduction: Unknown				
Upland buzzard (*Buteo hemilasius*)		Male: 950–1400 g Female: 970–2050 g	Rodents and occasionally small birds	Open, normally dry, grassy areas such as steppes and rocky outcrops

Continued

Name	Abbrev.	Weight range	Diet	Habitat
Reproduction: Small stick nest on rocky cliffs, under bushes, or in a rock pile. 3–4 eggs. Incubation for 28–30 days. Fledges at 42–45 days				
Ural owl	See Europe			
Verreaux's eagle (*Aquila verreauxii*)	See Africa			
Wallace's hawk-eagle (*Nisaetus nanus*)		510–610 g	Birds, bats, frogs, skinks, and lizards	Evergreen and semi-evergreen lowland forest
Reproduction: Nests in stick platforms lined with fresh, leafy branches. 1 egg				
Western marsh harrier	See Europe			
White-bellied sea eagle	See Australia			
White-eyed buzzard (*Butastur teesa*)		325 g	Small mammals, lizards, frogs, small snakes, crabs, and large insects	Dry, open country, wooded and cultivated areas in lowlands
Reproduction: Loose-twig platform nest in a tree fork. 3 eggs. Incubation for 19 days				
White-fronted scops owl (*Otus sagittatus*)		109–130 g	Insects (mostly moths)	Primary tropical forest, especially lowland evergreen forest
Reproduction: Nests in tree cavity. 3–4 eggs				
White-rumped falcon (*Neohierax insignis*)		84–112 g	Lizards and insects	Savannah and primary dipterocarp, mixed deciduous forest on plains and foothills
Reproduction: Nests in tree cavity. 2 eggs Note: Near-threatened				
White-rumped vulture (*Gyps bengalensis*)		3500–6000 g	Carrion	Open country near villages and towns
Reproduction: Small colonies build stick nests in large trees. 1 egg. Incubation for 45–48 days. Fledges at 3 months Note: Critically endangered				
White-tailed eagle	See Europe			

Australia

Name	Abbrev.	Weight range	Diet	Habitat
Australian hobby (*Falco longipennis*)	AUHO	Male: 132–380 g Female: 190–365 g	Small birds, bats, and flying insects	Open woodland and watercourses
Reproduction: Uses an old stick nest made by another species. 2–3 eggs. Incubation by female for 35 days. Fledges at 34–38 days				

Continued

Name	Abbrev.	Weight range	Diet	Habitat
Australian kestrel (*Falco cenchroides*)	AUKE	121–255 g	Small mammals, reptiles, and insects	Open habitats including urban parks. Prefers short grass
Reproduction: Nests in hollows, cliffs, nest of other species, or any ledge or cavity. 3–5 eggs. Incubation for 28 days. Fledges at 31–35 days				
Australian kite (*Elanus axillaris*)	AUKI		Small rodents, lizards, and insects	Grasslands and farm fields
Reproduction: Nests alone or in colonies. Platform of sticks lined with leaves. 3–4 eggs. Incubation mostly by female, for 31 days. Fledges at 36 days				
Australian masked owl (*Tyto novaehollandiae*)		660 g	Rodents, reptiles, small birds, and insects	
Reproduction: Nests in hollow trees. 2–3 eggs. Incubated by female only. Fledges at 2–3 months				
Barking/ Winking owl (*Ninox connivens*)		425–510 g		Wooded areas near rivers or swamps
Reproduction: Unknown Note: Characteristic voice like a barking dog or a shrill scream				
Barn owl	See North America			
Bat hawk (*Macheiramphus alcinus*)	BAHA	600–650 g	Primarily insectivorous bats but will also take insects and birds	Lowland clear spaces, forest edges, in urban areas. Often around limestone and areas where bats are found
Reproduction: Large stick nest in pale-barked trees such as eucalyptus. 1–2 eggs. Incubation for 42 days. Fledges at 67 days				
Black falcon (*Falco subniger*)	BLFA	Male: 510–710 g Female: 610–1000 g	Mammals, birds, reptiles, carrion. Sometimes hunts in groups	Open, flat country
Reproduction: Uses old stick nest of other species. 3–4 eggs. Incubation for 34 days. Fledges at 38–49 days				
Black kite (*Milvus migrans*)	BLKI	Male: 630–930 g Female: 750–940 g	Opportunistic, often feeding from roadkill and trash dumps	Wide range of habitats
Reproduction: Nests in trees, on cliffs and electrical towers. 2–3 eggs. Incubation for 28–30 days. Fledges at 42–48 days				
Black-breasted buzzard (*Hamirostra melanosternon*)	BBBU	Male: 1350 g Female: 1350 g	Mammals, carrion, and eggs which it breaks with a rock thrown with beak	Open plains and woodlands
Reproduction: Nest is large stick platform lined with leaves. 2 eggs. Incubation for 40 days. Fledges at 60 days				
Black-winged kite (*Elanus caeruleus*)	BWKI	Male: 230 g Female: 230 g	Mainly small rodents, reptiles, and insects	Open habitats, grasslands, and pastures

Continued

Name	Abbrev.	Weight range	Diet	Habitat
Reproduction: Flimsy stick nest in fork of small tree. 3–5 eggs. Incubation by female only				
Brahminy kite (*Haliastur indus*)	BRKI	320–670 g	Small birds, insects, fish snatched from the surface of water	Coastal areas, estuaries, and swamps
Reproduction: Nest is large stick platform lined with leaves and bark. 1–3 eggs. Incubation for 35 days. Fledges at 50–56 days				
Brown falcon (*Falco berigora*)	BRFA	Male: 316–590 g Female: 430–860 g	Mammals (rats), birds, reptiles, amphibians, fish, carrion, and large insects	Open, unforested areas. Cultivated fields and grasslands
Reproduction: Uses old nest from another species. 2–3 eggs. Incubation for 33 days. Fledges at 36–42 days				
Brown/Australian goshawk (*Accipiter fasciatus*)		Male: 250–415 g Female: 440–740 g	Mammals, birds, reptiles, insects, and carrion	Monsoon forest, forest edges, and lightly wooded cultivated areas
Reproduction: Nests on small stick platform lined with leaves. 3 eggs. Incubation for 30 days. Fledges at 28–37 days				
Collared sparrowhawk (*Accipiter cirrocephaus*)		Male: 105–155 g Female: 165–300 g	Small birds, lizards, insects, and mammals	Savannah, woods, and forest edges
Reproduction: Nests on small stick platform lined with leaves. 3–4 eggs. Incubation for 35 days. Fledges at 28–33 days				
Greater sooty owl (*Tyto tenebricosa*)		Male: 500–700 g Female: 750–1000 g	Birds, sugar gliders, and small mammals	Eucalyptus forests and tropical forests
Reproduction: Nests in hollow or cave. 1–2 eggs. Incubation for 42 days by female only. Fledges at 3 months				
Grey falcon (*Falco hypoleucos*)	GRFA	Male: 335 g Female: 500–624 g	Pigeons and parrots. Stoops to seize prey in flight	Inland drainage lowlands. Avoids desert habitats
Reproduction: Uses large stick nest of another species. 2–3 eggs. Incubation for 35 days. Fledges at 41–52 days				
Grey/Variable goshawk (*Accipiter novaehollandiae*)		Male: 238–470 g Female: 515–1050 g	Mammals, birds, reptiles, amphibians, and carrion	Tall, wet forests. Also open woodlands and urban areas
Reproduction: Nests on small stick platform lined with leaves. 2–3 eggs. Incubation for 31–34 days. Fledges at 30–42 days				
Letter-winged kite (*Elanus scriptus*)	LWKI	160–427 g	Rodents, particularly the long-haired rat	Dry, timbered watercourses and grasslands
Reproduction: Breeds in large colonies. Nest is a twig platform lined with leaves. 4–5 eggs. Incubation for 31 days. Fledges at 30–35 days Note: Primarily nocturnal. Roosts colonially during the day in coolabah trees				
Little eagle (*Aquila morphnoides*)	LIEA	Male: 530–810 g Female: 745–1250 g	Mammals, birds, lizards, and will steal fish from Whistling kites	Wooded habitats and rough, hilly country
Reproduction: Nests on stick platform lined with leaves. 2 eggs. Incubation for 36–40 days. Fledges at 54–66 days				

Continued

Name	Abbrev.	Weight range	Diet	Habitat
Orange-breasted falcon	See South America			
Osprey	See North America			
Pacific baza (*Aviceda subcristata*)	PABA	227–448 g	Omnivorous. Insects, frogs, lizards, and small fruits (figs)	Forest edges and scrub habitats
Reproduction: Nests on small stick platform lined with leaves. 2–3 eggs. Incubation for 29 days by both parents. Fledges at 32–35 days				
Peregrine falcon	See North America			
Powerful owl (*Ninox strenua*)	POOW	1050–1700 g	Small mammals, reptiles, amphibians, and insects	Forests, scrub, plantations, and urban parks
Reproduction: Nests in hollow trees. 1–3 eggs				
Red goshawk (*Erythrotriorchis radiatus*)		Male: 630–640 g Female: 1110–1370 g	Diet of mostly birds (parrots, pigeons, waterfowl)	Coastal forests
Reproduction: Nests on small stick platform lined with leaves. 2 eggs. Incubation for 40 days. Fledges at 51–53 days				
Rufous owl (*Ninox rufa*)	RUOW	Male: 1050–1300 g Female: 700–1050g	Wide variety. Beetles, crayfish, birds, and flying foxes	Tropical moist lowland forests
Reproduction: Nests in trunk of tree. 1–2 eggs. Incubation for 37 days. Young are dependent on parents often until the next breeding season				
Spotted harrier (*Circus assimilis*)	SPHA	Male: 407–537 g Female: 540–745 g	Small mammals, birds, reptiles, and large insects	Open fields, farmland, rice fields, and coastal fishponds
Reproduction: Nests on small stick platform lined with leaves. 3 eggs. Incubation for 33 days. Fledges at 36–42 days				
Square-tailed kite (*Lophoictinia isura*)		501–680 g	Eggs and bird nestlings. Also eats insects and frogs	Coastal forests
Reproduction: Nests on small stick platform lined with leaves. 2–3 eggs. Incubation for 40 days. Fledges at 59–65 days				
Swallow-tailed kite	See North America			
Swamp/Pacific marsh harrier (*Circus approximans*)		Male: 392–726 g Female: 622–1080 g	Mammals, birds and their eggs, reptiles, fish, amphibians, and insects	Swamps and wetlands
Reproduction: Nest made of sticks and grasses in tall grass or on the ground. 3–4 eggs. Incubation for 33 days. Fledges at 43–46 days				
Wedge-tailed eagle (*Aquila audax*)	WTEA	Male: 3.2–4.2 kg Female: 4.2–5.3 kg	Mammals, birds, reptiles, and carrion (especially roadkill)	Most terrestrial habitats away from urban or farmed areas
Reproduction: Nests on a huge stick platform in large tree or cliff. 2 eggs. Incubation for 42–44 days by both parents. Fledges at 79–90 days				

Continued

Name	Abbrev.	Weight range	Diet	Habitat
Whistling kite (*Haliastur sphenurus*)	WHKI	Male: 600–750 g Female: 760–900 g	Fish, mammals, birds, reptiles, crustaceans, insects, and roadkill	Swamps, lakes, or any place near water
Reproduction: Bowl-shaped nest of sticks in fork in tree. 2 eggs. Incubation for 35 days. Fledges at 44–54 days				
White-bellied sea eagle (*Haliaeetus leucogaster*)	WBSE	Male: 2.1–2.9 kg Female: 2.9–3.4 kg	Mammals, birds, reptiles, and fish	Coastal areas, estuaries, and rivers
Reproduction: Large stick nest lined with leaves and seaweed. Placed on the ground, on a cliff, or in a tree. 2 eggs. Incubation for 40 days. Fledges at 65–70 days				
White-tailed kite	See North America			

Europe

Name	Abbrev.	Weight range	Diet	Habitat
Barn owl	See North America			
Bearded vulture	See Africa			
Black kite	See Australia			
Booted eagle	See Africa			
Boreal owl	See North America			
Cinereous vulture	See Africa Longest breeding period of all raptors in Europe. One of the most endangered raptors in Europe			
Eastern imperial eagle	See Africa			
Egyptian vulture	See Africa			
Eurasian buzzard (*Buteo buteo*)	EUBU	525 g to 1.4 kg	Highly variable but primarily small mammals	Highly variable. Ideal habitat is forest edge
Reproduction: Builds nests in trees. 2–4 eggs. Incubation by both sexes for 33–35 days. Fledges at 2 months Note: Also called the Common buzzard, or just Buzzard				
Eurasian eagle owl (*Bubo bubo*)	EEOW	1.2–4.6 kg	Highly variable but mainly small mammals	Highly variable but are partial to irregular topography
Reproduction: They do not build nests but typically nest on the surface of rocks or boulders and have been reported to nest on the ground. 1–2 eggs. Incubation by female only for 31–36 days. Fledge at 5–6 weeks				

Continued

Name	Abbrev.	Weight range	Diet	Habitat
Eurasian griffon vulture (*Gyps fulvus*)		6–11 kg	Only carrion of large and medium-sized animals	Need cliffs for nesting and the landscape must support the production of thermals
Reproduction: Normally breeds in colonies on cliffs. 1 egg. Incubation by both sexes for 47–57 days. Fledges at 113–159 days				
Eurasian hobby (*Falco subbuteo*)		175–285 g	Birds and insects	Prefers lowlands
Reproduction: They do not build nests of their own. They use nests of other species such as crows. 2–4 eggs. Incubation by both sexes for 28–31 days. Fledges at 28–34 days. Note: It is a complete migrant that leaves Europe between August and October and returns in April or May. Winters in Africa				
Eurasian kestrel (*Falco tinnunculus*)	EAKE	163–290 g	Small rodents	Open areas with low vegetation
Reproduction: Nests in cliffs, buildings, or uses nests of other birds. 3–7 eggs. Incubation by both sexes for about 4 weeks. Fledges at 28–32 days				
Eurasian pygmy owl (*Glaucidium passerinum*)	EPOW	47–83 g	Primarily small birds but also small mammals	Prefers semi-open mature forest with clearings
Reproduction: Nest sites are normally cavities produced by the Great spotted or Three-toed woodpecker. 3–8 eggs. Incubation by both sexes for 28–29 days. Fledges at 30–34 days				
Eurasian sparrowhawk (*Accipiter nisus*)		110–342 g	Mainly birds	Nest in forests but often hunt in parks, gardens, and open country
Reproduction: Nests are often found in 20–40-year-old coniferous trees. 3–6 eggs. Incubation by both sexes for 31–36 days. Fledges at 26–30 days				
European honey buzzard (*Pernis apivorus*)		510 g to 1.1 kg	Most important food source is larvae of wasps and bees, but will also eat other small insects, eggs, and occasionally fruit	Mixture of open and woodland
Reproduction: Typically breeds in woodlands. 2 eggs. Incubation by both sexes for 30–37 days. Fledges at 35–48 days Note: Strictly migratory. Winters in Africa				
European scops owl (*Otus scops*)		60–135 g	Mainly insects but also small vertebrates	Semi-open or open country with scattered trees or small woods
Reproduction: Nest sites include natural cavities in trees, rocks or walls, woodpecker holes in tree trunks or thick branches, or holes in steep banks of ditches or sandpits, even under roofs. 3–4 eggs. Incubation by the female only for 20–31 days. Fledges at 3–4 weeks Note: Also called the Eurasian scops owl and the Common scops owl				
Golden eagle	See North America			
Great gray owl	See North America			

Continued

<table>
<tr><th>Name</th><th>Abbrev.</th><th>Weight range</th><th>Diet</th><th>Habitat</th></tr>
<tr><td>Greater spotted eagle
(Aquila clanga)</td><td>GSEA</td><td>1.6–3.1 kg</td><td>Mostly small mammals and birds</td><td>Prefers open areas with little to no human settlement</td></tr>
<tr><td colspan="5">Reproduction: Nests built in trees. Usually 2 eggs. Incubation by both sexes for 42 days. Fledges at 63–67 days
Note: Endangered. Fewer than 100 mating pairs outside Russia</td></tr>
<tr><td>Gyrfalcon</td><td colspan="4">See North America</td></tr>
<tr><td>Lanner falcon</td><td colspan="4">See Africa</td></tr>
<tr><td>Lesser kestrel</td><td colspan="4">See Africa</td></tr>
<tr><td>Lesser spotted eagle</td><td colspan="4">See Africa</td></tr>
<tr><td>Levant sparrowhawk</td><td colspan="4">See Africa</td></tr>
<tr><td>Little owl</td><td colspan="4">See Africa</td></tr>
<tr><td>Long-eared owl</td><td colspan="4">See North America</td></tr>
<tr><td>Long-legged buzzard</td><td colspan="4">See Africa</td></tr>
<tr><td>Merlin</td><td colspan="4">See North America</td></tr>
<tr><td>Montagu's harrier</td><td colspan="4">See Africa</td></tr>
<tr><td>Northern goshawk</td><td colspan="4">See North America</td></tr>
<tr><td>Northern harrier</td><td colspan="4">See North America</td></tr>
<tr><td>Northern hawk owl
(Surnia ulula)</td><td></td><td>215–392 g</td><td>Mainly small mammals but will take birds, frogs, and occasionally fish</td><td>Open boreal coniferous forest with clearings and moors in lowlands or mountains</td></tr>
<tr><td colspan="5">Reproduction: Nests in cavities. 5–13 eggs. Incubation by female for 25–30 days. Fledges at 23–30 days.
Note: A largely diurnal bird</td></tr>
<tr><td>Osprey</td><td colspan="4">See North America</td></tr>
<tr><td>Pallas's fish eagle
(Haliaeetus leucoryphus)</td><td></td><td>2.0–3.7 kg</td><td>Mainly fish but occasionally carrion</td><td>Near freshwater systems</td></tr>
<tr><td colspan="5">Reproduction: Nest is built out of sticks by both parents and placed in a tall tree close to water. 2–4 eggs. Incubation by both sexes for 40–45 days. Fledges at 70–105 days</td></tr>
<tr><td>Pallid harrier
(Circus macrourus)</td><td></td><td>235–550 g</td><td>Small mammals, birds, and locusts</td><td>Open country, marshes, and steppes</td></tr>
<tr><td colspan="5">Reproduction: Nests are typically built on the ground. 3–6 eggs. Incubation by female for 30 days. Fledges at 35–48 days
Note: Migratory. The most endangered of the European harriers</td></tr>
<tr><td>Peregrine falcon</td><td colspan="4">See North America</td></tr>
<tr><td>Red-footed falcon
(Falco vespertinus)</td><td></td><td>115–200 g</td><td>Mainly large insects</td><td>Open habitat like steppes or forest-steppes but also in cultivated landscape</td></tr>
</table>

Continued

Name	Abbrev.	Weight range	Diet	Habitat
Reproduction: Uses nests from other species such as magpies, crows, and especially rooks. 2–5 eggs. Incubation for about 4 weeks. Fledges at around 4 weeks Note: They are long-distance migrants. Winter in southern Africa				
Red kite (*Milvus milvus*)		750–1300 g	Highly variable but a renowned scavenger	Open country
Reproduction: Nest is normally built in a large tree close to the forest edge. It is constructed of dead twigs and lined with grass and sheep's wool. A couple of days prior to egg laying, kites decorate the nest with rubbish they find near the nest site. 1–3 eggs. Incubation by the female for 31–38 days. Fledges at 50–70 days Note: Saved from extinction by a reintroduction program				
Rough-legged hawk	See North America			
Saker falcon (*Falco cherrug*)	SAFA	700–1300 g	Medium-sized mammals and birds	Open habitat such as steppes or in open areas in mountains
Reproduction: Use nests in trees or cliffs from other large birds such as ravens, buzzards, or eagles. 3–5 eggs. Incubation by female for 36–38 days. Fledges at 48–50 days				
Shikra (*Accipiter badius*)		75–160g	Highly variable	Variable, including forests, farmland, and urban areas
Reproduction: The nest is a platform made of twigs and lined with grass. 2–4 eggs. Incubation for 18–21 days. Fledges at around 1 month Note: Migratory				
Short-eared owl	See North America			
Short-toed snake eagle (*Circaetus gallicus*)		1.2–2.3 kg	Snakes. Sometimes other reptiles	Open cultivated plains, arid stony deciduous scrub areas and foothills, and semi-desert areas
Reproduction: Builds nests in trees, occasionally on cliffs. 1 egg. Incubation by both sexes for 45–47 days. Fledges at 60–80 days				
Snowy owl	See North America			
Spanish imperial eagle (*Aquila adalberti*)		2.5–3.5 kg	Most important prey is rabbit. Will also eat other small mammals and carrion	Woodland, plains, and marshes; sometimes found along mountain slopes
Reproduction: Nests normally built in trees. 1–4 eggs. Incubation by the female for 39–42 days. Fledges at 69–83 days				
Steppe eagle (*Aquila nipalensis*)		2.4–3.9 kg	Small mammals, birds, reptiles, and carrion	Occurs in steppe, desert, semi-desert, open savannah, pastures, agricultural fields, paddy fields, grassland, and open woodland

Continued

Name	Abbrev.	Weight range	Diet	Habitat
Reproduction: Builds a flat stick nest lined with scraps of skins and placed on the ground, rock columns, power poles, or in anthropogenic locations, including abandoned cars. 1–4 eggs. Incubation by both sexes for 45 days. Fledges at 55–60 days Note: Nearly always found in groups in winter, sometimes numbering more than 100 birds, and often in association with other raptors, especially Black kites and Lesser spotted eagles Note: Migratory				
Tawny eagle (*Aquila rapax*)		2.0–2.5 kg	Mammals, birds, reptiles, insects, amphibians, fish, and carrion	Most often found along open wooded savannah and steppe; avoids deserts and dense woodland areas
Reproduction: The nest is made in a tree with sticks and occasionally animal bones. Lined with grass, leaves, and fur. 1–2 eggs. Incubation by both sexes for 39–45 days. Fledges at 75–76 days Note: There are several morphologic forms of this species				
Tawny owl (*Strix aluco*)		325–716 g	Rabbits and small rodents. Also earthworms, insects (especially beetles), birds, frogs, fish, lizards, mollusks, and crustaceans	Though woodland is their preferred habitat, they are adaptable and have even taken up residence in cities
Reproduction: Typically nests in cavities but has been reported to use ledges of old buildings and chimneys. 2–6 eggs. Incubation by female for 28–29 days. Fledges at 28–37 days Note: There are multiple morphologic forms of this species				
Ural owl (*Strix uralensis*)		500–1300 g	Wide variety of mammals, birds, insects, and reptiles	Mature, deciduous, and mixed forest with clearings
Reproduction: Nests in cavities but will sometimes use stick nests of other birds. 3–4 eggs. Incubation by female for 28–35 days. Fledges at 35 days Note: Light and dark morphologic forms are known to occur, with the light being more common				
Western marsh harrier (*Circus aeruginosus*)		400–800 g	Feeds primarily on frogs but will also eat small mammals, insects, reptiles, and eggs	Open areas
Reproduction: Nests on the ground, preferably in reed beds. Typically 4–5 eggs. Incubation for 35–38 days. Fledges at 38–45 days				
White-tailed eagle (*Haliaeetus albicilla*)		3.1–6.9 kg	Highly variable but includes fish, birds, mammals, carrion, and offal	Wide range, though most commonly found close to water and in lowlands
Reproduction: Nests built in trees or on cliffs, typically close to water. They are made of sticks and lined with vegetation, seaweed, and/or wool and fur. 1–2 eggs. Incubation for 34–46 days. Fledges at 70–90 days Note: Largest raptor in Europe				

North America

<table>
<tr><th>Name</th><th>Abbrev.</th><th>Weight range</th><th>Diet</th><th>Habitat</th></tr>
<tr><td>American kestrel
(Falco sparverius)</td><td>AMKE</td><td>80–165 g</td><td>Insects, small rodents, and birds</td><td>Meadows, grasslands, parks, and suburbs</td></tr>
<tr><td colspan="5">Reproduction: Uses existing cavity in tree. 4–5 eggs. Incubation for 29–30 days mostly by female. Fledges at 28–31 days. Sexually dimorphic. Breeding season: Early March in south, May in north</td></tr>
<tr><td>Aplomado falcon
(Falco femoralis)</td><td>APFA</td><td>Male: 208–305 g
Female: 271–460 g</td><td>Invertebrates and small birds</td><td>Dry grasslands, savannahs, and marshes</td></tr>
<tr><td colspan="5">Reproduction: Uses existing nests. 2–3 eggs. Incubation for 31–32 days by both sexes. Fledges at 28–35 days
Note: Mostly found in the southern United States</td></tr>
<tr><td>Bald eagle
(Haliaeetus leucocephalus)</td><td>BAEA</td><td>3.0–6.3 kg
Male: 4100 g
Female: 5300 g</td><td>Fish, waterfowl, and scavenged carcasses/carrion</td><td>Most wetlands (rivers, lakes, coastal) with old-growth trees for perching and nesting</td></tr>
<tr><td colspan="5">Reproduction: Uses very large stick nest that is reused each year. Usually 2 eggs. Incubation by both sexes for 35–46 days. Fledges at 8–14 weeks. Sexually mature at 4–5 years. Nesting pair requires relative freedom from disturbance during nesting season. Breeding season: Late fall/November in south, May in north
Note: A relatively high-stress species. Lead poisoning is a serious concern</td></tr>
<tr><td>Barn owl
(Tyto alba)</td><td>BNOW</td><td>250–480 g</td><td>Small rodents</td><td>Variable but prefers open woodland with structures for nesting</td></tr>
<tr><td colspan="5">Reproduction: Breeds year-round. Nests in tree-hollows or buildings. 4–7 eggs. Incubation for 32–34 days by female only. Fledges at 50–55 days. Breeding season: January in south, March in north
Note: Produces a horrible, rasping scream when frightened. Very "grabby" with talons so never carry more than one bird in the same box. A delicate species with long, fragile legs</td></tr>
<tr><td>Barred owl
(Strix varia)</td><td>BDOW</td><td>500–1050 g</td><td>Small mammals, birds, insects, small fish, frogs, and reptiles</td><td>Deep forests, wooded swamps, and woodlands near rivers</td></tr>
<tr><td colspan="5">Reproduction: Cavity nester. 2–3 eggs. Incubation for 28–33 days by female only. Fledges at 35–40 days. Breeding season: December in south, March in north
Note: Incredibly versatile, resilient species. They do very well in captivity and seem to be able to heal from almost any injury. Can be very unpredictable when being grabbed from a confined space such as a dog kennel. Consider wearing goggles when grabbing this species</td></tr>
<tr><td>Black vulture
(Coragyps atratus)</td><td>BLVU</td><td>1600–2200 g</td><td>Carrion</td><td>Open land interspersed with woods. Does well in urban settings</td></tr>
<tr><td colspan="5">Reproduction: Eggs laid on ground, usually in some sort of cavity or structure. 2 eggs. Incubation by both sexes for 32–39 days. Fledge at 11 weeks but are dependent on parents for another 8–12 weeks. Breeding season: Late January
Note: Chicks are very imprintable. Very dangerous beak so restrain head at all times. A very intelligent, curious species</td></tr>
<tr><td>Boreal owl
(Aegolius funereus)</td><td>BOOW</td><td>Male: 90–113 g
Female: 126–194 g</td><td>Small rodents, frogs, and insects</td><td>Old-growth forests</td></tr>
</table>

Continued

Name	Abbrev.	Weight range	Diet	Habitat
Reproduction: Cavity nester. 3–8 eggs. Incubation for 26–36 days by female. Fledges at 30–36 days. Mature at 9 months				
Broad-winged hawk (*Buteo platypterus*)	BWHA	265–560 g	Highly variable: small mammals, frogs, lizards, and insects	Deciduous forests, wetlands, and meadows
Reproduction: Stick nest in deciduous trees. 2–3 eggs. Incubation for 28–31 days mostly by female. Fledges at 37–46 days. Independent at 56 days. Breeding season: April in south, June in north Note: Migrate in massive groups to Central and South America. Have a tendency to get overweight in captivity				
Burrowing owl (*Athene cunicularia*)	BUOW	147–240 g	Small mammals and insects	Open, dry grasslands or deserts associated with burrowing animals
Reproduction: Use abandoned burrows or will dig their own. 5–6 eggs. Incubation for 27–30 days. Leaves nest at 44 days. Starts hunting at 49–56 days. Breeding season: March in south, May in north Note: Diurnal				
California condor (*Gymnogyps californianus*)	CALC	7.0–9.9 kg	Carrion	Rocky shrubland, cliffs, and oak savannahs
Reproduction: No nest built. Eggs laid on ground in caves or cliffs. 1 egg every other year. Incubation by both sexes for 53–60/42–50 days. Fledges at 5–7 months. Stays with parents into 2nd year Note: Critically endangered				
Common black hawk (*Buteogallus anthracinus*)	CBHA	Male: 793 g Female: 1199 g	Crabs and small vertebrates	Coastal. Mangrove swamps and estuaries
Reproduction: Stick nest often 100 feet up in mangrove. 1–2 eggs. Incubation by both sexes for 38 days. Fledges at 43–50 days. Independent at 15 weeks				
Cooper's hawk (*Accipiter cooperii*)	COHA	Male: 220–440 g Female: 330–700 g	Small to mid-sized birds, and small mammals	Wooded areas but also common in urban environments and backyard bird feeders
Reproduction: Stick nest in tree. 4 eggs. Incubation by female for 36 days. Fledges at 30–34 days. Independent at 8 weeks. Breeding season: Late February in south, April in north Note: A very high-stress species. Prone to damaging the cere and tail feathers if not protected and housed properly. Digit 3 is longer than the other digits and it has a pronounced protuberance on the plantar surface (Fig. 13.23). These birds are escape artists, so be careful when handling!				
Crested caracara (*Caracara cheriway*)	CRCA	1050–1300 g	Insects, reptiles, small mammals, eggs, and carrion	Arid, open country, semi-desert, and pastureland
Reproduction: Nests in trees or cacti, on rock ledges, or on ground. 2–3 eggs. Incubation by both sexes for 28 days. Fledges at 42–56 days				
Eastern screech owl (*Megascops asia*)	EASO	100–200 g	Almost anything suitably sized	Variable, but prefer open forests along edges of open fields or wetlands

Continued

Name	Abbrev.	Weight range	Diet	Habitat
Reproduction: Cavity nester. 4–5 eggs. Incubation by female for 26 days. Fledges at 31 days. Breeding season: March to May Note: Will play dead: sometimes difficult to tell if still alive! Cannibalism is not uncommon. There are several color morphs. Generally very hardy and more resilient than would be expected based on their size				
Elf owl (*Micrathene whitneyi*)	ELOW	Male: 36–44 g Female: 41–48 g	Arthropods (insects and scorpions)	Arid deserts
Reproduction: Nests in cavities in trees and cacti. 3 eggs. Incubation for 14–24 days. Fledges at 28–33 days				
Ferruginous hawk (*Buteo regalis*)	FEHA	977–2267 g	Small to medium-sized mammals, birds, and reptiles	Open, arid grasslands and prairie
Reproduction: Nests almost anywhere: trees, ledges, the ground, power poles. 2–3 eggs. Incubation by both sexes for 32 days. Fledges at 44–48 days. Breeding season: Early May				
Flammulated owl (*Otus flammeolus*)	FLOW	45–63 g	Insects and spiders	Coniferous mountain forest
Reproduction: Nests in woodpecker cavities. 2–4 eggs. Incubation by female for 21–28 days. Fledges at 4–5 weeks				
Golden eagle (*Aquila chrysaetos*)	GOEA	Male: 3.6 kg Female: 5.1 kg	Large rodents	Mountainous regions with deep canyons. Open or semi-open areas
Reproduction: Nests on cliffs or man-made structures. 2 eggs. Incubation for 43–45 days usually by female or both. Fledges at 66–81 days. Breeding season: February in south, June in north				
Gray hawk (*Buteo plagiatus*)	GRHA	475 g	Lizards, snakes, birds, and small mammals	Forest edges, river edges, clear cuts, and farmland
Reproduction: Stick nest built in trees. 1–3 eggs. Incubation by female for 32–33 days. Fledges at 6 weeks				
Great gray owl (*Strix nebulosa*)	GGOW	790–1454 g	Small mammals	Forests. Forages in open areas
Reproduction: Uses existing stick nests. 3–5 eggs. Incubation by female for 28–30 days. Fledges at 8 weeks. Breeding season: March				
Great-horned owl (*Bubo virginianus*)	GHOW	900–1800 g	Variable: rodents, reptiles, and other birds (including chickens)	Dense forests, open fields, and golf courses
Reproduction: Uses existing stick nests of other species. 2–3 eggs. Incubation by female for 26–35 days. Young stay with family until the fall. Breeding season: November to January in south, April in north Note: Very strong and dangerous talons. Generally do well in captivity but return to silent flight can be difficult to achieve even with no identifiable feather damage				
Gyrfalcon (*Falco rusticolus*)	GYRF	Male: 800–1350 g Female: 1200–2100 g	Mammals and birds	Tundra and mountains
Reproduction: Nests on bare cliff ledge or uses abandoned nest. 3–4 eggs. Incubation by female for 35–36 days. Fledges at 46–49 days but dependent for another month Note: Found mostly in northern regions of Canada and Alaska				
Harris's hawk (*Parabuteo unicinctus*)	HRSH	Male: 546–850 g Female: 766–1633 g	Birds, lizards, small mammals, and insects	Sparse woodland, desert as well as marshes

Continued

<table>
<tr><th>Name</th><th>Abbrev.</th><th>Weight range</th><th>Diet</th><th>Habitat</th></tr>
<tr><td colspan="5">Reproduction: Builds stick nests in trees, shrubs, or cacti. 2–4 eggs. Incubation by both sexes for 31–36 days. Fledges at 45–50 days. Young may stay with parents for up to 3 years. Breeding season: Early February
Note: Hunts in packs</td></tr>
<tr><td>Hook-billed kite
(Chondrohierax uncinatus)</td><td>HBKI</td><td>Male: 253 g
Female: 255–360 g</td><td>Tree snails, amphibians, and insects</td><td>Wide variety of forest habitats from swamps to coffee plantations</td></tr>
<tr><td colspan="5">Reproduction: Builds flimsy stick platform or shallow cup. 1–3 eggs. Incubation by both sexes for 34–35 days. Fledges at 38–39 days</td></tr>
<tr><td>Long-eared owl
(Asio otus)</td><td>LEOW</td><td>210–430 g</td><td>Small mammals</td><td>Open woodlands and forest edges</td></tr>
<tr><td colspan="5">Reproduction: Uses existing stick nests from other species. 4–5 eggs. Incubation normally by female for 25–30 days. Independent at 2 months. Breeding season: March in south, April in north</td></tr>
<tr><td>Merlin
(Falco columbarius)</td><td>MERL</td><td>Male: 150–210 g
Female: 189–255 g</td><td>Small songbirds and shorebirds</td><td>Variable habitat depending on subspecies. Often nests near water</td></tr>
<tr><td colspan="5">Reproduction: Reuses existing nest, or nests in cavity or on the ground. 5–6 eggs. Incubation by female for 28–32 days. Fledges at 30 days. Breeding season: Mid-May</td></tr>
<tr><td>Mississippi kite
(Ictinia mississippiensis)</td><td>MIKI</td><td>214–388 g</td><td>Insects, particularly cicadas and dragonflies captured in flight</td><td>Open woodlands and riverine forest</td></tr>
<tr><td colspan="5">Reproduction: Nests in colonies. 1–3 eggs. Incubation by both sexes for 30–32 days. Fledges at 30–35 days
Note: Despite their unusual natural diet, these birds do surprisingly well in captivity fed a diet of minced mice, crickets, and superworms</td></tr>
<tr><td>Northern goshawk
(Accipiter gentilis)</td><td>NOGO</td><td>Male: 500–1200 g
Female: 820–2200 g</td><td>Small mammals and birds</td><td>Deciduous and coniferous, old-growth forests</td></tr>
<tr><td colspan="5">Reproduction: Bulky stick nests. 2–3 eggs. Incubation mostly by female for 36–41 days. Fledges at 45–56 days. Independent at 70 days. Breeding season: March in south, June in north</td></tr>
<tr><td>Northern harrier
(Circus cyaneus)</td><td>NOHA</td><td>Male: 290–400 g
Female: 390–750 g</td><td>Small mammals and birds</td><td>Meadows and open marshland (salt- or freshwater)</td></tr>
<tr><td colspan="5">Reproduction: Nests on ground. 4–6 eggs. Incubation by female for 29–39 days. Fledges at 36 days but not independent until 45–66 days. Breeding season: March in south, May in north
Note: Also known as the Marsh hawk. One male mates with several females</td></tr>
<tr><td>Northern hawk owl
(Surnia ulula)</td><td>NHOW</td><td>Male: 215–375 g
Female: 323–392 g</td><td>Small mammals</td><td>Coniferous forest with clearings</td></tr>
<tr><td colspan="5">Reproduction: Cavity nester. 5–13 eggs. Incubation by female for 25–30 days. Independent by August</td></tr>
<tr><td>Northern pygmy owl
(Glaucidium californicum)</td><td>NOPO</td><td>62–73 g</td><td>Small prey (mammals, birds, reptiles)</td><td>Open coniferous and mixed forests</td></tr>
<tr><td colspan="5">Reproduction: Cavity nester. 3–4 eggs. Incubation for 29 days. Fledges at 30 days</td></tr>
</table>

Continued

Name	Abbrev.	Weight range	Diet	Habitat
Northern saw-whet owl (*Aegolius acadicus*)	NSWO	54–124 g	Small mammals and birds	Deciduous forests
Reproduction: Uses old woodpecker cavities. 5–6 eggs. Incubation by female for 26–28 days. Fledges at 4–5 weeks. Breeding season: March to April				
Osprey (*Pandion haliaetus*)	OSPR	Male: 1200–1600 g Female: 1600–2000 g	Exclusively fish	Near any expanse of shallow water (lakes, rivers)
Reproduction: Large stick nests on platforms or trees are reused each year. Usually 3 eggs. Incubation by both for 32–33 days. Fledges at 51–59 days. Breeding season: March typically but as early as December in the south Note: Very graceful in the air but quite ungainly on land. Sometimes very difficult to get to eat in captivity (they eat better when in small groups) and they are prone to self-induced injury and feather damage				
Peregrine falcon (*Falco peregrinus*)	PEFA	530–1600 g	Mostly birds	Open landscapes with cliffs or in urban settings with artificial nest sites and pigeons
Reproduction: Nest built on ledge. 3–4 eggs. Incubation mainly by female for 28–29 days. Fledges at 35–42 days but dependent for another 2 months. Breeding season: Early March in south, May in north Note: Stoops at 200 mph (320 km/h) when hunting. Not possible to recondition or evaluate flight in a flight cage or on a creance line. Need to utilize a falconer for evaluation and training in free flight. Very prone to bumblefoot				
Prairie falcon (*Falco mexicanus*)	PRFA	Male: 500–650 g Female: 700–975 g	Small mammals and birds caught in flight	Open country (tundra, prairie, high desert)
Reproduction: Nests on cliffs. 4–5 eggs. Incubation by female for 29–31 days. Fledges at 36–41 days. Breeding season: Mid-April				
Red-shouldered hawk (*Buteo lineatus*)	RSHA	460–930 g	Small mammals, amphibians, reptiles, and insects	Forests, deciduous swamps. Also in suburban wooded areas
Reproduction: Stick nest in major fork of tree. 2–3 eggs. Incubation mainly by female for 23–25 days. Fledges at 6 weeks but not independent until 17–19 weeks. Breeding season: Late January in south, April in north Note: Very vocal and this can be used to differentiate the species when a nestling/hatchling				
Red-tailed hawk (*Buteo jamaicensis*)	RTHA	800–1600 g	Small mammals, reptiles, and birds	Variable from farm fields to forests to urban areas
Reproduction: Large stick nest in tree. 2–3 eggs. Incubation mostly by female for 28–32 days. Fledges at 42–46 days. Independent at 3–4 months. Breeding season: Mid-February in south, April in north Note: A very tough, strong species. They generally fall into two categories: either very calm or very stressed. Some can be very food aggressive and others can be completely anorectic and difficult to manage. Many geographically separated subspecies. Large variations in size and plumage are common. Young birds (hatch year and second year) are very susceptible to Aspergillosis				
Rough-legged hawk (*Buteo lagopus*)	RLHA	Male: 800–1000 g Female: 1080–1300 g	Small mammals (lemmings, voles)	Tundra and taiga

Continued

Name	Abbrev.	Weight range	Diet	Habitat
Reproduction: Nests on cliff, bluff, or in tree. 2–3 eggs or 5–7 in good lemming years. Incubation by both sexes for 28–31 days. Fledges at 41 days				
Sharp-shinned hawk (*Accipiter striatus*)	SSHA	Male: 80–110 g Female: 150–220 g	Small birds	Wooded areas
Reproduction: Stick nest in conifer. 4–5 eggs. Incubation by both sexes for 30–35 days. Fledges at 23 days and independent 3–4 weeks later. Breeding season: April Note: Similar to a Cooper's hawk but much smaller. The males are very delicate and often do not survive in a rehabilitation environment				
Short-eared owl (*Asio flammeus*)	SEOW	Male: 206–396 g Female: 260–475 g	Small mammals and birds	Grasslands, agricultural fields, and estuaries
Reproduction: Nests on ground. 4–8 eggs. Incubation by female for 24–28 days. Fledges at 14 weeks Breeding season: April Note: Diurnal				
Short-tailed hawk (*Buteo brachyurus*)	STHA	Male: 450–470 g Female: 530 g	Small birds	Wooded savannah, woodlands near water, and swamps
Reproduction: Large stick nest in a tree. 1–3 eggs. Incubation by female for 34 days. Fledge age unknown				
Snail kite (*Rostrhamus sociabilis*)	SNKI	300–570 g	Apple snails	Freshwater wetlands
Reproduction: Nests in bush or on ground. Usually in colony. 3–4 eggs. Incubation by both sexes for 27 days. Fledges at 23–34 days. Independent at 10 weeks				
Snowy owl (*Bubo scandiacus*; formerly *Nyctea scandiaca*)	SNOW	1100–2000 g	Voles and other mammals, gamebirds, and will even catch fish	Arctic tundra and open grasslands
Reproduction: Nests on ground. 4–10 eggs. Incubation by female for 32–37 days. Fledges at 50–60 days. Breeding season: May to June				
Spotted owl (*Strix occidentalis*)	SPOW	520–760 g	Small mammals, snakes, and insects. All suitable-sized prey	Dense, old-growth coniferous forests
Reproduction: Nests in cavities or using old stick nests. 2 eggs. Incubation by female for 28–30 days. Fledges at 9–10 weeks. Breeding season: Early April				
Swainson's hawk (*Buteo swainsoni*)	SWHA	Male: 810 g Female: 1150 g	Mostly insects but diet varies during breeding season	Prairie and dry grasslands
Reproduction: Stick nest in a tree or shrub or on a ledge. 2–3 eggs. Incubation by both sexes for 34–35 days. Fledges at 38–46 days Note: Migrates to Argentin				
Swallow-tailed kite (*Elanoides forficatus*)	STKI	310–600 g	Small reptiles, frogs, and insects	Woodlands and forested wetlands. Near fresh water
Reproduction: Nests made from broken twigs in trees. 2–4 eggs. Incubation mostly by female for 28 days. Fledges at 36–42 days				

Continued

Name	Abbrev.	Weight range	Diet	Habitat
Turkey vulture (*Cathartes aura*)	TUVU	2000 g	Carrion	Open land interspersed with wood
Reproduction: Eggs laid on ground, usually in some sort of cave or structure. Usually 2 eggs. Incubation by both sexes for 37–41 days. Fledges at 10–11 weeks. Breeding season: Late January in south, April in north Note: Chicks are very imprintable. Very dangerous beak so restrain head at all times. Can cohabit with large hawks and Black vulture in the same enclosure. Regurgitates when stressed				
Western screech owl (*Megascops kennicottii*)	WESO	90–250 g	Small rodents and insects	Variable, but prefers open forests along edges of open fields or wetlands
Reproduction: Cavity nester. 2–4 eggs. Incubation for 21–30 days. Fledges at 35 days. Breeding season: March to June				
White-tailed hawk (*Buteo albicaudatus*)	WTHA	880–1240 g	Rabbits, lizards, or other small prey	Arid, open, or semi-open areas with few trees
Reproduction: Nest built from twigs or thorny plants. 1–3 eggs. Incubation by both sexes for 31 days. Fledges at 49–53 days				
White-tailed kite (*Elanus leucurus*)	WTKI	250–380 g	Small mammals, lizards, and insects	Savannahs, pastures, marshes, and agricultural areas
Reproduction: Twig and grass nest. 4–5 eggs. Incubation by female for 28–30 days. Fledges at 35–40 days Note: Roosts in communal groups of up to 100 individuals				
Zone-tailed hawk (*Buteo albonotatus*)	ZTHA	565–900 g	Small birds, mammals, and lizards	Highly variable
Reproduction: Stick nest in top or main fork of tree. Usually 2 eggs. Incubation by both sexes for 28–35 days. Fledges at 42–50 days but may be fed by adults for a few more weeks Note: Appearance mimics Turkey vulture				

South/Central America

Name	Abbrev.	Weight range	Diet	Habitat
American kestrel	See North America			
Andean condor (*Vultur gryphus*)		Male: 11–15 kg Female: 8–11 kg	Mostly carrion but will kill helpless newborn prey	Canyons and peaks throughout the Andes. Open grasslands
Reproduction: No nest is built. A natural cavity in a rock pile or cliff is used instead. 1 egg. Incubation for 54–58 days by both parents. Fledge at 6 months but remain with parents until aged 2 years when parents start a new clutch				
Aplomado falcon	See North America			

Continued

Name	Abbrev.	Weight range	Diet	Habitat
Austral pygmy owl (*Glaucidium nanum*)		55–100 g	Insects make up half the diet	Open woodlands with thorn shrubs
Reproduction: Nests in tree-hollows or rodent burrows. 3–6 eggs. Incubation for 15–17 days				
Band-bellied owl (*Pulsatrix melanota*)		590–1250 g	Unknown	Dense, humid mountain forests
Reproduction: Unknown				
Bare-shanked screech owl (*Megascops clarkii*)		123–190 g	Large insects, spiders, and small invertebrates	Dense mountain and cloud forests
Reproduction: Nests in natural cavity?				
Barn owl	See North America			
Barred forest falcon (*Micrastur ruficollis*)		Male: 161–167 g Female: 196–232 g	Mostly lizards. Also prey on insects caught in an ant swarm	Understory of humid primary forest
Reproduction: Nests in natural cavities. 2–3 eggs. Incubation for 33–35 days. Fledges at 35–44 days				
Barred hawk (*Leucopternis princeps*)		1000 g	Mostly snakes but will also eat frogs, large insects, and crabs	Inside canopy or edges of mountain or cloud forests
Reproduction: Nests in stick platform on rocky cliffs. 1 egg. Fledges at 80 days				
Bat falcon (*Falco rufigularis*)		Male: 108–148 g Female: 177–242 g	Bats and birds, small mammals, and insects (moths). Will crash into canopy to flush bumblebees	Open habitats, savannahs, and agricultural fields
Reproduction: Nests in tree cavity. 2–4 eggs. Incubation for 30 days by female. Fledges at 35 days				
Bicolored hawk (*Accipiter bicolor*)			Mostly smaller birds. Flushes prey in the tree canopy. Follows monkey troops to capture flushed insects	Variable but prefers wooded areas
Reproduction: Small cup-shaped platform of sticks. 1–3 eggs. Incubation for 34 days by female				
Black caracara (*Daptrius ater*)		330–354 g	Insect larvae, amphibians, reptiles, nestling birds, and fish. Will also eat certain fruits and carrion, and pick ticks off tapirs and deer	Forest edges, especially along rivers and swamps
Reproduction: Unknown Note: Can be quite tame around people				
Black hawk-eagle (*Spizaetus tyrannus*)		Male: 950 g Female: 1120 g	Mammals (marmosets, squirrels) and birds, lizards, and snakes	Forested and semi-open areas

Continued

Name	Abbrev.	Weight range	Diet	Habitat
Reproduction: Stick platform placed in dense tangle of vines near trunk of tree. 1 egg. Incubation by the female only. Fledges at 71 days				
Black solitary eagle (*Buteogallus solitarius*)		3000 g	Mostly snakes	Heavily forested areas in hilly or mountainous terrain
Reproduction: Large stick structure in main crotch of tree. Possibly just 1 egg				
Black vulture	See North America			
Black-and-chestnut eagle (*Spizaetus isidori*)			Large arboreal birds (guans) and squirrels	Wet cloud forest on slopes at higher elevations
Reproduction: Huge stick structure in tree. 1 egg. Fledges at 4 months				
Black-and-white hawk-eagle (*Spizaetus melanoleucus*)		850 g	Medium-sized birds, small mammals, reptiles, and toads	Edges and gaps in wet forests
Reproduction: Nest is a large cup-shaped stick structure. 2 eggs				
Black-and-white owl (*Ciccaba nigrolineata*)		404–535 g	Mostly insects but also small mammals, bats, and tree frogs. Can hunt prey in the air	Rainforest and swampy, flooded deciduous woodlands and mangroves
Reproduction: Usually nests in a tree cavity or among epiphytes and orchids on large trees. 1–2 eggs				
Black-banded owl (*Ciccaba huhula*)		397 g	Mainly insects	Lowland rainforests, but also plantations
Reproduction: Unknown				
Black-capped screech owl (*Megascops atricapilla*)		115–160 g	Insects and spiders	Rainforest with dense undergrowth
Reproduction: Unknown				
Black-chested buzzard-eagle (*Geranoaetus melanoleucus*)		2000 g	Small mammals, birds, snakes, lizards, and carrion. Domestic pigeons are a favorite	Open, dry habitats in rugged terrain
Reproduction: Bulky stick nest on ledge or cliff. 1–3 eggs. Incubation for 37–42/27–30 days by both sexes				
Black-collared hawk (*Busarellius nigricollis*)		Male: 695 g Female: 796 g	Perches overlooking water. Fish, frogs, aquatic insects, and crustaceans	Lowlands, mangroves, marshes, ponds, and flooded fields
Reproduction: Large stick platform in upper mangrove tree. 1–2 eggs. Fledges at 55–66 days				

Continued

Name	Abbrev.	Weight range	Diet	Habitat
Black-faced hawk (*Leucopternis melanops*)		297–317 g	Mostly reptiles, birds, and insects	Lowland mangroves and along rivers and streams
Reproduction: Unknown				
Broad-winged hawk	See North America			
Buckley's forest falcon (*Micrastur buckleyi*)			May follow army ant swarm to feed on flushed reptiles and insects	Interior of humid forest and lowland forest edges
Reproduction: Nests in tree cavity. 2 eggs Note: Semi-crepuscular				
Buff-fronted owl (*Aegolius harrisii*)		104–155 g	Unknown	Mountain, cloud, and alpine forests
Reproduction: Unknown				
Burrowing owl	See North America			
Caruncalated caracara (*Phalcoboenus carunculatus*)			Carrion and live prey including rodents and rabbits, lizards, frogs, and insects	Open grasslands and bushy pastures
Reproduction: Nest is a stick structure on rock ledges. 2 eggs				
Chaco owl (*Strix chacoensis*)		360–500 g	Small vertebrates and insects	Dry, semi-open scrub on hills or mountain slopes
Reproduction: Unknown				
Chilean hawk (*Accipiter chilensis*)			Variable but mostly birds and flying insects	Prefers a patchwork of open land and forest
Reproduction: Oval-shaped twig platform in upper canopy. 2–3 eggs. Incubation for 20–21 days				
Chimango caracara (*Milvago chimango*)		Male: 289 g Female: 300 g	Opportunistic. Feeds on carrion, ticks picked off the back of cattle, turtle and bird eggs. May forage in city dumps	Open lowlands, savannahs, farm fields, marshes, and beaches
Reproduction: Stick nest lined with grass, wool, or rags. 2–4 eggs. Incubation for 32 days. Fledges at 32–41 days				
Cinereous harrier (*Circus cinereus*)		Male: 340 g Female: 500 g	Rodents, small birds, frogs, and insects. Carrion	High mountains but also lowland grasslands and marshes
Reproduction: Nests in grass or reeds in marsh. 3–4 eggs				
Cinnamon screech owl (*Megascops petersoni*)		88–119 g	Unknown	Moist cloud forests rich in epiphytes and moss
Reproduction: Unknown				

Continued

Name	Abbrev.	Weight range	Diet	Habitat
Cloud-forest pygmy owl (*Glaucidium nubicola*)		73–80 g	Insects and small vertebrates	Humid cloud forest on Andean slopes
Reproduction: Unknown				
Collared forest falcon (*Micrastur semitorquatus*)		Male: 584 g Female: 820 g	Large lizards, snakes, rodents, birds, and large insects	Heavily wooded areas, typically near forest edges in tangled thickets
Reproduction: Nests in cavities. 1–3 eggs. Incubation for 46–48 days by the female only. Fledges at 50 days Note: Crepuscular. Has large eyes and well-developed sense of hearing. Can produce a high-pitched vocalization to attract passerines				
Colombian screech owl (*Megascops colombianus*)		150–210 g	Larger insects and arthropods	Cloud forest with epiphyte and dense undergrowth
Reproduction: Unknown				
Common black hawk	See North America			
Crane hawk (*Geranospiza caerulescens*)		Male: 225–358 g Female: 273–353 g	Rodents, bats, lizards, snakes, small birds, and insects	Tropical lowlands. Wooded swamps and mangroves
Reproduction: Nests high in trees, often in clumps of orchids. 1–2 eggs Note: Can bend legs backward at the tarsal joint to assist in reaching into crevices and tree cavities				
Crested caracara	See North America			
Crested eagle (*Morphnus guianensis*)		1750 g	Birds, mid-sized mammals (small monkeys and opossums), snakes, and frogs	Undisturbed, lowland, wet primary forest
Reproduction: Huge stick platform in the central fork of a large tree. 1–2 eggs. Incubation for 40–50 days by female only. Fledges at 103–114 days				
Crested owl (*Lophostrix cristata*)		425–620 g	Large insects and some vertebrates	Lowland rainforest but also mid-level forested areas
Reproduction: Cavity nester				
Crowned eagle (*Buteogallus coronatus*)		2950 g	Mostly armadillos and other medium-sized mammals such as skunks	Open country including grasslands and savannahs
Reproduction: Huge stick platform in main fork of tree. Single egg. Incubation for at least 39–40 days by female only Note: Semi-crepuscular. Also known as the Crowned solitary eagle				
Cryptic forest falcon (*Micrastur mintoni*)			Generalist. Will eat a variety of reptiles and small invertebrates	*Terra firme* forest
Reproduction: Unknown				

Continued

Name	Abbrev.	Weight range	Diet	Habitat
Double-toothed kite (*Harpagus bidentatus*)		168–229 g	Lizards, insects, and small birds	Upland forest edges
Reproduction: Nests in shallow cup of twigs in fork of tree. 1–2 eggs. Incubation for 42–45 days by female only. Fledges at 27–37 days Note: Has double "tooth" in maxillary beak				
Elf owl	See North America			
Ferruginous pygmy owl (*Glaucidium brasilianum*)		46–107 g	Insects and small birds. Able to catch prey larger than itself	Lowland forests but also pastures and parks in urban areas
Reproduction: Unknown				
Flammulated owl	See North America			
Galapagos hawk (*Buteo galapagoensis*)		Male: 844 g Female: 1223 g	Generalist but rodents are largest part of diet	All island habitats from barren lava fields and shoreline to deciduous forest and mountain peaks
Reproduction: Stick nest lined with leaves and bark on rocky outcrop or in low tree. 1–3 eggs. Incubation for 37–38 days. Fledges at 50–60 days Note: The only diurnal raptor on the islands				
Gray hawk	See North America			
Gray-backed hawk (*Leucopternis occidentalis*)		Female: 660 g	Varied but reptiles/snakes are a major part of the diet	Deciduous and evergreen forests. Also found in agricultural lands
Reproduction: Nests in trees on steep slopes near water. 1 egg. Incubation for 36 days by female. Fledges at 76+ days Note: Breeding occurs throughout the year				
Gray-bellied hawk (*Accipiter poliogaster*)			Hunts in canopy for small birds	Lowland humid forest, dense woodlands
Reproduction: Unknown				
Gray-headed kite (*Leptodon cayanensis*)		416–605 g	Snakes, frogs, lizards, eggs, nestlings, and insects (wasps, hornets, ants)	Mature forest. Often in canopy and in vicinity of water
Reproduction: Nests on shallow stick cup in fork of tree. 1–2 eggs Note: Siblicide may be common				
Gray-lined hawk (*Buteo nitidus*)		Male: 465 g Female: 554 g	Lizards, small snakes, and birds	Lowland tropical and subtropical forest to arid, open country
Reproduction: Small stick nest high in tree. 1–3 eggs. Incubation for 32 days. Fledges at 42 days				

Continued

Name	Abbrev.	Weight range	Diet	Habitat
Great black hawk (*Buteogallus urubitinga*)		Male: 853–996 g Female: 900–1250 g	Almost anything from mammals to frogs and fish	Frequently found around lakes, marshes, but also around pastures and fields
Reproduction: Bulky flat stick platform. 1 egg. Incubation for 35–37 days. Fledges at 55–60 days				
Great-horned owl	See North America			
Greater yellow-headed vulture (*Cathartes melambrotus*)		1650 g	Carrion, especially of forest mammals	Mature forest
Reproduction: Nests in tree cavity. 2 eggs.				
Harpy eagle (*Harpia harpyja*)		Male: 4.0–4.8 kg Female: 7.6–9.0 kg	Mammals such as monkeys, sloths, and armadillos	Lowland and foothill rainforests
Reproduction: Nests on a huge stick platform in a high crotch in tree. 1–2 eggs. Incubation for 56 days. Fledges at 140+ days				
Harris's hawk	See North America			
Hook-billed kite	See North America			
King vulture (*Sarcoramphus papa*)	KIVU	3000–3750 g	Carrion. Usually the dominant species at a carcass	Clear or partly forested areas
Reproduction: Single egg laid in a rock crevice or the hollow of a tree stump. Incubation for 50–58 days by both parents. Fledges at 130 days. May only breed every other year				
Laughing falcon (*Herpetotheres cachinnans*)		Male: 567–686 g Female: 626–800 g	Mostly snakes. Small snakes are swallowed whole	Open country and savannahs. Rarely enters dense woods
Reproduction: Usually nests in tree cavity or at the base of palm fronds. Usually 1 egg. Incubation for 40–45 days by the female only. Fledges at 65–72 days				
Least (Pernambuco) pygmy owl (*Glaucidium minutissimum*)		51 g	Insects	Lowland rainforests
Reproduction: Unknown Note: Very rare. Critically endangered. Entire population lives in a protected reserve				
Lesser yellow-headed vulture (*Cathartes burrovianus*)		950–1550 g	Fish and reptiles. May forage behind moving farm equipment	Lowlands in marshes, grasslands, mangroves
Reproduction: No nest. Eggs are laid on the ground in dense grass or in hollow of tree. 2 eggs. Incubation for 40 days. Fledges at 70–75 days				
Lined forest falcon (*Micrastur gilvicollis*)		172–223 g	Small mammals, birds, reptiles, and insects	Lowland interior humid forest
Reproduction: Unknown				

Continued

Name	Abbrev.	Weight range	Diet	Habitat
Long-winged harrier (*Circus buffoni*)		Male: 397 g Female: 605 g	Mainly frogs and small mammals	Marshlands and wet pastures
Reproduction: Nests on ground in wet grassy area. 3–4 eggs				
Mantled hawk (*Pseudastur polionotus*)			Mostly birds and snakes. Some rodents	Mixed woodland
Reproduction: Unknown				
Merlin	See North America			
Mississippi kite	See North America			
Mottled owl (*Strix/Ciccaba virgata*)		235–307 g	Small mammals, birds, snakes, and frogs	Humid lowland forests
Reproduction: Nests in tree cavity or nest built by other species. 1–2 eggs				
Mountain caracara (*Phalcoboenus megalopterus*)		795 g	Lizards, rodents, carrion, and will scavenge at city dumps	Open grasslands, heavily grazed pastures, and in recently plowed farm fields
Reproduction: Large nest on rock ledges made from dried guano. 2–3 eggs				
Northern harrier	See North America			
Orange-breasted falcon (*Falco deiroleucus*)		Female: 654 g	Captures medium- to large-sized birds in flight	Mature, heavily forested areas with openings with cliffs
Reproduction: Nests on cliffs and Mayan temples. 2–4 eggs. Incubation for 30 days. Fledges at 40 days				
Ornate hawk-eagle (*Spizaetus ornatus*)		Male: 1000 g Female: 1450 g	Birds mostly but also hunts mammals, lizards, and snakes	Rainforest or pine forest
Reproduction: Bulky stick platform in the fork or top of tree. 1 egg. Incubation for 47–50 days mostly by female. Fledges at 79 days				
Osprey	See North America			
Pearl kite (*Gampsonyx swainsonii*)		Male: 94 g	Lizards, frogs, and insects	Open woodlands, savannahs, farm fields, and even in suburbs
Reproduction: Small twig platform. 1–4 eggs. Incubation for 34–35 days mostly by the female. Fledges at 5 weeks				
Peregrine falcon	See North America			
Peruvian pygmy owl (*Glaucidium peruanum*)		58–65 g	Insects, arthropods, and small birds	Riparian thickets, mesquite, and semi-arid areas with cacti and thorny shrubs
Reproduction: Unknown				

Continued

Name	Abbrev.	Weight range	Diet	Habitat
Plain-breasted hawk (*Accipiter ventralis*)			Small birds	Humid forests, woodlands, and in partially cleared agricultural areas
Reproduction: Unknown				
Plumberous forest falcon (*Micrastur plumbeus*)			Small ground-dwelling mammals, reptiles, and insects	Wet lowlands and foothills
Reproduction: Nests in tree cavities.				
Plumberous hawk (*Leucopternis plumbeus*)			Frogs, crabs, and snakes. Hunts along riverbanks	Lowland humid, tropical rainforests
Reproduction: Unknown				
Plumberous kite (*Ictinia plumbea*)		Male: 190–267 g Female: 232–280 g	Insects like ants and termites but also large flying insects	Forest patches, pastures, savannahs, and mangroves
Reproduction: Cup-shaped stick platform in tree. 1–2 eggs. Incubation for 31–32 days. Fledges at 36–38 days				
Red-tailed hawk	See North America			
Red-throated caracara (*Ibycter americanus*)		510–680 g	Tears open the nests of arboreal bees, wasps, and hornets to feed on larvae. Also seeds, palm fruit, and turtle eggs	Lowlands, semi-open areas, and edges of humid forests
Reproduction: Nesting behavior unknown. 2–3 eggs Note: Often moves in noisy groups				
Roadside hawk (*Buteo magnirostris*)		Male: 251 g Female: 303 g	Mostly large insects. Nestling birds, small mammals/bats, snakes, and scorpions	Forest edges, scrub, savannahs with scattered trees. Also found in parks in urban areas
Reproduction: Small stick nest lined with bark, leaves, lichen. 1–3 eggs. Incubation for 35–37 days Note: Can be very tame and approachable				
Rufescent screech owl (*Megascops ingens*)		134–223 g	Large insects and spiders	Humid forest on mountain slopes
Reproduction: Cavity nester				
Rufous-banded owl (*Strix/Ciccaba albitarsis*)			Unknown	Cloud and mountain forests with dense undergrowth
Reproduction: Unknown				

Continued

Name	Abbrev.	Weight range	Diet	Habitat
Rufous crab hawk (*Buteogallus aequinoctialis*)		Male: 595 g Female: 796 g	Feeds exclusively on crabs	Mangroves and coastal swamps
Reproduction: Twig nest. 1–2 eggs				
Rufous-legged owl (*Strix rufipes*)		350 g	Small mammals, birds, reptiles, frogs, and insects	Moist forest on mountain slopes
Reproduction: Cavity nester. 2–3 eggs				
Rufous-tailed hawk (*Buteo ventralis*)		950 g	Rabbits and small rodents	Generalist. Reported in dense forest and open coastal grasslands
Reproduction: Stick nest. Up to 3 eggs?				
Rufous-thighed hawk (*Accipiter erythronemius*)			Small to mid-sized birds	Arid or wet lowland forest but also in suburban areas
Reproduction: Small stick platform. 2–3 eggs. Incubation by female				
Rufous-thighed kite (*Harpagus diodon*)			Primarily large insects such as cicadas	Lowland forests
Reproduction: Nest in shallow stick cup. 1–2 eggs				
Rusty-barred owl (*Strix hylophia*)		285–395 g	Insects, voles, mice, and small birds	Forests with dense undergrowth
Reproduction: Cavity nester. Incubation for 29 days. Fledges at 5 weeks				
Savannah hawk (*Buteogallus meridionalis*)		825–1069 g	Small mammals, birds, snakes, lizards, frogs, toads, eels, crabs, and large insects. May forage while walking on the ground	Lowland savannahs, open dry country but also along mangroves and roadways
Reproduction: Large platform of sticks lined with grass or lichen. 1–2 eggs. Incubation for 35–36 days. Fledges at 48–55 days				
Semi-collared hawk (*Accipiter collaris*)			Exclusively birds	Humid forests with large trees
Reproduction: Unknown				
Semiplumbeous hawk (*Leucopternis semiplumbeus*)		Male: 250 g Female: 325 g	Reptiles, frogs, and small mammals	Lowland forests. Prefers the understory and lower canopy
Reproduction: Unknown				
Short-eared owl	See North America			
Short-tailed hawk (*Buteo brachyurus*)	STHA	Male: 450–470 g Female: 530 g	Small birds	Wooded savannah, woodlands near water, and swamps

Continued

Name	Abbrev.	Weight range	Diet	Habitat
Reproduction: Large stick nest in a tree. 1–3 eggs. Incubation by female for 34 days. Fledge age unknown				
Slate-colored hawk (*Buteogallus schistaceus*)		Female: 455 g	Snakes, lizards, frogs, crabs, fish, insects. Follows monkey troops to capture flushed insects	Lowlands near rivers, lakes, and swamps
Reproduction: Unknown				
Slaty-backed forest falcon (*Micrastur mirandollei*)		556 g	Preys mostly on birds	Interior of lowland wet forests
Reproduction: Unknown Note: Produces a high-pitched vocalization that attracts passerines				
Slender-billed kite (*Helicolestes hamatus*)		Male: 377–448 g Female: 367–485 g	Freshwater snails and crabs	Lowland swamps, lagoons, and ponds
Reproduction: Twig platform high in a tree in flooded forest. 2 eggs. Incubation for 30 days. Fledges at 35–40 days				
Snail kite	See North America			
Solitary eagle (*Buteogallus solitarius*)		3000 g	Mostly snakes	Forested mountain slopes and cloud forest
Reproduction: Unknown				
Southern caracara (*Caracara plancus*)			Carrion, roadkills. Follows tractors to feed on exposed prey. Turtle and bird eggs. Even eats vegetable matter such as peanuts and avocados	Open country
Reproduction: Bulky stick structure in tree or cliff ledge. Lined with wool or animal hair. 2–3 eggs. Incubation for 28–32 days. Fledges at 50–56 days				
Spectacled owl (*Pulsatrix perspicillata*)	SPOW	590–982 g	Small mammals and birds, crabs, insects, and spiders	Lowland tropical and subtropical forests
Reproduction: Cavity nester. 2–3 eggs. Fledges at 5–6 weeks				
Spot-winged falconet (*Spiziapteryx circumcincta*)		150 g	Wide variety of insects, lizards, and birds	Lowland savannahs and mesquites
Reproduction: Nests in unoccupied Monk parakeet or Ovenbird nest. 2–4 eggs. Fledges at 33 days?				
Striated caracara (*Phalcoboenus australis*)		1187 g	Feeds on colonial nesting seabirds (especially penguins and albatross) and their eggs. Carrion. Will attack injured sheep	Lowlands, particularly rocky coasts

Continued

Name	Abbrev.	Weight range	Diet	Habitat
Reproduction: Bulky nest of grass and twigs on cliff ledges and rocks. 1–3 eggs. May have 3 adults caring for a nest				
Striped owl (*Asio clamator*)		335–556 g	Small vertebrates and large insects	Savannahs and grasslands. Avoids dense forest
Reproduction: Nests on ground on a flattened grassy clump. 2–4 eggs				
Swainson's hawk	See North America			
Swallow-tailed kite	See North America			
Tawny-bellied screech owl (*Megascops watsonii*)		114–155 g	Insects and small vertebrates	Lowland subtropical and tropical forests and swamps
Reproduction: Cavity nester. 3–4 eggs. Incubation for 25–26 days. Fledges at 1 month				
Tawny-browed owl (*Pulsatrix koeniswaldiana*)		481 g	Unknown	Tropical and subtropical forests
Reproduction: Unknown				
Tiny hawk (*Accipiter superciliosus*)		Male: 75 g Female: 115–134 g	Small passerines, hummingbirds, and insects	Lowland rainforest. Woodlands
Reproduction: Stick nest in tall tree				
Tropical screech owl (*Megascops choliba*)		100–160 g	Insects, spiders, and small vertebrates	Open forest, clearings, farmlands, and urban parks
Reproduction: Cavity nester. 1–4 eggs. Incubation by female. Fledges at 30 days				
Turkey vulture	See North America			
Variable/Puna hawk (*Geranoaetus polyosoma*)		1000 g	Rats, rabbits mostly but also birds and insects	Dry, open country with scattered vegetation. Farmlands and also rugged mountains in the Andes
Reproduction: Large, bulky nest in tree, cactus, or ledge. 1–3 eggs				
White hawk (*Pseudastur albicollis*)		Male: 600–650 g Female: 710–855 g	Mostly snakes and lizards	Lowlands and foothills with forested, hilly terrain
Reproduction: Nest is cupped stick platform. 1 egg. Incubation for 35 days. Fledges at 65–88 days				
White-browed hawk (*Leucopternis kuhli*)			Snakes, lizards, and insects	Humid, lowland forests
Reproduction: Unknown				

Continued

Name	Abbrev.	Weight range	Diet	Habitat
White-collared kite (*Leptodon forbesi*)		Male: 580 g Female: 550 g	Unknown	Atlantic coastal rainforest
Reproduction: Unknown				
White-necked hawk (*Buteogallus lacernulatus*)			Invertebrates including large insects and spiders	Dense, lowland forest
Reproduction: Unknown				
White-rumped hawk (*Parabuteo leucorrhous*)		Male: 290 g	Small mammals, frogs, and insects	Humid forest edges near clearings
Reproduction: Cup-shaped stick nest. 2 eggs				
White-tailed hawk	See North America			
White-tailed kite	See North America			
White-throated caracara (*Phalcoboenus albogularis*)			Feeds on carrion, at garbage dumps, but also hunts small rodents and insects	Open habitat. Often seen perched on cliffs, hillsides, and fences
Reproduction: Stick nest on rock ledge. 2–3 eggs				
White-throated hawk (*Buteo albigula*)			Birds, rodents, snakes, and lizards	Variable forested areas
Reproduction: Stick nest on cliff or in tree. 1–2 eggs. Incubation for 30 days. Fledges at 6 weeks				
Yellow-headed caracara (*Milvago chimachima*)		Male: 315 g Female: 335 g	Opportunistic. Feeds on carrion, garbage, small live animals including mammals, lizards, snakes, and insects. Eats ticks off the back of cattle	Open country, savannahs, pastures, and farm fields
Reproduction: Substantial stick platform on top of a tree or in a palm tree. 2 eggs				
Zone-tailed hawk	See North America			

Bibliography

Baicich, P. and Harrison, C. (2005) *Nests, Eggs and Nestlings of North American Birds*, 2nd edn. Princeton University Press, Princeton, NJ, USA.

del Hoyo, J., Elliot, A. and Sargatal, J. (1994) *Handbook of the Birds of the World*. Vol. 2. Lynx Edicions, Barcelona, Spain.

Jimenez, J. (1989) Biology of the austral pygmy owl. *Wilson Bulletin* 101(3), 377–389.

Johnsgard, P. (1988) *North American Owls: Biology and Natural History*. Smithsonian Institution Press, Washington, DC, USA.

Johnsgard, P. (1990) *Hawks, Eagles & Falcons of North America*. Smithsonian Institution Press, Washington, DC, USA.

Mikkola, H. (2014) *Owls of the World: A Photographic Guide*, 2nd edn. Firefly Books, Buffalo, NY, USA.

Santillán, M.A., Travaini, A., Procopio, D.E., Zanón, J.I., Yaya, M., de la Cruz Martinez, J. and Peck, R.M. (2009) New records indicate that Austral pygmy owl Glaucidium nanum breeds in eastern Patagonia. *Contiga* 32.

Scott, D. (2015) *Medical records in RaptorMed™ database*. Carolina Raptor Center, Huntersville, NC, USA.

Sibley, D.A. (2000) *The Sibley Guide to Birds*. Alfred A. Knopf, Inc., New York, NY, USA.

Sibley, D.A. (2001) *The Sibley Guide to Bird Life & Behavior*. Alfred A. Knopf, Inc., New York, NY, USA.

Online Sources

Beauty of Birds. Available at: www.beautyofbirds.com (accessed December 2015).

BirdLife International. Available at: www.birdlife.org (accessed December 2015).

Birds of India. Available at: https://indianbirds.thedynamicnature.com (accessed December 2015).

Birds of the World—An Online Bird Book. Available at: https://carolinabirds.org (accessed December 2015).

Cornell Lab of Ornithology. Available at: www.allaboutbirds.org (accessed July 2015).

The Eagle Directory. Available at: http://www.eagleencyclopedia.org (accessed December 2015).

Eagle Watch. Available at: www.eaglewatch.nl (accessed December 2015).

European Raptors—Biology and Conservation. Available at: www.europeanraptors.org (accessed December 2015).

Handbook of Birds of the World. Available at: https://birdsoftheworld.org/bow/home (accessed December 2015).

Oiseaux-Birds.com. Available at: www.oiseaux-birds.com (accessed December 2015).

Owling.com. Available at: www.owling.com (accessed December 2015).

The Owl Pages. Available at: www.owlpages.com (accessed July 2015).

The Peregrine Fund: Global Raptor Information Network (GRIN). Available at www.globalraptors.org (accessed December 2015).

South African National Biodiversity Institute. Available at: www.sanbi.org (accessed December 2015).

Taylor and Francis Online. Available at: www.tandfonline.com (accessed December 2015).

Wikipedia. Available at: https://www.wikipedia.org/ (accessed July 2015).

4 Fluid Therapy and Treatments

There are many commonly performed treatments and procedures used in avian medicine. Raptors are very tolerant and usually cooperative, but it is important to become proficient. Practicing with cadavers is always a good idea before attempting to work with a live patient.

Learning Objectives

1. How to provide fluid therapy.
2. Various bandages including the figure-8 wrap.
3. Advanced procedures such as blood transfusions.
4. Humane euthanasia.

Fluid Therapy: Routes of Administration

The maintenance requirement is *50 ml/kg/day* and this volume can be administered in many ways including orally, subcutaneously, intravenously, or intraosseously. The route depends on many factors, the most important being the patient's clinical condition.

Oral Fluids and Formula

Oral fluids and/or dietary supplementation are appropriate when the patient is able to stand, is able to keep its head elevated, and when there is little chance of regurgitation or aspiration. The stomach volume can be roughly estimated as 50 ml/kg of BW (Table 4.1).

Red-rubber feeding tubes work well for both fluids and nutritional formula when used with a syringe with the proper tip (Fig. 4.1). Obviously, the bird should be held upright when administering anything orally and should not be laid on its back for any other treatments once completed.

The bird's esophagus follows along the right side of the neck so it is best to pass the tube with your right hand into the back right side of the oral cavity. The goal is to pass the tube through the crop (if present) and into the proventriculus. This can be difficult at times as the tube can get misdirected and coil around in the crop. It is very helpful to have the person holding the bird use their right hand to help direct the tube through the crop. The glottis is quite large in some species so you must visualize the tube passing behind the glottis before beginning to inject fluids or formula.

Note that oral fluids can be difficult (and stressful) to administer in smaller patients such as the screech owl or sharp-shinned hawk so other routes (i.e. SQ) should be considered.

Most raptors do best on a whole-prey diet. In cases of inappetence, a whole-prey diet can be easily force-fed with a pair of long, smooth-tipped forceps. When force-feeding, introduce the food into the

Table 4.1. Oral fluid volumes. Psittacines are included to aid in estimating the stomach volume in other raptor species.

Species	Stomach volume (ml)	Tube volume (ml)
Budgie	1–3	0.5–1.0
African grey	15–35	–
Cockatoo	20–40	8–12
Macaw	35–60	25–35
Red-tailed hawk	50	30–40
Peregrine falcon	–	25

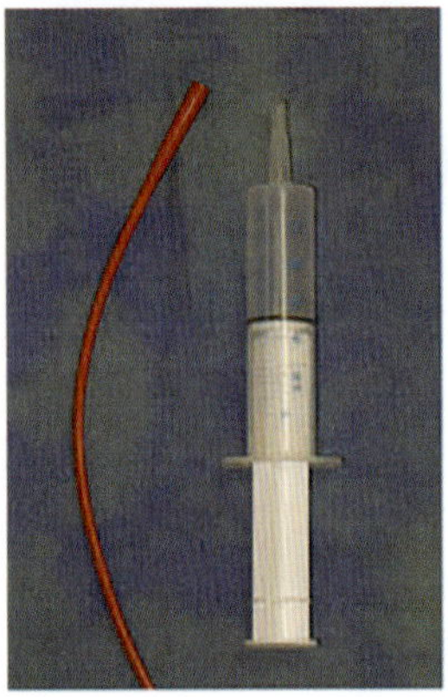

Fig. 4.1. Feeding tube.

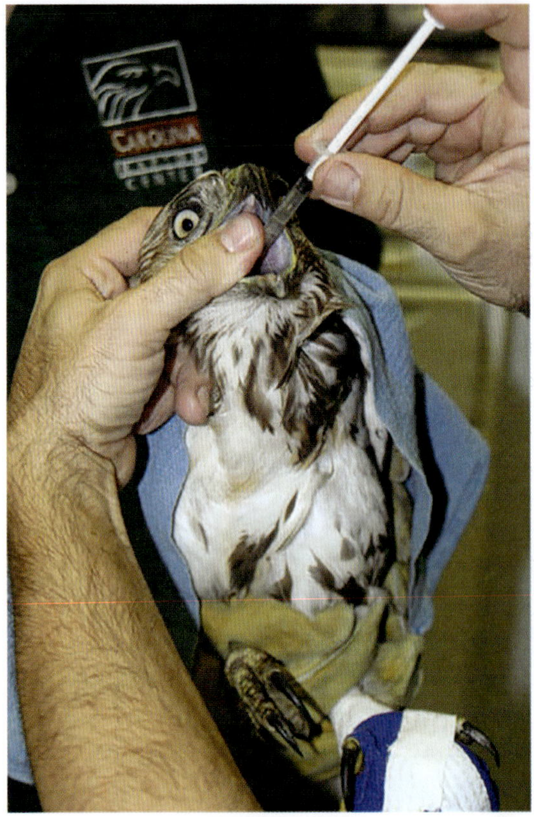

Fig. 4.2. Proper restraint for oral medications.

crop in one smooth motion using care to avoid traumatizing the oral cavity, esophagus, or mandible.

When force-feeding either medications or food, the bird must be properly restrained in an upright position by an assistant and the bird's head is grasped with the left hand with two fingers behind the head and the thumb in the right commissure of the mouth. This ensures good control of the patient's head. Keep your thumb away from the tip of the beak to avoid getting bitten. The right hand is then free to force-feed the bird, pass a tube, or provide medications (Fig. 4.2).

In cases when whole food is regurgitated or in emaciated birds, dietary supplementation with a liquid formula diet may be indicated. There are several commercial carnivore formula diets but blenderized furless, whole-prey diet seems to be the most effective.

> **Raptor Tip**
>
> Using live mice can sometimes stimulate anorectic birds (especially hawks) to start eating.

Oral Medications

If a bird is eating consistently, oral medications should always be given in the food since this reduces the need to be handled. This approach requires that the daily food amount be split into the appropriate number of feedings to match the requirements of the medications being administered. Liquid medications should be injected into the food, and pills should be ground and poured into the abdominal cavity of the prey item through a small opening made in the body wall. Medications should not simply be applied to the fur as it is impossible to guarantee delivery of the entire dose. This is especially important since some birds pluck or skin their prey before eating. Birds that are not eating reliably need to be medicated manually.

Subcutaneous Fluids

The subcutaneous route can be very effective and is probably the most common route of administration used (Fig. 4.3); however, it will not be appropriate for patients that are critically ill or in shock. Fluids can be administered in either the leg webs over the medial thigh or between the shoulder blades. You should be able to easily administer *30–35 ml per kg in each* leg web. Fluids should always be warmed to match the body temperature of the patient (typically around 40°C/105°F). Although important for all routes of administration, it is critical to ensure the fluids are not too warm since severe burns and necrosis will occur. When giving fluids subcutaneously, use a 22- or 23-gauge needle (25-gauge in smaller species) and inject the fluid until the pocket is somewhat firmly distended (but not too tight, as this can also lead to necrosis of the skin). Hyaluronidase can be added to the fluids to speed the absorption. Do not give fluids with a concentration of greater than 2.5% dextrose subcutaneously.

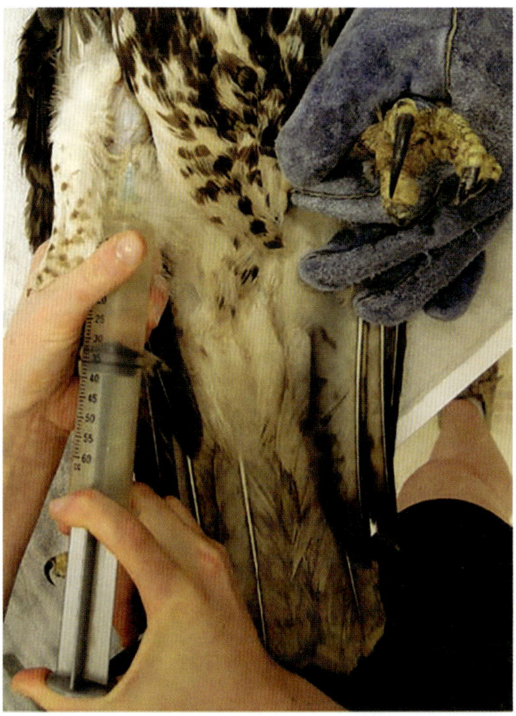

Fig. 4.3. When giving SQ fluids, your assistant restrains the bird from the cranial end. As shown in this picture, it is safest to grip the bird's leg AND the syringe in the same hand. If you do this, there is very little chance of accidentally jabbing the bird if it jerks its leg.

Raptor Tip

You can give 30–35 ml per kg SQ in each leg web.

Intravenous Fluids

Intravenous catheters can be placed in the medial metatarsal vein or the basilic vein but placement can be technically challenging and, once placed, the catheter can be difficult to maintain. IV catheters are best used for temporary venous access during surgery. A 24-gauge, 1.5″ catheter works well in the basilic vein of larger birds (Fig. 4.4).

Intraosseous Fluids

Intraosseous catheters are easy to place and are extremely effective (Fig. 4.5). Spinal needles with a stylet are used and can be placed in the distal ulna or proximal tibiotarsus. *Never* place one in the femur or humerus as these bones communicate with the air sacs. Larger needles (20-gauge) are best and are ideal for patients greater than 500 g. Smaller needles (22-gauge) can be used in birds as small as screech owls. Shorter needles (1.5″ or 2.5″) are suggested since longer ones can be more difficult to place. Placement is quick but can be painful, so a short duration of anesthesia is usually indicated.

To place an IO catheter in the ulna

Always use good sterile techniques and swab all ports with alcohol before use.

- Aseptically prepare the dorsal surface of the distal ulna. There is a small transverse notch that you can place your fingernail in. This is your entry point. There is a shiny white ligament that runs just adjacent to the notch (Figs 4.5 and 4.6a). Avoid this ligament when placing the catheter.

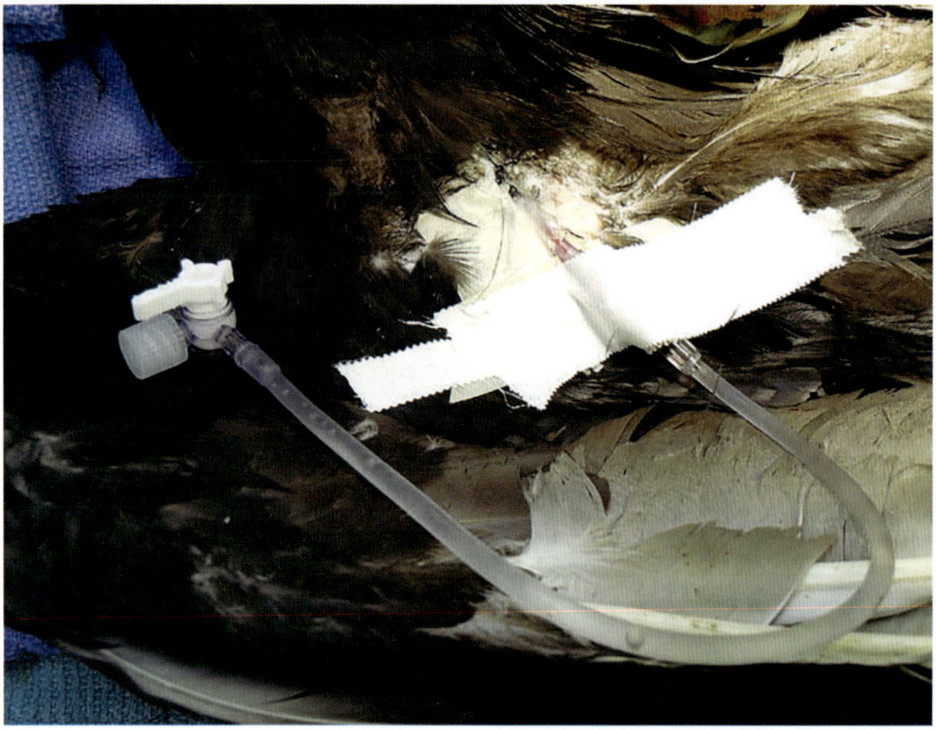

Fig. 4.4. IV catheter in the basilic vein of a black vulture.

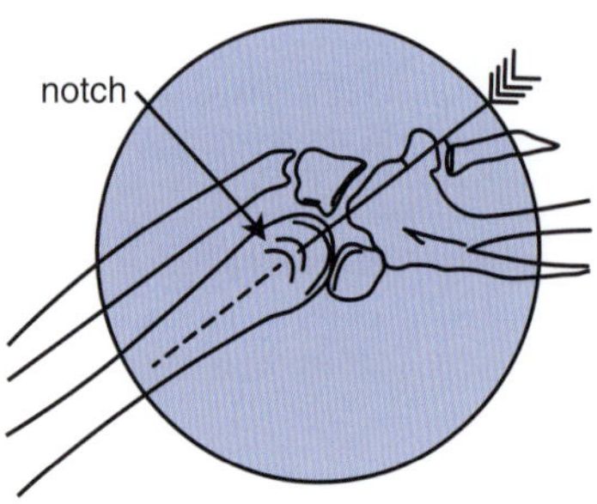

Fig. 4.5. IO catheter placement in the distal ulna.

- Grasp the ulna and radius with the thumb and index finger of one hand. Make sure that you are aware of the direction that the bones are running as it is easy to enter the ulna and then exit accidentally through the opposite cortex.
- Grasp the spinal needle with your other hand. Make sure that the stylet is firmly held in place with your index finger and start drilling the needle just behind the notch. Avoid any unnecessary wobbling when placing the needle as this will lead to leakage of fluid when it is administered.
- You should quickly feel a pop as the needle penetrates the cortex. Continue to insert the catheter by rotating back and forth as this ensures that the tip does not dig into the endosteal surface of the medullary canal.
- Remove the stylet then test the catheter by injecting a few milliliters of warm saline or LRS. It should flow freely with little pressure. You may need to apply pressure in a few small pulses to dislodge any blockages that may have formed when the catheter was placed.
- Attach an injection port, secure the catheter with tape, and immobilize the catheter and the wing with a figure-8 wrap. Tongue depressors should be used on the dorsal and ventral sides to protect the catheter from being bent (Fig. 4.7).

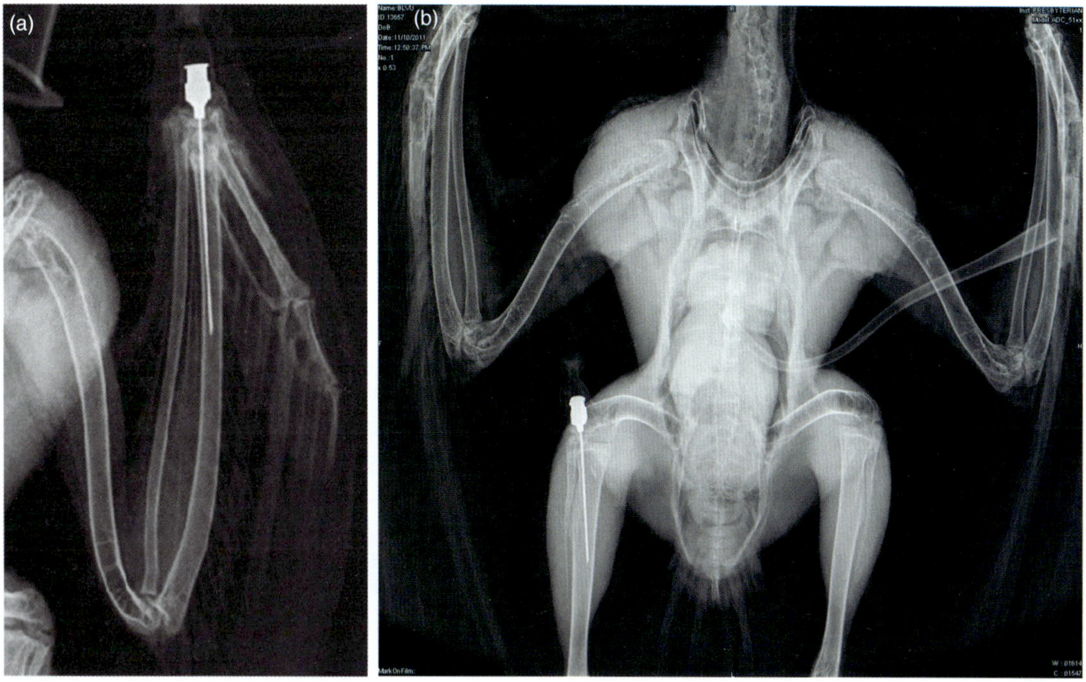

Fig. 4.6. (a) IO catheter placement in the distal ulna. (b) This black vulture has an IO catheter in the right tibiotarsus and an air sac tube placed in the left caudal thoracic air sac.

To place a catheter in the tibiotarsus

Aseptically prepare the stifle joint.

- Flex the joint fully.
- Locate the tibial plateau and drill the spinal needle in as described above. Note that the patellar tendon is a wide band of connective tissue and it is very difficult or impossible to avoid when placing the catheter. The proximal tibiotarsus flares out to form the tibial plateau so be sure to start a few millimeters back from the cranial edge to avoid missing the medullary canal and ending up subcutaneously (Figs 4.6b and 4.8).
- Place an injection port and secure the catheter with a wrap made of gauze, elastic wrap, and tape.

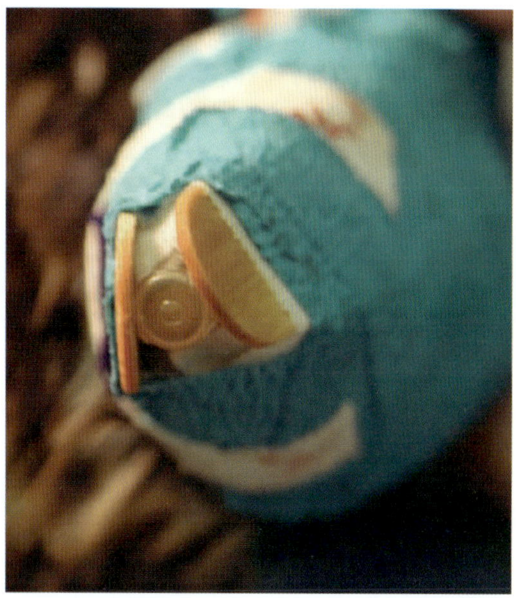

Fig. 4.7. The injection port of the IO catheter can be protected with tongue depressors integrated into the figure-8 wrap.

Note that significant pressure can be generated inside the ulna when administering IO fluids. This pressure is not only painful but can make fluid

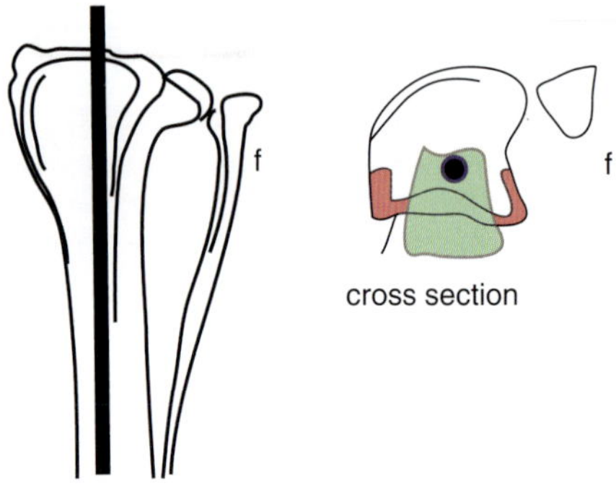

Fig. 4.8. When placing an IO catheter in the tibiotarsus, place the spinal needle (black dot) back from the edge of the tibial plateau to avoid going through the flared bony margin (red). Fibula (f). Patellar tendon (green).

administration difficult. To avoid this, small syringes (5–10 ml) should be used when administering IO fluids. The catheter should be flushed with heparin (see Formulary) only once per day as it is easy to over-heparinize smaller patients. An IO catheter can be maintained for a maximum of 3 days before being removed. If placed carefully, it causes little or no damage and does not seem to cause much discomfort once in place.

Fluid Therapy: What and How Much to Give?

Raptor Tip

Maintenance is 50 ml/kg/day.

Here are some pointers and facts to remember when giving fluids:

- Maintenance requirements = 50 ml/kg/day.
- Replace all fluid deficits over 48 h. If in doubt, assume all sick or debilitated patients are 10% dehydrated for the purposes of the fluid deficit calculation.
- For shock therapy, the maximum IV/IO bolus = 25 ml/kg in a slow bolus (over 1–2 min).
- 30 ml/kg can be easily administered subcutaneously into each leg web.
- Do not give fluids with greater than 2.5% dextrose subcutaneously.

Some recipes for shock therapy:

- Hetastarch 5 ml/kg + crystalloids (LRS, NaCl) 15 ml/kg.
- Crystalloids 10–20 ml/kg over 1 min followed by 90 ml/kg over next 1 h.
- Hypertonic saline 3 ml/kg + hetastarch 3–5 ml/kg slow bolus followed by LRS 10 ml/kg until systolic blood pressure = 90–120 mmHg.
- When giving crystalloids, you can give half the volume as LRS and half as D5W.
- 50% dextrose can be given at 1.0 ml/kg IV *slowly* in cases of hypoglycemia and sepsis. Ideally it should be diluted before administration.

Example 4.1

A 1200 g hawk is 10% dehydrated. What would be a reasonable fluid therapy protocol?

- Maintenance requirements = 1.2 kg × 50 ml/kg/day = 60 ml/day.
- The deficit = 1200 × 10% = 120 ml.

We want to replace the deficit over 48 h so this bird would need 60 + 60 + 120 = 240 ml over the next 2 days. Depending on the bird's condition, a reasonable plan might be 40 ml SQ TID × 2 days. You can also try to replace more of the deficit on the first day.

Blood Collection

You can safely collect blood in a volume equivalent to 1% of the patient's BW (*10 ml/kg*). Luckily, only about 0.3 ml is required to run a complete blood panel on most machines and with most labs. In many cases, a 1 ml syringe with a 25- or 27-gauge needle is sufficient. Once collected, two microhematocrit tubes should be filled and two blood smears should be made. Samples for chemistries should be collected into lithium heparin (green top) Microtainer® vials (Becton, Dickinson and Co., Franklin Lakes, NJ, USA); they require 0.3–0.4 ml of whole blood (Fig. 4.9). Restraint under general anesthesia is helpful but is not necessary in most cases.

Blood can be collected from one of three locations:

1. The jugular vein. The right vein is generally larger in most species. This is the preferred site when large volumes are needed (e.g. for transfusions). This vein can be difficult to stabilize for collection as it is highly mobile. Getting it to fill and "rise up" can be highly dependent on the position of the bird and the way the neck is positioned. The vein is located in a featherless tract and is more dorsal than the typical jugular furrow in a mammal.
2. The basilic vein (Fig. 4.10) crosses the ventral surface of the ulna and radius just distal to the elbow joint. It is easily accessible when the bird is in dorsal recumbency. It is critical to apply pressure following venipuncture to avoid large hematomas. In larger species (>300–400 g) this vein is large enough for most diagnostic blood collection, but it may not be sufficient in smaller birds.
3. The medial metatarsal/caudal tibial vein can also be used. This vein lies on the medial side of the tibiotarsus directly over the hock joint and along the medial side of the tarsometatarsus. This can be very useful in vultures but can be a very difficult vein to access in some birds with heavy feathering (owls) or thick scales (hawks).

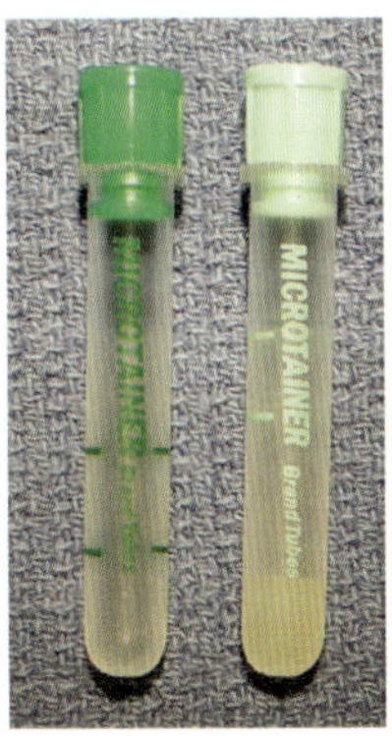

Fig. 4.9. Blood collection vials.

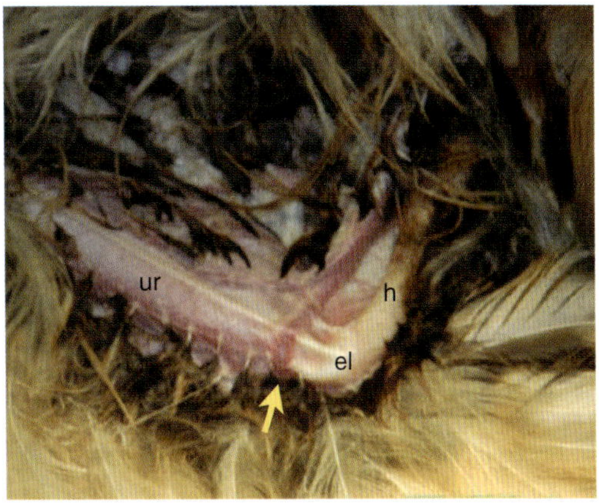

Fig. 4.10. Basilic vein: humerus (h), elbow (el), ulna and radius (ur), basilic vein (arrowhead).

Blood Transfusions

Blood transfusions are indicated in cases of extreme blood loss or in chronic cases where the PCV is below 20%. Conspecific (i.e. same species) transfusions seem to be more effective but it has been reported that blood can be transfused between species if necessary.

> **Example 4.2**
>
> - A 1500 g donor can donate 15 ml of whole blood.
> - A 1100 g recipient has 88 ml blood (assume 8% of BW).
>
> We would like to transfuse 15% of this or 13 ml. So, we preload a 15 ml syringe with 1.95 ml ACD, collect 13 ml blood into it, and transfer it to the recipient through a 20-gauge IO catheter and a blood filter into the distal ulna.

The blood volume of a healthy bird ranges from *6% to 10% of BW or 60–100 ml/kg.* A healthy bird can safely donate around 1% of BW or around 10 ml/kg. The goal of a transfusion is to replace 10–20% of the recipient's blood volume or around 10–20 ml/kg.

Blood should be collected from the donor's jugular vein while the donor is under inhalant anesthesia. Since you will need access to the neck, the donor may need to be intubated. Otherwise, the anesthesia mask will be in the way. Blood should be collected with a 23-gauge butterfly catheter into a syringe preloaded with anticoagulant. The recommended anticoagulant is anticoagulant citrate dextrose (ACD) at a rate of *0.15 ml per ml of blood*. The blood should be kept warm and administered through a blood filter (Hemo-Nate®, Jorgensen Laboratories, Inc., Loveland, CO, USA) and catheter (IV or IO). The donor should receive SQ fluids after donation at a volume of approximately 3 to 4 times the amount donated.

Intramuscular Injections

Intramuscular injections should generally be given in the pectoral muscles while the bird is restrained in dorsal recumbency. The thigh muscles should be avoided since there is risk of traumatizing the sciatic nerve and potentially nephrotoxic drugs may damage the kidneys due to alternate blood flow through the renal portal system.

When giving IM injections it is important that the patient is firmly restrained on its back and the needle is directed parallel to the table top (not perpendicular) in order to avoid injury and deep penetration if the patient jerks.

Air Sac Tube Placement

Air sac tubes can be placed in the caudal air sacs in cases of severe dyspnea (Fig. 4.6b and 4.11). They can also be used temporarily to provide an alternate airway when doing endoscopy of the trachea. Note that air sac tube placement will only be helpful in resolving dyspnea due to upper airway (i.e. trachea or syrinx) obstruction. It will not be useful in cases of primary lung disease, air sacculitis, or any other lower airway problem.

Tubes can be placed on the left or right side and typically enter into the caudal thoracic or abdominal air sac. Flexible red-rubber feeding tubes or endotracheal tubes are often used for this purpose. To place a tube:

- The patient is placed in lateral recumbency.
- The upper leg is pulled back.

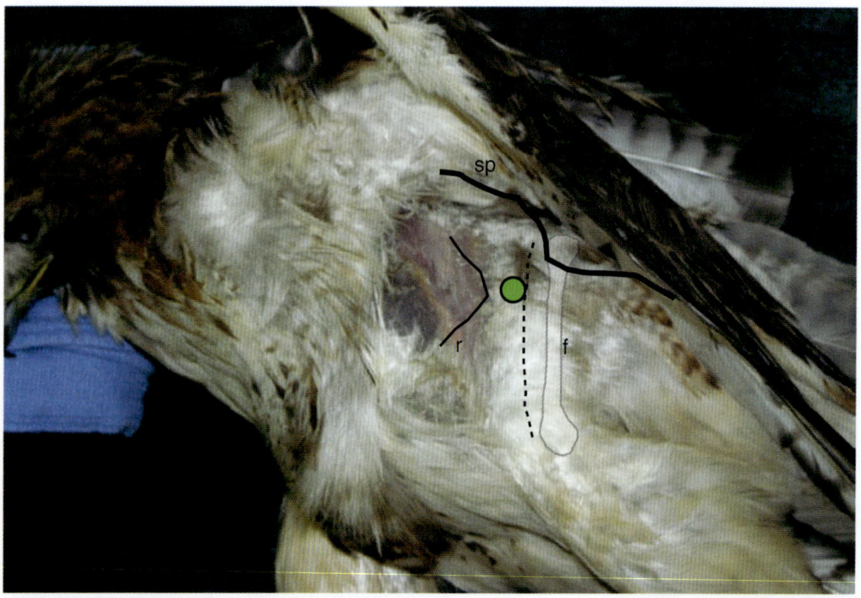

Fig. 4.11. Air sac tube placement. Spine and pelvis (sp), femur (f), last rib (r), cranial extent of thigh (dotted line). The entry point is indicated by the green circle.

- The area caudal to the last rib and cranial to the thigh muscles is aseptically prepared. Note that there may not be time for a full surgical preparation in emergency situations. This area is generally bare, so feathers rarely need to be plucked.
- A small skin incision is made cranial to the thigh muscle approximately one-third of the way between the hip and stifle joints.
- A hemostat is used to bluntly dissect through the body wall. It is important that you brace your hand so the hemostat cannot penetrate too deeply as this can cause serious injury.
- The hemostats are opened and the tube is inserted into the gap between the jaws of the hemostat.
- The airway is tested by holding a downy feather in front of the tube. If properly placed, the feather should move in response to each breath.
- Once properly placed, the tube is secured with tape tabs and sutured to the skin.

If you plan to administer anesthesia via the air sac tube, have an endotracheal tube adapter available in order to connect to the anesthesia machine.

Bandages

Many injuries require some type of bandage to immobilize a limb or protect and cover a wound. In general, elastic wrap (e.g. VetWrap®, 3M, St. Paul, MN, USA) is ideal for avian bandages. In addition, rolled cotton or cast padding may sometimes be necessary below the outer layer.

Figure-8 wrap

The figure-8 wrap is the most commonly needed wrap. It is used to immobilize the wing for any fracture distal to the elbow (ulna, radius, metacarpal) or for injuries to the elbow or carpus. In addition, this type of bandage is used in combination with a body wrap for humeral, coracoid, and clavicle fractures. To place a figure-8 wrap:

- Place the bird in dorsal recumbency.
- Unroll and re-roll the bandage material to ensure it will not be too tight when placed.
- Fold the wing up towards the body in a natural position.
- Place the free end underneath the wing, as high up into the axilla as possible. It is very important to include the long scapular feathers in the wrap since this allows the bandage to be placed as far as possible up into the axilla (Fig. 4.12a).
- Pull it back over the ulna, radius, and metacarpal bone to the dorsal side (Fig. 4.12b).
- Take the roll end and loop it over the ventral side of the metacarpal bones and the ulna and radius, around the patagium to the dorsal side (Fig. 4.12c).
- The bandage should now form an "X" or figure-8 around the wing. Complete the bandage by repeating the process with one more loop (Fig. 4.12d).

For humerus fractures, a body wrap is required, so continue the bandage material from the dorsal side of the wing, across the chest, under the axilla on the opposite side, and back around to the original side. Be sure not to include the scapular feathers on the opposite side when going under the axilla. Pull the legs downward when crossing the chest to ensure a secure fit (Fig. 4.12e). Note that the body wrap should only be tight enough to minimize movement of the wing but not so tight it inhibits respiration. You should be able to easily slide a finger under the body wrap if the wrap is placed correctly.

A few other details and things to watch out for:

- The bandage must be placed well up into the axilla. Otherwise it may slip off past the elbow. It should only cover about ⅔ of the distance down the humerus to the elbow (unless it needs to cover a wound or fracture of the distal humerus).
- The carpal joint should not be over-flexed as this can potentially decrease the blood supply to the distal wing. When over-flexed, the primary and secondary flight feathers will be criss-crossed.
- A well-placed bandage should only require two passes of bandage material.
- An underlayer of rolled cotton gauze (Conform, Kendall/Covidien, Dublin, Republic of

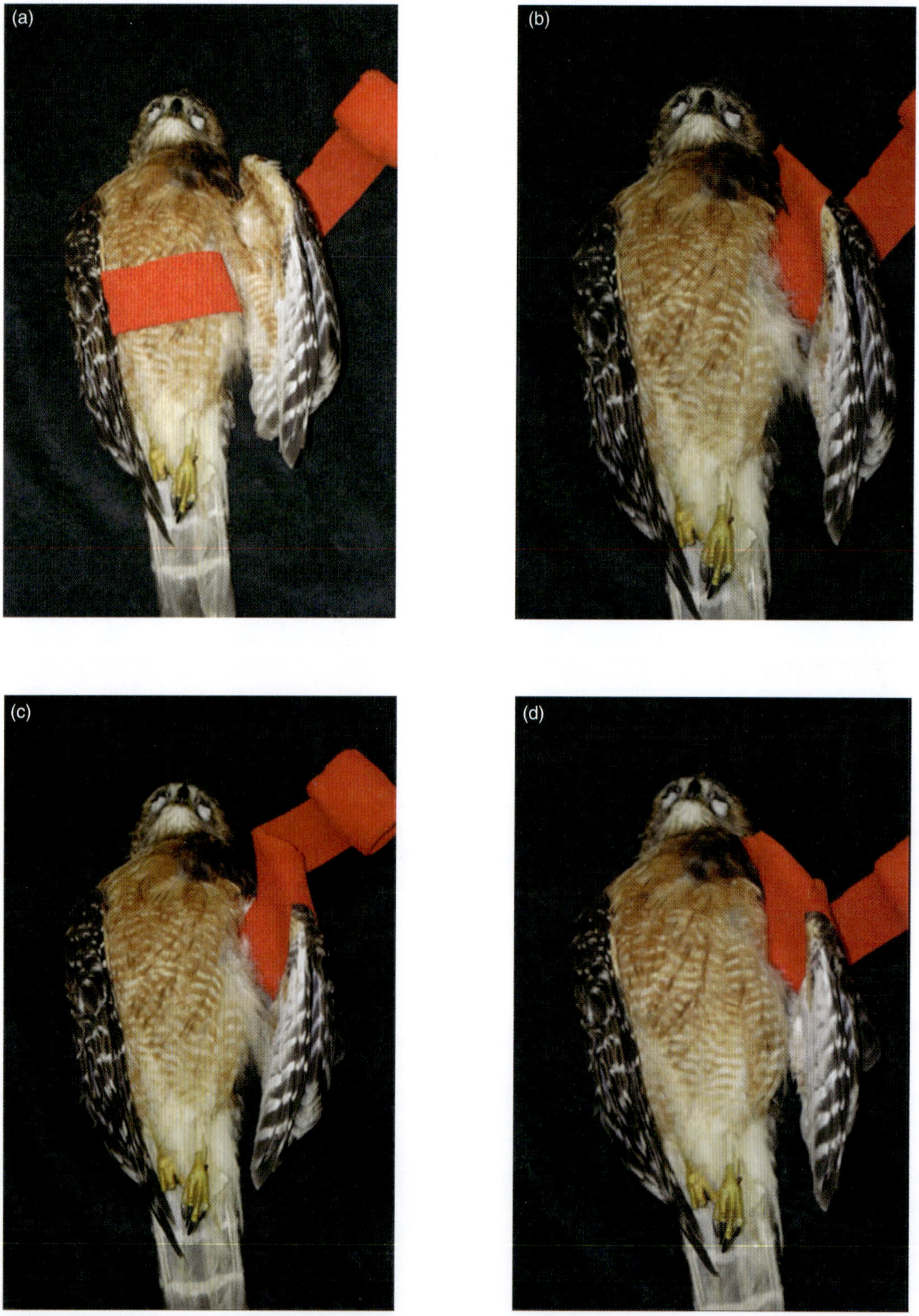

Fig. 4.12. Figure of 8: (a) step 1, (b) step 2, (c) step 3, (d) step 4, (e) step 5.

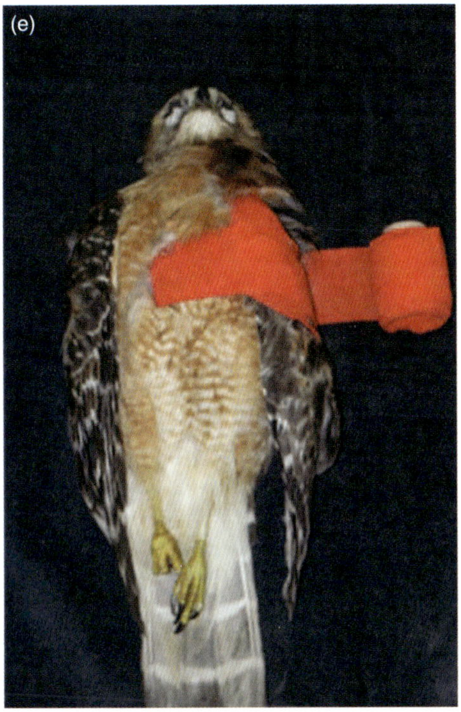

Fig. 4.12. Continued.

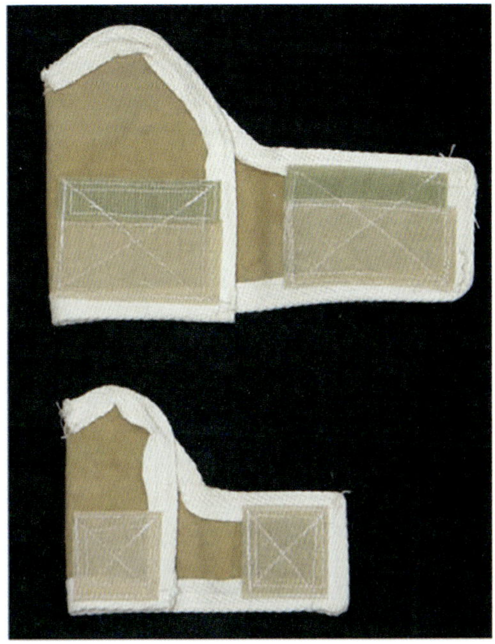

Fig. 4.13. Velcro® wraps.

Ireland) under the elastic wrap can provide additional padding and stabilization.

- Some birds (such as great-horned owls) can be very destructive and the bandages should be reinforced with duct tape.
- Accipiters do not tolerate figure-8 wraps as well as other species. They are often able to slip out of even a well-placed wrap and it is not uncommon to see significant elbow swelling and/or thickening of the patagium when a wrap is in place.
- Reusable and washable wraps made of sturdy canvas material and Velcro® (Velcro® USA Inc., Manchester, NH, USA) (Figs 4.13 and 4.14; Fig. 8.3) can be used instead of a traditional figure-8 wrap. They are easy to place and remove. They are also not as snug and this can be important when bandaging a wing with blood feathers as the Velcro® wrap will allow the feathers to slide and grow underneath. See Appendix D for a pattern that you can use to make your own.

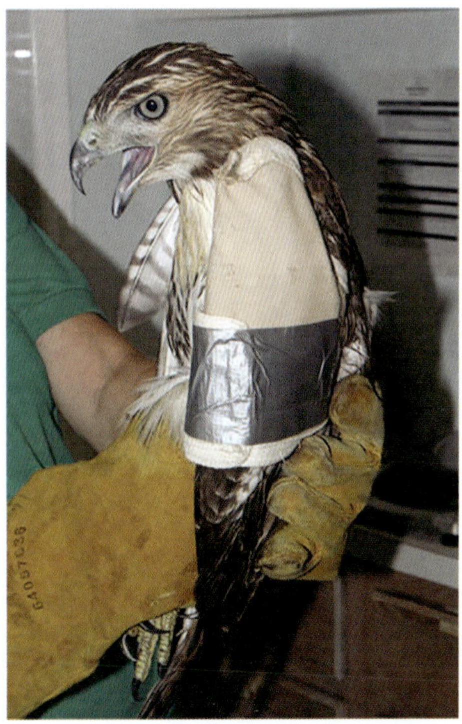

Fig. 4.14. Velcro® wrap in use.

Leg Splint

Most leg fractures require surgical stabilization for the best outcome. However, fractures below the stifle joint should be *temporarily* stabilized with a modified Robert Jones bandage. Any wounds should be cleaned and covered with a non-adherent dressing and cotton cast padding should be applied without creases or wrinkles, since these can lead to pressure sores. The cast padding is then covered with elastic wrap.

For tibiotarsus fractures, the padding should extend above the stifle and well below the hock. Note that most birds have a short femur and a leg web that extends to the stifle, so getting much above the stifle with a bandage can be difficult.

For metatarsal fractures, the padding should extend to the midshaft tibiotarsus and can be incorporated into a foot wrap below the fracture (see below).

If additional stiffness is required, a sidebar of coat hanger wire can be applied on top of the elastic wrap on the lateral and cranial aspects of the leg. Placing wire on the medial aspect can help stiffen the splint but can also lead to abdominal wounds if the proximal end of the wire is not carefully covered. Other materials such as padded tongue depressors or molded thermoplastic also work very well.

Fractures of the femur are very difficult to splint effectively, and surgical repair should be carried out as soon as possible.

Foot Wraps and Shoes

Foot wraps and shoes are very effective for immobilizing fractures of the digits, for treating bumblefoot, and when incorporated into leg splints for fractures of the tarsometatarsus. Temporary wraps made from a ball of gauze and elastic wrap are also useful to spread the toes when radiographs of the digits are required (Fig. 1.8). A shoe is most easily made from a slice of pool "water noodle" (Fig. 4.15). Since it is flat, it provides for much more comfort and balance than a traditional "ball" bandage. The diameter of the foam shoe should be of sufficient size to position the digits such that they are in a natural position and so that the talon tips are not curled underneath. Realize

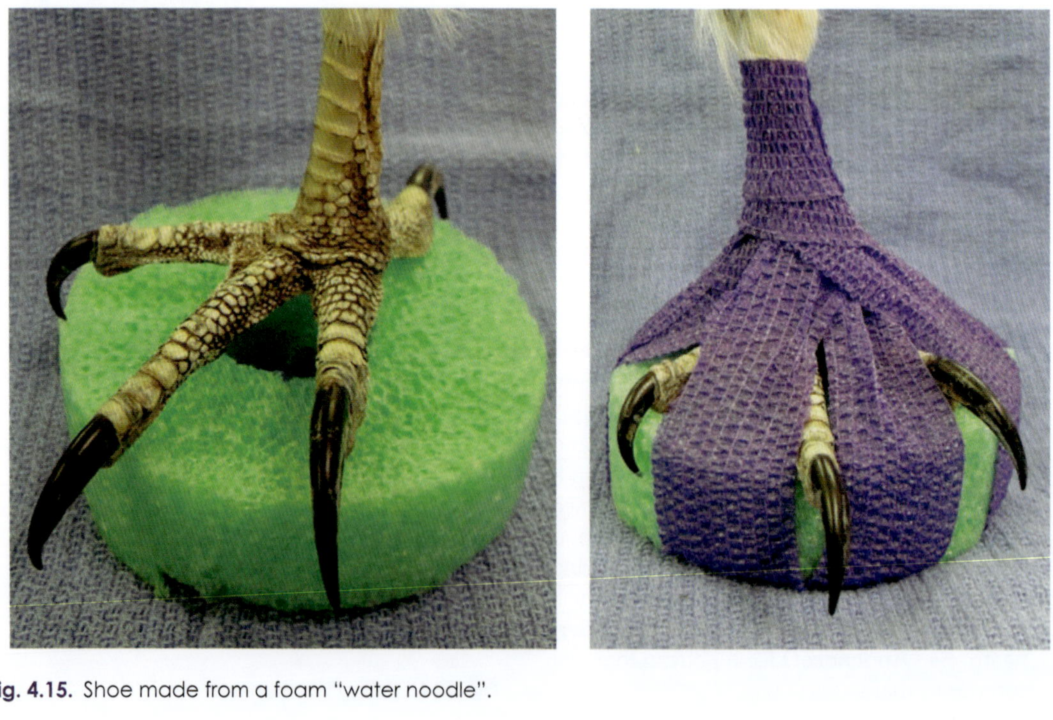

Fig. 4.15. Shoe made from a foam "water noodle".

that the shoe will compress over time, so it is best to make it a bit thicker than needed to compensate for this.

The ball is then secured with 1″ (2.5 cm) elastic wrap wrapped around the ankle. It is best to keep the digits at least partially uncovered so any potential swelling can be quickly identified and treated.

Tail Wrap

Tail wraps are used to prevent damage to the tail feathers. They can be made from many materials, but one easy method uses a manilla folder (Fig. 4.16):

- Cut the manilla folder to fit the tail and round the edges nearest the body to prevent discomfort from rubbing.
- Stiffen the folder with wooden tongue depressors attached with masking tape on the inside.
- Slide the folder over the tail.
- Wrap around the tail and attach it with 2″ (5 cm) wide masking tape to the upper covert feathers and lower downy feathers. Make sure that feathers from the ventral abdomen are not taped down over the vent.
- Cover the tip of the tail wrap with duct tape to make it more waterproof.

These wraps are easy to place and remove and can last up to 2 weeks before needing to be replaced. They should always be replaced if they become soiled or wet.

Carpal Bandages

Carpal bandages are very important for preventing self-inflicted damage to the wrist and are especially helpful in species that are prone to this type of injury such as bald eagles and ospreys. See "Wrist/Carpal Wounds" in Chapter 7.

Temporary Identification Bands

Aluminum identification (ID) bands (National Band and Tag Co., Newport, KY, USA) are used to positively identify each bird. They fit around the tarsometatarsus and can easily be placed and removed (Fig. 4.17).

All species except vultures can be banded. Vultures eliminate on their legs in order to regulate

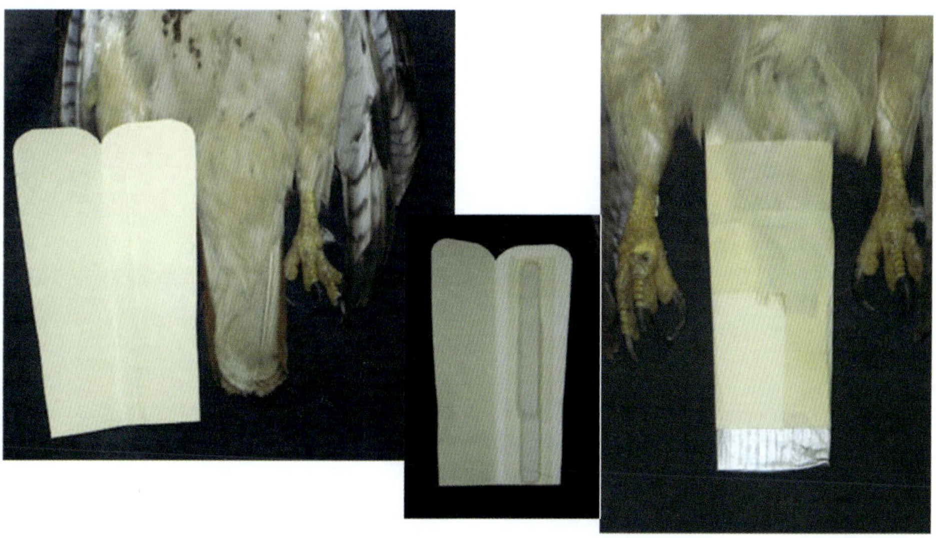

Fig. 4.16. Tail wrap made from a manilla folder.

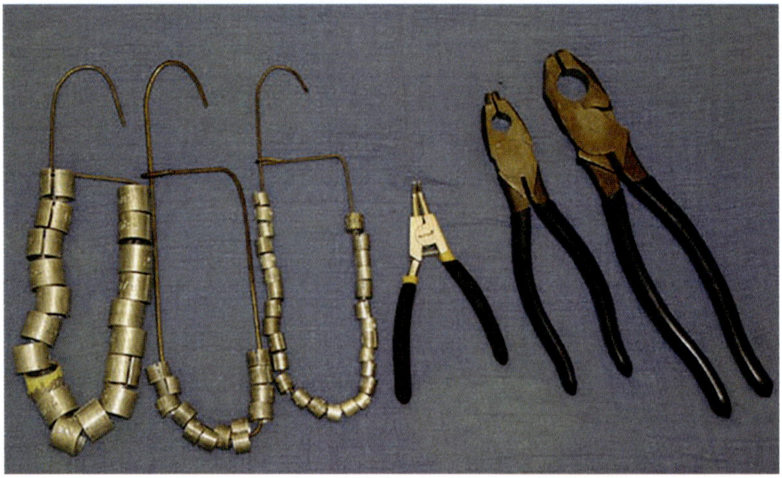

Fig. 4.17. Temporary ID bands in different sizes with spreader and crimper tools.

temperature, so a band would become soiled and this could lead to sores and other complications.

Bands are well tolerated by most birds. However, there will be individuals that will attempt to remove them, leading to severe soft tissue wounds with tendon and bone exposure. Because of this, any signs of inflammation or a wound associated with the band should be immediately addressed and the band should be removed (Fig. 4.18).

Oxygen Chambers

A combination oxygen chamber/intensive care unit is very handy to have for many types of cases. Oftentimes birds are so stressed that even a simple intake exam can prove fatal. In these cases, 30 min in an oxygen chamber can be very helpful (Fig. 4.19). In addition, a chamber that can control heat and humidity is critical in the treatment of emaciation cases.

Euthanasia

Unfortunately, euthanasia is an important part of raptor rehabilitation. Pentobarbital is a humane and

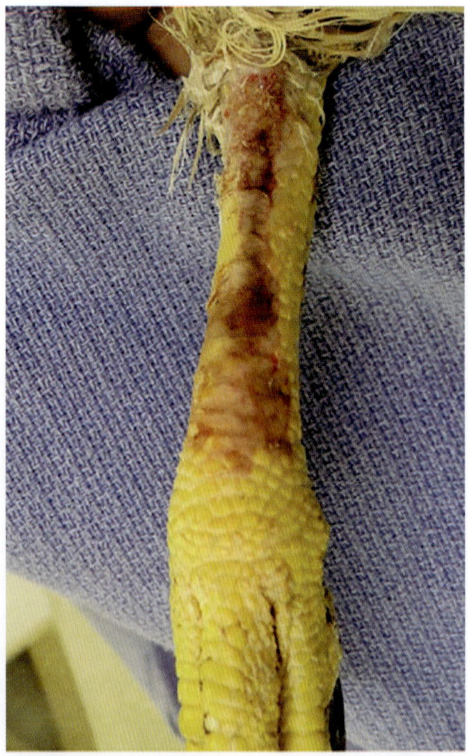

Fig. 4.18. A typical band-induced injury on the tarsometatarsus of a hawk. This is relatively minor, but these wounds can be extremely severe if not discovered in time.

effective method for euthanasia when administered intravenously. For larger birds, the basilic vein or medial metatarsal vein can be used. For smaller birds, an IC injection is often the easiest route (Fig. 4.20). When doing an IC injection, the bird should be fully anesthetized with isoflurane. The needle is introduced on the midline in the clavicular hollow. Gentle suction is applied to the syringe and the needle is slowly advanced towards the heart until a flash of blood is seen and the solution is then injected. It is important to direct the needle parallel to the spine and dorsal to the keel. A 1.5–2.5″ (4–6 cm), 21-gauge needle works best.

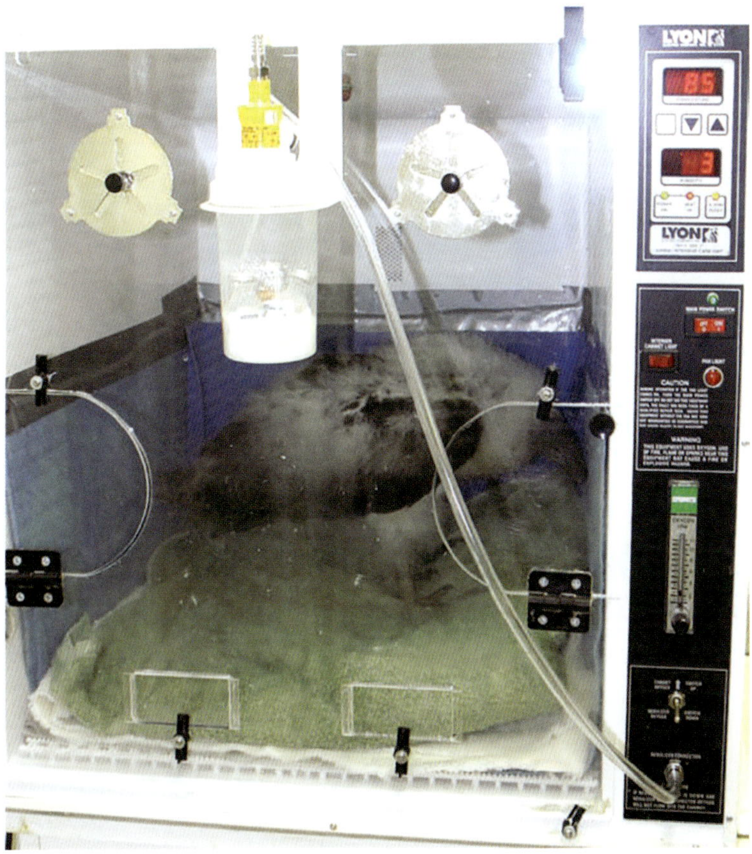

Fig. 4.19. A neonatal vulture with severe dyspnea was stabilized after a short stay in the oxygen chamber.

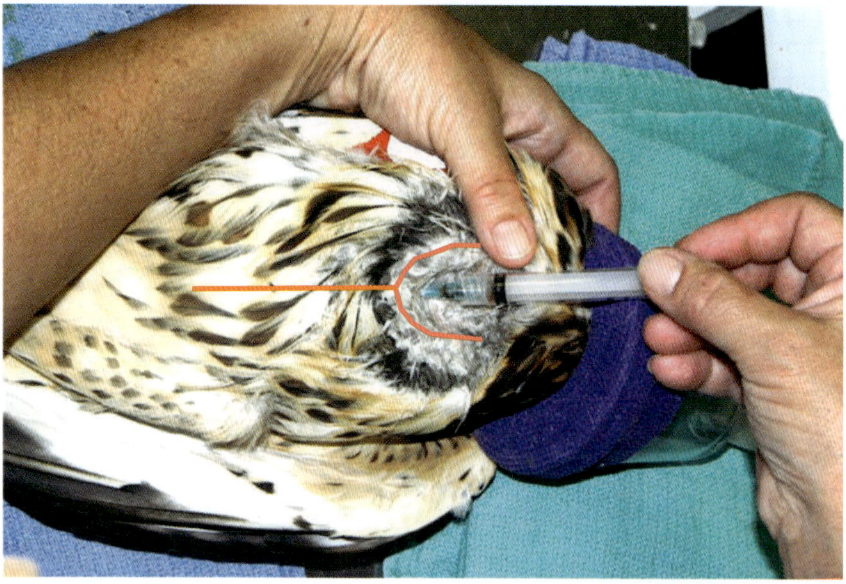

Fig. 4.20. Euthanasia via IC injection. The keel and clavicles are outlined by the orange lines. The needle is directed on the midline parallel to the spine. The head is to the right in an anesthetic cone.

Bibliography

Altman, C. and Dorrestein, Q. (1997) *Avian Medicine and Surgery*. W.B. Saunders Company, Philadelphia, PA, USA.

Bartges, J. and Ritchie, B.W. (1999) Calculating the required volume of nutritional products for birds. *Compendium on Continuing Education for the Practicing Veterinarian* 21(8), 694–695.

Chitty, L. (2008) *BSAVA Manual of Raptors, Pigeons and Passerine Birds*. BSAVA, Gloucester, UK.

Ritchie, B.W., Harrison, G.J. and Harrison, L.R. (1994) *Avian Medicine: Principles and Application*. Wingers Publishing, Inc., Lake Worth, FL, USA.

5 Ophthalmology

A careful examination of the eyes is absolutely required during all intake exams. It is very easy to focus on an obvious fracture, for instance, and miss serious unilateral or bilateral eye damage. Eye trauma is actually very common in birds of prey. At Carolina Raptor Center, 40% of all birds admitted had damage to one or both eyes in the period 2010–2014 (Scott, 2015a) so it is critical that a thorough exam (including the posterior chamber) be done. Bayón *et al.* (2007) is an excellent overview of avian ophthalmology.

It does not take much to do a complete exam. All that is required is a good light source and a direct ophthalmoscope (Fig. 5.1). Induction of mydriasis is rarely needed but can sometimes be induced with general anesthesia if necessary.

Learning Objectives

1. Avian ocular anatomy.
2. Commonly encountered problems.
3. Recognizing damage in the posterior chamber/retina.
4. One-eyed raptors and potential for release.

Anatomy and Physiology

The avian eye is huge in comparison to the rest of the head (Fig. 5.2). The globe has one of three shapes:

- Anterior–posterior flattened: psittacines, pigeons.
- Conical: hawks.
- Tubular: owls.

The eye's shape is maintained by a series of 10–18 scleral ossicles. These ossicles help maintain the shape of the eye while focusing and may also help protect the eye, as the actual socket is quite shallow (Fig. 5.3).

The extraocular muscles are under-developed. Thus, the eye cannot move within the orbit.

The iris contains striated muscle allowing voluntary control of pupil size. This makes evaluation of the pupillary light reflex (PLR) less reliable, and also means that mydriasis cannot be achieved with topical atropine. When a bird is stressed, the PLR can be essentially absent.

There is a complete decussation (crossover) of the optic nerve at the optic chiasm and, therefore, there is no indirect PLR. However, there is a very

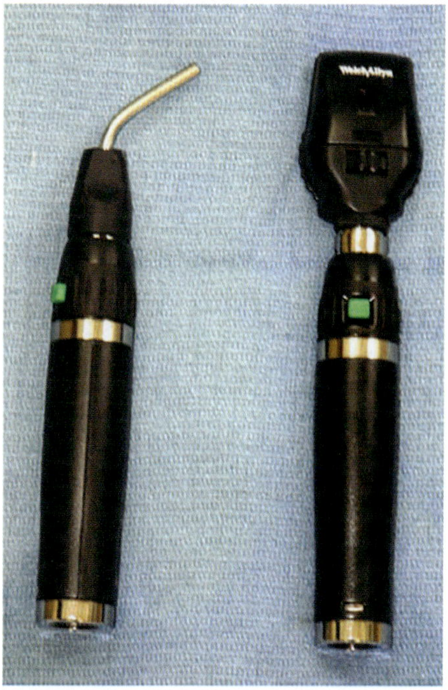

Fig. 5.1. Direct ophthalmoscope and transilluminator.

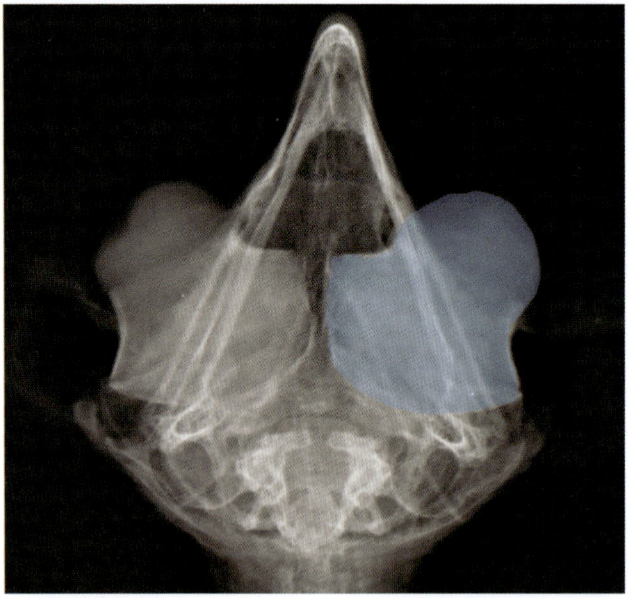

Fig. 5.2. The globes fill most of the space in the head of this barred owl.

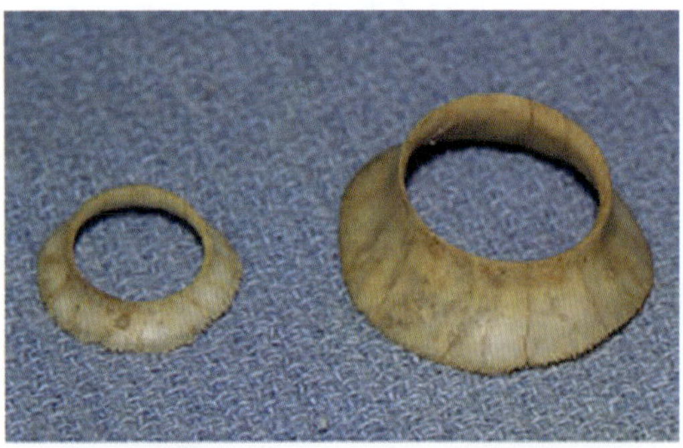

Fig. 5.3. The scleral ossicles from a barn owl (left) and a barred owl (right).

thin bony septum between the eyes, so a bright light shined in one eye may elicit a PLR in the other eye. This may give the appearance of an indirect PLR when, in fact, it is not.

Raptor Tip

Birds have voluntary control of their iris so the PLR can be difficult to evaluate.

As with the PLR, the menace response is also very difficult to assess reliably in birds. Do not consider a bird to be blind based on these simple tests alone.

The lower lid is more mobile, contains a cartilaginous plate in diurnal birds, and covers more of the eye when blinking.

The membrana nictitans is very thin and translucent, and moves from dorsonasal to ventrotemporal. The harderian gland is the major source of tears and is located at the base of the nictitans.

Birds can detect light into the ultraviolet (UV) range and it is believed that they see UV emissions from their prey's urine. Therefore, it seems logical that artificial light in kennel areas should be "full spectrum" and include the UV wavelengths. In addition, the "flicker fusion frequency" in birds is much greater than that of humans (120 versus 18 frames/s) so the light source should also be flicker-free if possible. Note that incandescent bulbs do not flicker, but neither do they provide the UV wavelengths. Conversely, fluorescent bulbs can provide UV wavelengths, but they do flicker. Direct, natural sunlight is always best.

Retina

The retina is avascular and lacks a tapetum lucidum. Avian eyes may contain one, two (diurnal raptors), or no foveas (areas of increased visual acuity). The optic disk is covered by the pecten, a vascular prominence projecting from the underlying choroid. The pecten is responsible for nourishment of the posterior segment and production of intraocular fluid, as well as maintaining physiologic homeostasis. A subtle head and eye "shivering" is considered normal and it is believed that these oscillations shake the pecten and agitate the vitreous fluid (Fig. 5.5).

The retina is unpigmented in owls and the pattern that can be seen during a fundic exam reflects the appearance of underlying choroidal vasculature. In owls, this pattern appears as alternating linear stripes of pink and gray. In hawks, the retina is heavily pigmented and this obscures the choroidal vessels, giving the retina a grayish-pink, ground-glass appearance.

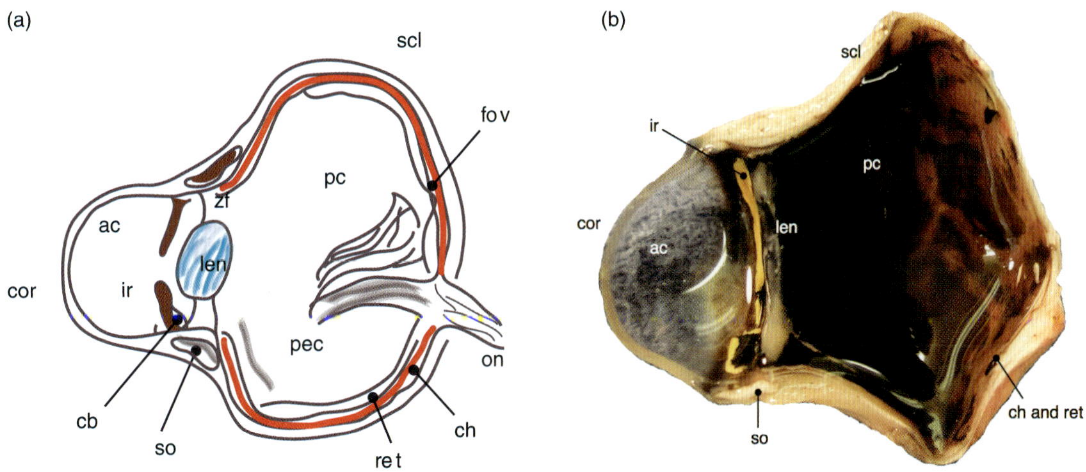

Fig. 5.4. (a) Eye anatomy: cornea (cor), anterior chamber (ac), iris (ir), ciliary body (cb), scleral ossicle (so), lens (len), zonular fibers (zf), posterior chamber (pc), pecten (pec), sclera (scl), fovea (fov), optic nerve (on), choroid (ch), retina (ret). (b) A cross section of an eye from a great-horned owl (*Bubo viginianus*). The tubular structure is clearly evident. The pecten is not visible.

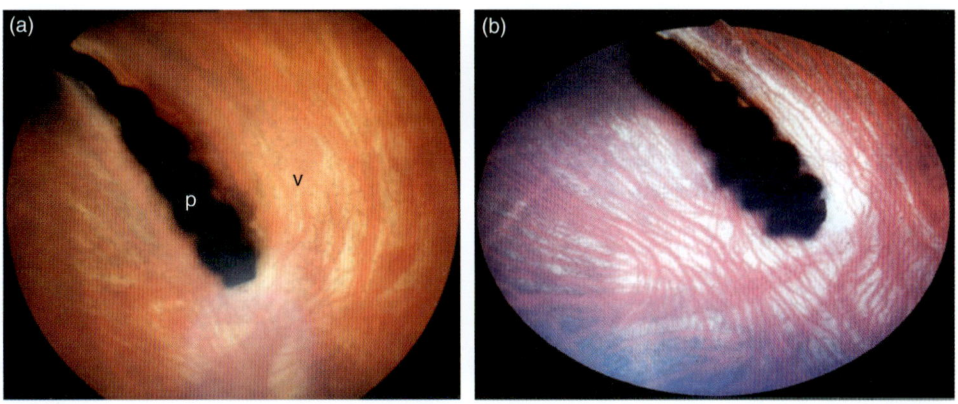

Fig. 5.5. (a) Normal owl retina: pecten (p), choroidal vessels (v). Image from Michelle Hawkins and the University of California-Davis, Veterinary Ophthalmology Service Collection. (b) Another normal retina. Image from Ralph Hamor from the University of Illinois, Comparative Ophthalmology Service.

Common Problems

Keratitis

Corneal ulcers are commonly seen in raptors, and often blepharospasm is the only hint of a problem. Fluorescein stain is used, just as in mammals, to diagnose the condition. Ulcers can be very expansive and cover large areas of the cornea. Topical treatment with triple-antibiotic ointment BID or TID is usually effective and most ulcers heal within 3–4 days (Fig. 5.6). Repeat stain every 3 days until negative. Eyes with ulcers should never be treated with topical corticosteroids.

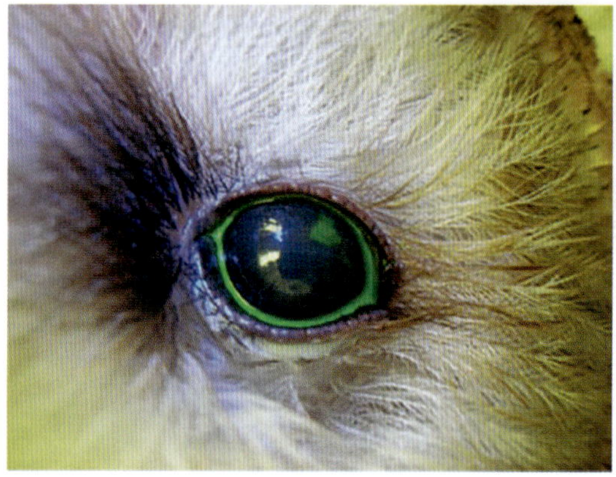

Fig. 5.6. Corneal ulcers are commonly seen in raptors. They are usually superficial and heal rapidly.

Terms

blepharospasm—closure of the eyelids, usually secondary to pain

chorioretinitis—inflammation of the choroid and retina, usually due to trauma or infection

hyphema—blood in the anterior chamber

hypopyon—inflammatory exudate (i.e. pus) in the anterior chamber

keratitis—damage to the cornea, usually from trauma

synechia—attachment of the iris to the cornea or lens

uveitis—inflammation of the iris and adjacent structures in the anterior chamber

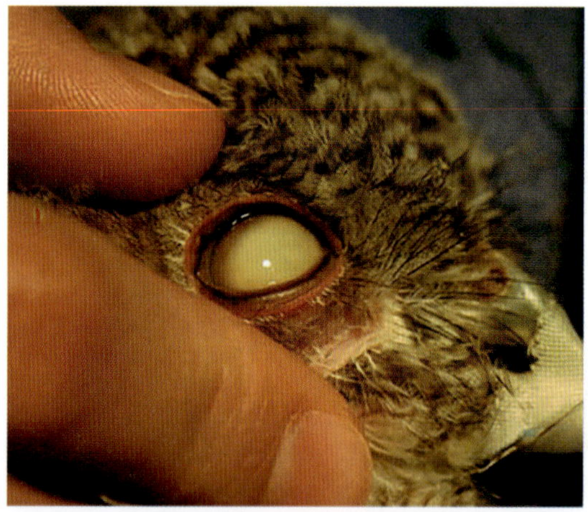

Fig. 5.7. Hypopyon in an eastern screech owl. This required evisceration.

Uveitis

Uveitis is common secondary to trauma. Both anterior and posterior synechias are seen, as are blepharospasm, hypopyon, hyphema, hemorrhage, and luxation of the lens. Low intraocular pressure is also a common sequela to trauma and uveitis. In many cases, the anterior chamber may be completely or partially collapsed, but it is not uncommon for the globe to re-inflate if the damage is not severe. Because of this, it is best to wait before considering anything drastic. Note that an eye may re-inflate and look good for a few weeks, only to collapse again up to 3–4 weeks later (Figs 5.7–5.14).

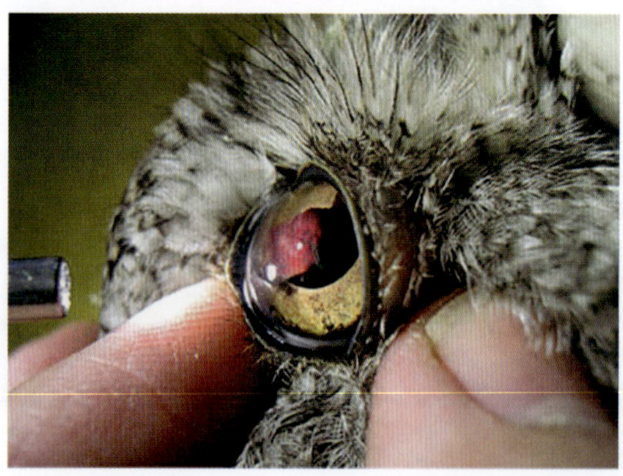

Fig. 5.8. A large, fresh blood clot in the anterior chamber.

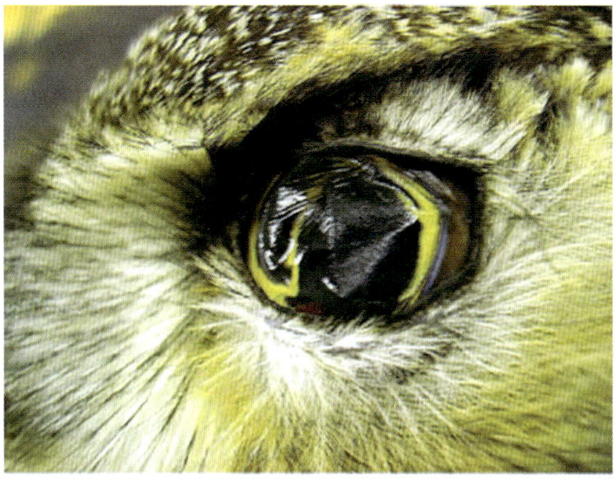

Fig. 5.9. Partially collapsed globe.

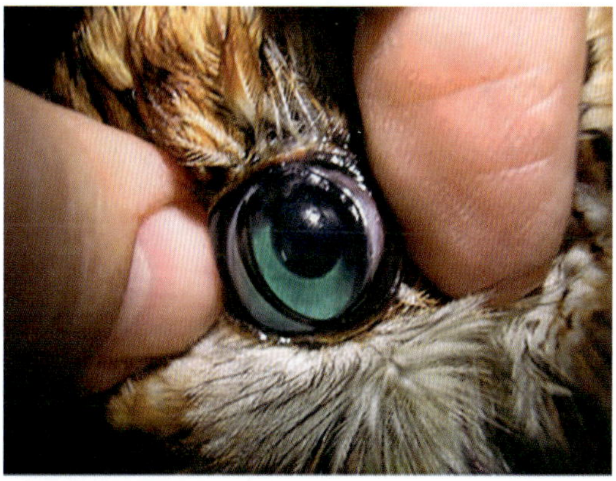

Fig. 5.10. Traumatic uveitis with a resolving hyphema (note the green coloration).

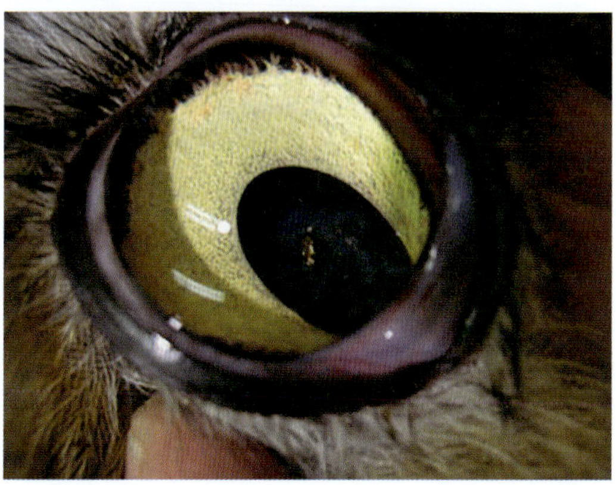

Fig. 5.11. Posterior synechia.

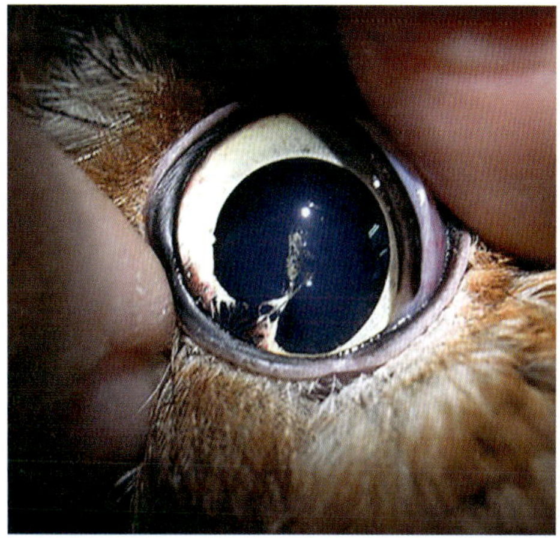

Fig. 5.12. Anterior synechia.

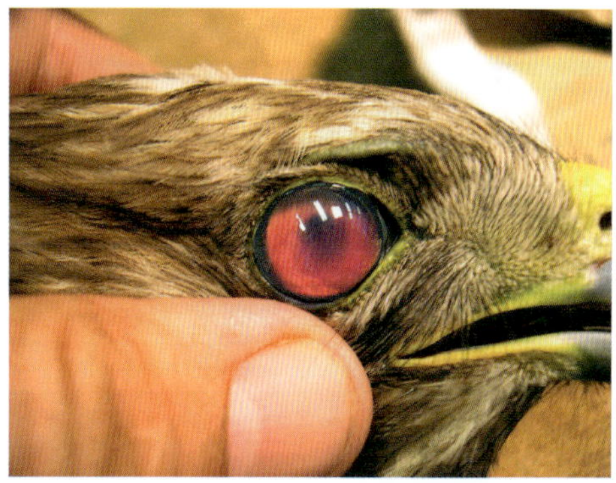

Fig. 5.13. Acute traumatic uveitis and hyphema in a hawk.

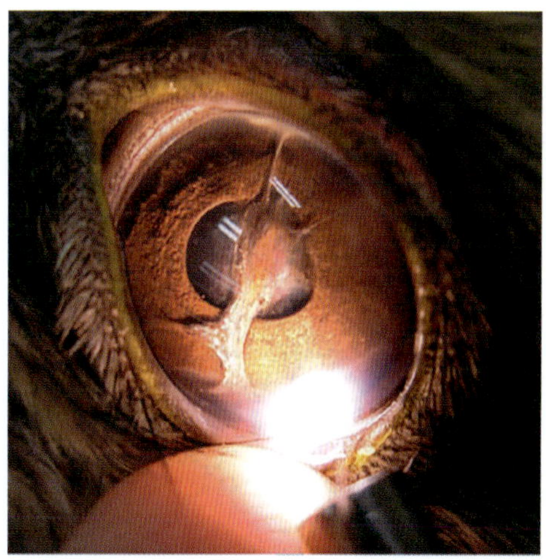

Fig. 5.14. Chronic uveitis with mature fibrin strands stretched across the iris.

Birds do not commonly get primary glaucoma due to the normally wide drainage angle, but glaucoma can result secondary to uveitis. Intraocular pressure can be difficult to measure in small eyes but it can be measured in corneas greater than 9 mm in diameter (Table 5.1). Note that the measurement is highly dependent on the device used.

Treatment for uveitis can include topical corticosteroid (as long as no ulcers are present) or NSAID drops. Remember that mydriasis cannot be achieved with atropine drops.

Table 5.1. Intraocular pressure in healthy birds ([1]Reuter *et al.*, 2011; [2]Bayón *et al.*, 2007; [3]Bayón *et al.*, 2006—using a TonoVet® (Kruuse, Langeskov, Denmark)).

Species	Normal pressure (mmHg)
Psittacines[2]	12–15, 20–25
Birds of prey[2]	11–16
Hawks/diurnals	12–17
Falcons[2]	15–17
Owls/nocturnals	8–12
Small raptors[3]	9
Large raptors[3]	40
Eurasian eagle owl (*Bubo bubo*)	14 ± 2.4
Barn owl[1] (*Tyto alba*)	10.8 ± 3.8
Common buzzard[1] (*Buteo buteo*)	26.9 ± 7.0
Common kestrel[1] (*Falco tinnunculus*)	9.8 ± 2.5
Eurasian sparrowhawk[1] (*Accipiter nisus*)	15.5 ± 2.5
Northern goshawk[1] (*Accipiter gentilis*)	18.3 ± 3.8
Long-eared owl[1] (*Asio otus*)	7.8 ± 3.2
Peregrine falcon[1] (*Falco peregrinus*)	12.7 ± 5.8
Red kite[1] (*Milvus milvus*)	13.0 ± 5.5
Tawny owl[1] (*Strix aluco*)	9.4 ± 4.1
White-tailed sea eagle[1] (*Haliaeetus albicilla*)	26.9 ± 5.8

Cataracts

Cataracts are common and are thought to occur for many reasons including trauma and malnutrition (Fig. 5.15). Vision loss depends on the extent of the cataract and the level of opacity. Phacoemulsification is a realistic option for birds with cataracts.

While actual cataracts do occur in young birds, they must be differentiated from the normal appearance of the juvenile eye, which may appear hazy or cloudy for the first 6–8 weeks.

Lens luxation may also occur secondary to trauma (Fig. 5.16).

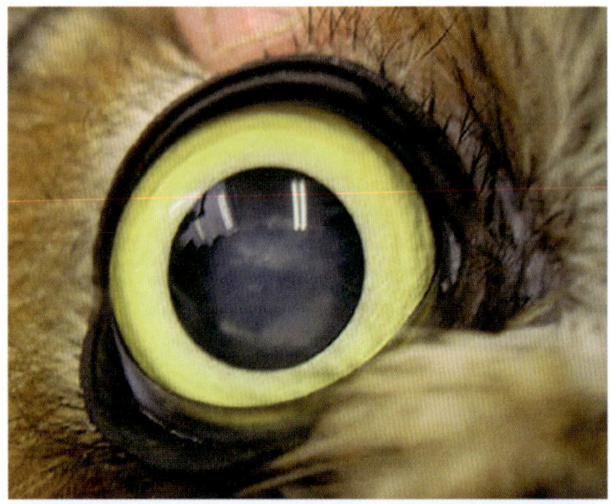

Fig. 5.15. A mature, mostly opaque cataract.

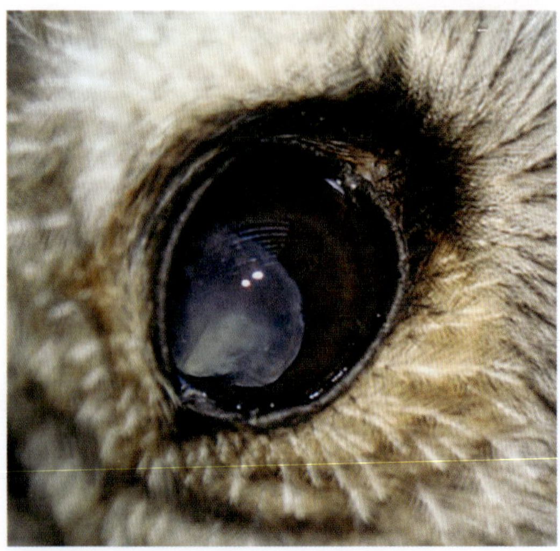

Fig. 5.16. Lens luxation in a barred owl.

Chorioretinitis

Inflammation of the choroid, retina, and pecten is very common as a result of head trauma (Figs 5.17–5.21). Vision loss ranges from minimal to total. There may be a large amount of floating debris and fresh blood obscuring the view of retina. Also, the normal retinal pattern as described above may be replaced by a very chaotic appearing field.

- Retinal detachments typically appear as white, smooth areas with well-demarcated boundaries. They may appear wavy and there may actually be full-thickness tears visible (Figs 5.17–5.19).
- Irregular white patches can also be seen and may result from the sclera showing through tears or defects in the retina and choroid.
- Black craters and irregular blotchy areas are typically the result of old, chronic inflammation and scarring. Smooth circular clusters of craters are often the result of an infectious agent.
- Hemorrhage appears bright red and typically comes from around the base of the pecten.

Treatment for chorioretinitis includes meloxicam and simply giving the eye enough time to heal. A single dose of dexamethasone (2 mg/kg IM) can

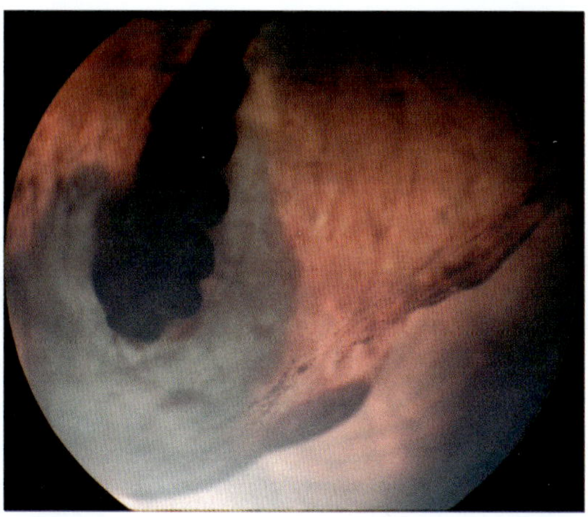

Fig. 5.17. Acute, traumatic chorioretinitis in a nocturnal bird. Note the large gray area of retinal detachment around the base of the pectin and the loss of visibility to the retina due to inflammatory exudate. Compare to Fig. 5.5. Image provided by Michelle Hawkins and the University of California-Davis, Veterinary Ophthalmology Service Collection.

be effective if given within 24 h of the trauma. Actual damage to the retina is unlikely to heal in a functional way. However, if there is a large amount of floating debris and blood that obscures the view of the retina, it is recommended that the patient be given adequate time (2–3 weeks) before any decisions are made. It is often surprising how much floating debris can resolve and be resorbed, especially in diurnal species (Scott, 2015b). Damage to the ventral fundus is less important since the foveas are located dorsally. Frequent fundic exams will allow progress to be gauged and it is important to thoroughly test vision with obstacle courses and live prey before considering release.

Evisceration

Eye trauma severe enough to warrant removal of the eye is common, especially in owls. Consider removal of the eye when the globe is collapsed (and has not re-inflated) or when the eye is clearly non-functional and there is evidence of discomfort or infection. Enucleation is possible but can be difficult and risky in birds. Another option is to simply eviscerate the ocular contents while leaving the sclera and scleral ossicles intact (Fig. 5.22). This procedure is much easier and safer, and maintains the weight and shape of the entire head much better than an enucleation.

To eviscerate an eye:

- Intubate to protect the airway. This is very important as fluids used to flush the surgical site may enter the oral cavity.
- Pluck feathers along the lid margins and surgically prepare the area.
- Make a stab incision through the cornea.
- With iris scissors, remove the entire cornea right at the margin with the sclera.
- Remove the contents of the eye including the lens, iris, and all the posterior chamber contents including the retina and choroid. It is critically important that all the potentially secretory tissue be removed. When complete, you should see the inside of the sclera and it should appear white, shiny, and will often have deep folds or wrinkles.

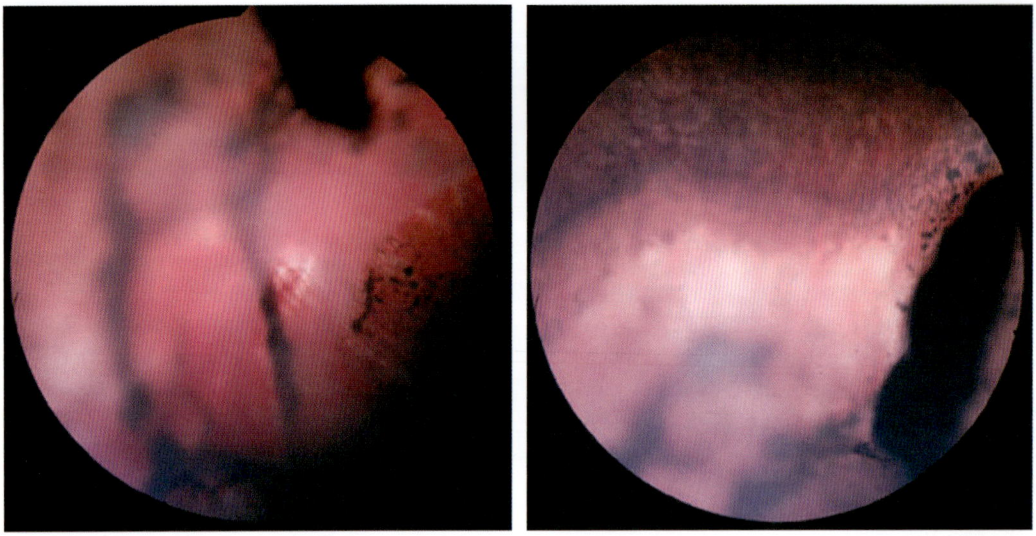

Fig. 5.18. Retinal detachment. The dark, linear streaks are hyperpigmentation of the retinal pigmented epithelium. Image provided by Ralph Hamor from the University of Illinois, Comparative Ophthalmology Service.

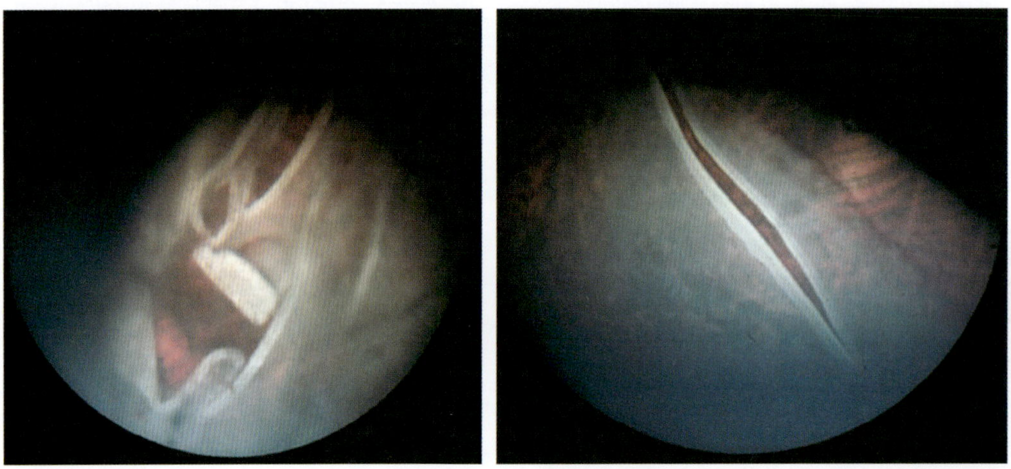

Fig. 5.19. Diffuse retinal detachment with obvious retinal tears. Note that all of the visible retina is elevated and has a white, smooth appearance. Image provided by Ralph Hamor from the University of Illinois, Comparative Ophthalmology Service.

- Flush repeatedly but try to limit the amount of fluid escaping into the oral cavity by packing the area with gauze.
- Pack the globe with gauze to prevent or stop any bleeding.
- With iris scissors, carefully remove the entire nictitans.
- Flush the eye again and pack the globe with one or two absorbable, hemostatic sponge cubes (Vetspon®, Elanco, Greenfield, IN, USA).
- Remove a 1 mm margin from the edges of both lids.
- Close the lids in two layers with 4-O or 5-O Vicryl® (Ethicon, Somerville, NJ, USA).
- The globe itself is not closed in any way.
- Treat with antibiotics, anti-inflammatories, and analgesics.

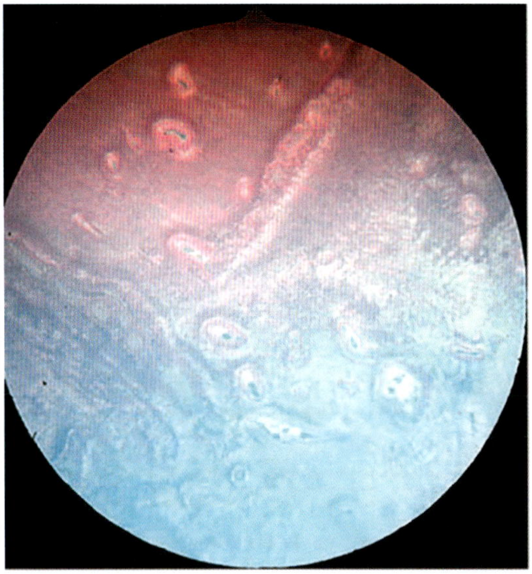

Fig. 5.20. Chronic chorioretinitis. Note the irregular, cratered appearance. Image provided by Ralph Hamor from the University of Illinois, Comparative Ophthalmology Service.

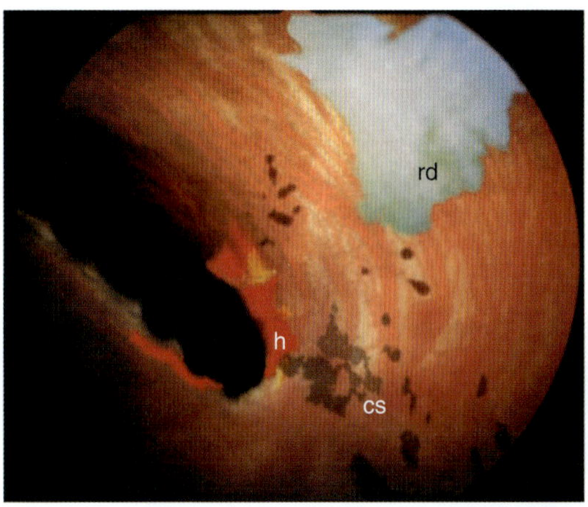

Fig. 5.21. This nocturnal retinal image has been edited to demonstrate some commonly seen traumatic lesions. The red area around the pecten is fresh hemorrhage (h). The dark, irregular craters are chronic scarring (cs) and the white area with the sharp margin is an example of retinal detachment (rd). Note the normal choroidal vascular pattern in the background. Original image provided by Michelle Hawkins and the University of California-Davis, Veterinary Ophthalmology Service Collection.

There may be some initial post-op swelling but there should not be any drainage from the suture line. The socket should start to become concave within 1 week.

Releasing One-eyed Birds

A one-eyed bird is at a major disadvantage so releasing a bird with this condition is not always advisable. However, at Carolina Raptor Center, we do release one-eyed owls after they successfully pass various vision tests. The reasoning behind this is that owls hunt by pouncing on prey from short distances and they rely heavily on hearing to capture prey. In addition, owls do not migrate and generally stay in the same, familiar location year-round. Note that this practice is highly controversial and valid arguments can be made against the release of any raptor with less-than-perfect vision. Recent band return data, however, have shown that one-eyed owls do survive and can do quite well once released (Scott, 2013). *In cases with less-than-perfect vision, the bird should always be released in a remote, rural area, far from the danger of car traffic and busy roads.*

One test utilizes an obstacle course in a flight cage with strips of plastic sheeting hanging from the ceiling. The birds must be able to navigate successfully and consistently around the strips (Fig. 5.23). Although this test is helpful, it can be difficult to interpret as some birds with full vision will fly into the strips when stressed. In addition, some birds will tap them with their wing tips as they learn that they are not dangerous. Because of this, it is helpful to move or change the obstacles periodically so the bird does not simply memorize the course.

Besides the vision strip test, these birds must also pass a live-prey test in which they must maintain their BW for 1 week when provided live prey. These tests are performed in a large flight cage with natural ground covering. See Chapter 12 for more details about live-prey testing.

Diurnal birds of prey such as hawks, falcons, eagles, and osprey, on the other hand, often hunt from high up and rely more on binocular, stereoscopic vision for hunting. In addition, many hawks

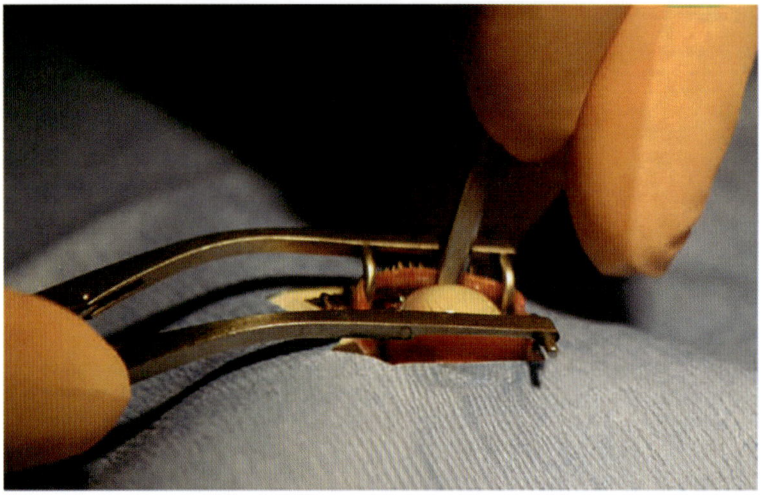

Fig. 5.22. Evisceration procedure. The eyelids are separated with a retractor and a stab incision is made through the cornea.

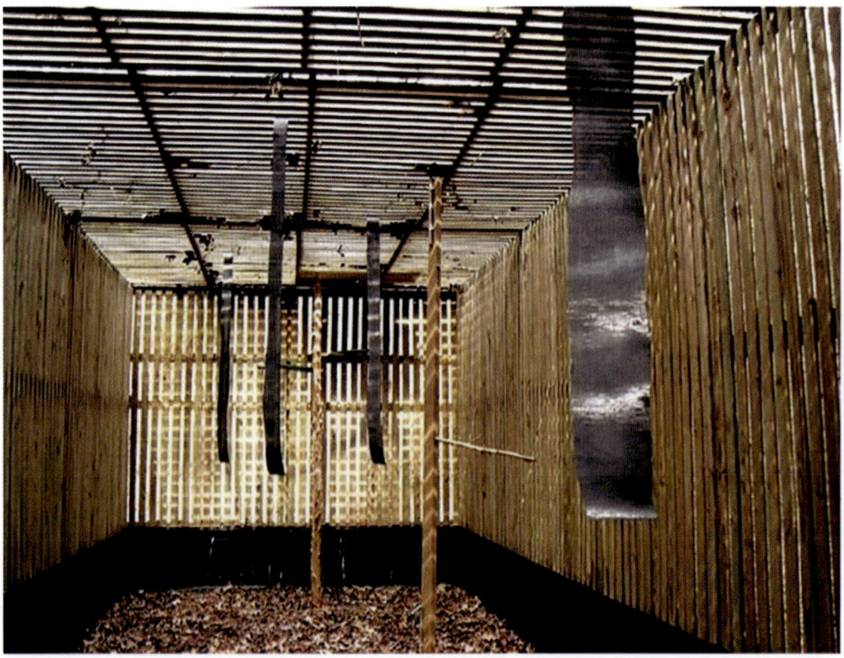

Fig. 5.23. Vision strips.

migrate and will therefore encounter new and unfamiliar territory. For these reasons, it is not advisable to release a one-eyed hawk. The rare exception is when a hawk is admitted with an eye problem that is clearly chronic and is likely unrelated to its current situation. Even in those cases, these birds are always flown and evaluated by an experienced falconer prior to release. In general, hawks with vision loss in an eye should be considered non-releasable.

Bibliography

Bayón, A., Vecino, E., Albert, A., Almela, R.M., Cozzi, A., Talavera, J. and Fernandez del Palacio, M.J. (2006) *Evaluation of intraocular pressure obtained by two tonometers and their correlations with corneal thickness obtained by pachymetry in raptors. Proceedings of the 2006 ESVO-ECVO Meeting, Bruges, Belgium*. European Society of Veterinary Ophthalmology–European College of Veterinary Ophthalmologists, p. 154.

Bayón, A., Almela, R.M. and Talavera, J. (2007) Avian ophthalmology. *EJCAP* 17(3), 253–265.

Meekins, J.M., Stuckey, J.A., Carpenter, J.W., Armbrust, L., Higbie, C. and Rankin, A.J. (2015) Ophthalmic diagnostic tests and ocular findings in a flock of captive American flamingos (*Phoenicopterus ruber ruber*). *Journal of Avian Medicine and Surgery* 29(2), 95–105.

Murphy, C.J. (1987) Raptor ophthalmology. *Compendium on Continuing Education for the Practicing Veterinarian* 9, 241–260.

Reuter, A., Müller, K., Arndt, G. and Eule, J.C. (2011) Reference intervals for intraocular pressure measured by rebound tonometry in ten raptor species and factors affecting the intraocular pressure. *Journal of Avian Medicine and Surgery* 25(3), 165–172.

Scott, D. (2013) A retrospective look at the survival of birds of prey released from a rehabilitation center in North Carolina. *Proceedings of the 2013 Association of Avian Veterinarians Annual Conference, Jacksonville, FL, USA*. Association of Avian Veterinarians, Teaneck, NJ, USA, p. 359.

Scott, D. (2015a) Medical records in RaptorMed™ database. Carolina Raptor Center, Huntersville, NC, USA.

Scott, D. (2015b) A retrospective look at outcomes of raptors with ocular trauma. *Proceedings of the 2015 Association of Avian Veterinarians Annual Conference, San Antonio, TX, USA*. Association of Avian Veterinarians, Teaneck, NJ, USA, p. 103.

6 Infectious Diseases

Symbol key	
Zoonotic	z
Contagious	c
Reportable	r

There are several infectious diseases that affect raptors. Some are easy to recognize but others can be very difficult and expensive to diagnose definitively. Aspergillosis is probably the most important infectious disease affecting birds of prey and should almost always be on your differential diagnosis list until ruled out.

Learning Objectives

1. Diagnosis and treatment of Aspergillosis.
2. The clinical signs commonly seen with each infectious agent.
3. How to diagnose or rule out various diseases.

Aspergillosis

Etiology: *Aspergillus fumigatus*

This fungal organism is:

- Ubiquitous. It is everywhere in the environment and there is constant exposure. This is usually not a problem in a healthy animal but can be a major issue in certain circumstances.
- Saprophytic. It grows in decaying organic matter. It is very important to avoid organic bedding such as mulch, straw, or leaves in enclosures housing raptors.
- Opportunistic. The organism flourishes in a host with a compromised immune system (stress, injury, other illness, prolonged antibiotic use) or in an animal excessively exposed (poor ventilation, improper bedding). In addition, some species such as goshawks, gyrfalcons, rough-legged hawks and, especially, young red-tailed hawks, seem to be highly susceptible.
- Not contagious between animals, so isolation protocols do not need to be followed.
- Not zoonotic. However, special care should be taken when doing necropsies as there can be a dangerous exposure when examining the air sacs of a heavily infected bird (Fig. 6.1a).

Clinical signs

- Chronic form: this is the most common and is usually secondary to immunosuppression or an otherwise weakened state. Depression and emaciation are common presenting signs. Anorexia and regurgitation are also common. Surprisingly, respiratory signs are not typically seen until very late in the disease. Prognosis is generally poor as massive granulomas and fungal masses are usually present in the air sacs and lungs.
- Acute form: this occurs after a massive inhalation of spores and results in multiple, miliary nodules in the lungs and air sacs. This is a rare clinical presentation and the prognosis is very poor.
- Tracheal form: this results when a granuloma forms in the lumen of the trachea or in the syrinx (Fig. 6.1b). Typical signs include dyspnea and a change or loss of voice. This form can progress alarmingly fast and can become

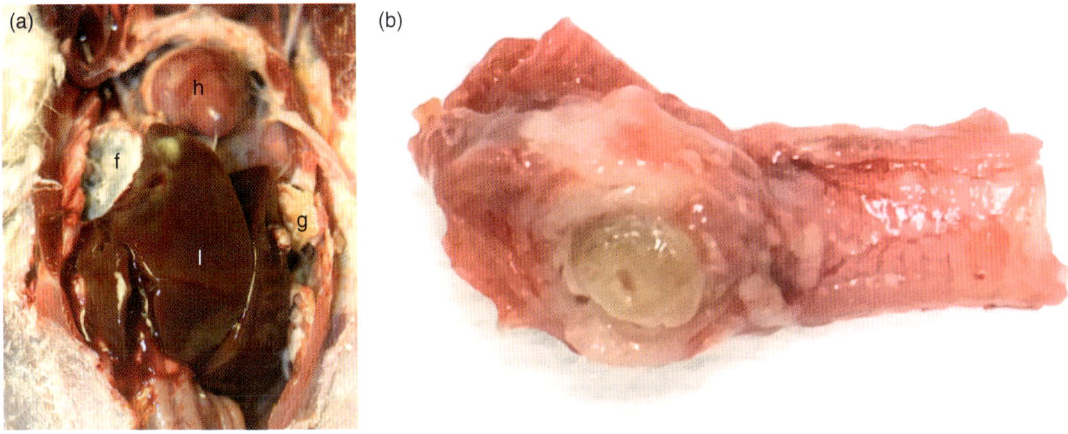

Fig. 6.1. (a) Necropsy of bird with severe Aspergillosis infection: heart (h), liver (l), fungal plaque (f), granuloma filling the left thoracic air sac (g). The syrinx is completely obstructed by a granuloma in (b).

an emergency requiring the placement of an air sac tube. This form is rarely seen in wildlife and it is presumed that they die acutely and do not make it to a rehab facility.

Diagnosis

Diagnosis can be difficult and includes multiple methodologies:

- CBC. A leukocytosis with a toxic heterophilia and monocytosis is common in the systemic form, but rare in the tracheal form.
- As with many inflammatory conditions in birds, an elevation in TS/TP may be a good indication of infection.
- Radiographs may show masses or opacities in the lungs and/or air sacs in advanced cases (Fig. 6.2). Prognosis is very poor if there is radiographic evidence of the disease. May also see hyper-inflated air sacs secondary to obstruction of outflow.
- Cytology of active fungal lesions will show the classic fungal conidiophore when stained with lactophenol cotton blue (Fig. 6.3).
- Tracheal culture directly from a lesion may be useful but can take 36 h for results. Also, since this organism is ubiquitous, false positives are common.
- Serology (ELISA Ab + galactomannan Ag + EPH) is available but may not be useful due to questionable sensitivity and specificity, as well as the cost.

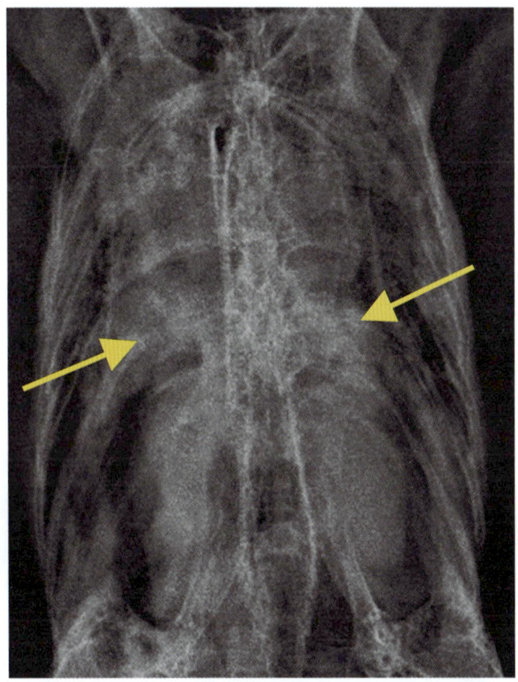

Fig. 6.2. Radiograph of bird in Fig. 6.1. The arrows are pointing to large fungal masses and, overall, there is a massive increase in air sacs' opacity. Compare to Fig. 2.7 left.

- Endoscopy is the gold standard as it is quick and can be the most cost effective.

Lesions as shown in Figs 6.4 and 6.5 are commonly seen.

Treatment

Do not wait for all your lab results before starting treatment. It is best to start treating if the index of suspicion is high, even if you do not have a definitive diagnosis.

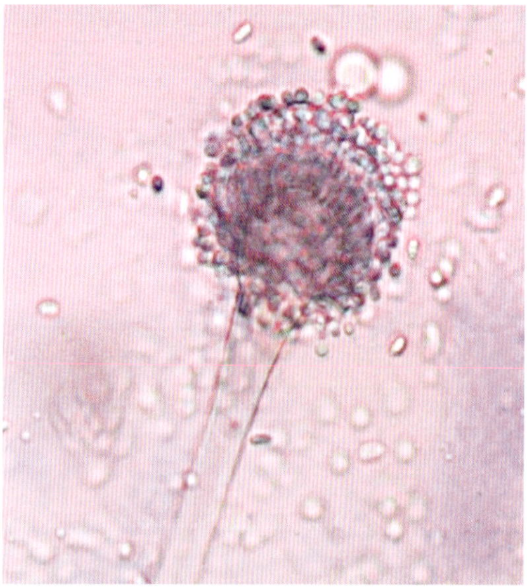

Fig. 6.3. Microscopic view of *Aspergillus fumigatus* stained with lactophenol cotton blue.

The acute form with obstruction of the syrinx or trachea is a true emergency and an air sac tube should be placed immediately. Once the bird is stabilized, you can attempt to alleviate the obstruction by physically removing the granuloma (via endoscopy or directly through a tracheotomy). Topical treatments of lesions with antifungals such as amphotericin B can also be tried.

> **Raptor Tip**
>
> Emaciation and depression are the most common clinical signs in Aspergillosis cases.

Treatment for the chronic form can be complicated, expensive, and often unrewarding as the patient's overall condition can be very poor at the time of diagnosis. In addition, clinical improvement can be obtained, only to have the disease recur.

However, treatment can be successful and should be attempted if possible. Voriconazole, a relatively new antifungal, has become the treatment of choice (12.5 mg/kg PO BID × 21 days). It is

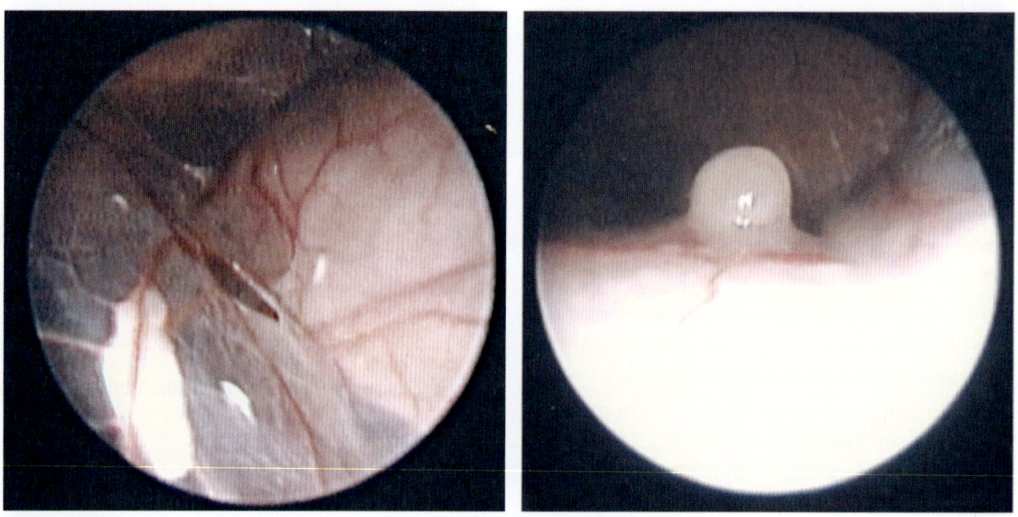

Fig. 6.4. Endoscopic views of Aspergillosis lesions on the air sacs (a, b).

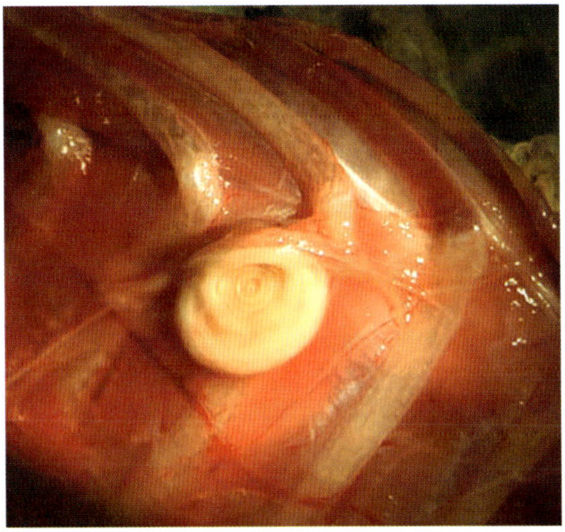

Fig. 6.5. A classic "bulls-eye" fungal lesion on the surface of an air sac. These can be seen during necropsy or endoscopically.

somewhat expensive but is safe, can be very effective, and is simple to administer. Depending on the severity of the case, supportive care and careful patient monitoring may still be required in many cases. Nebulization may also still be helpful.

Before voriconazole was available, protocols using amphotericin B were commonly used. Success rates varied and the treatment was resource-intensive and stressful to the patient. A typical protocol was as follows:

- Supportive care with fluids, force-feeding, tube-feeding, etc.
- Metoclopramide or other anti-emetics as needed for regurgitation.
- Amphotericin B: 1.5 mg/kg via IV or IO catheter TID × 3 days. The drug should be diluted in 15 ml/kg of D5W and administered as a slow bolus since it is potentially nephrotoxic.
- Nebulize TID for 20 min with saline, clotrimazole, or F10® (Health & Hygiene, Gauteng, South Africa).

> **Raptor Tip**
>
> Itraconazole alone is not an effective treatment for Aspergillosis.

Other treatment considerations include:

- After resolution of clinical signs, prolonged treatment with an oral antifungal such as itraconazole or terbinafine should be considered. Note: studies have shown that compounded itraconazole has very poor bioavailability. Therefore, only the name-brand Sporonox® (Ortho Biotech, Raritan, NJ, USA) oral suspension should be used. Treatment should be continued for 2–3 months (if possible) beyond resolution of clinical signs and normalization of white counts. Note that itraconazole can have side effects including hepatotoxicity. Therefore, serum biochemistries should be run periodically to check for this and the drug should be discontinued if the bird becomes anorexic or starts to regurgitate.
- Treat potential secondary bacterial infections with broad-spectrum antibiotics.
- Monitor progress with serial CBCs. The total white count, the monocyte count, and TS/TP can often be good indicators of the disease state.
- Surgical debulking of large lesions has been described and can sometimes be achieved endoscopically.
- Topical treatment of lesions with amphotericin B can also be accomplished endoscopically.
- Terbinafine is an inexpensive, antifungal drug that has also shown to have promise. It is fungicidal so may have potential benefits when used alone or in combination with the other drugs. In this author's experience, it is much more effective and much less expensive than itraconazole.

Prevention

This is one disease that is better to avoid than to treat. You can go a long way by simply avoiding the risk factors mentioned above.

To address the risk factors:

- Birds should be housed in well-ventilated enclosures with non-organic bedding (smooth pea gravel works very well).
- Birds should be kept in good health and on a good diet.

- Birds should be removed from an enclosure before it is cleaned due to the risk of inhaling fungal spores.
- Patient stress should be kept to a minimum. Therefore, treatment protocols should be tailored to minimize the number of times a bird must be handled.
- Patients at high risk (young red-tailed hawks, for instance) should be treated prophylactically on admission with itraconazole or terbinafine for 21 days. This includes any captive birds that are going to be undergoing a stressful change such as a relocation or a major change in their daily life.

Avian Influenza (AI)

z c r

Etiology: Influenza type A orthomyxovirus

Migratory birds, especially waterfowl and poultry, can act as a reservoir but can also become clinically ill after infection. The virus is spread by aerosolization of respiratory secretions, fecal material, and by ingestion of infected waterfowl and poultry. Several strains of highly pathogenic avian influenza (HPAI) have been identified that are related to the Asian bird flu isolated in China in 2005 (Krautwald-Junghanns *et al.*, 2008). A particularly severe outbreak occurred in the USA in 2015 and the primary wildlife vector was determined to be a species of duck. This disease is potentially zoonotic, contagious, and can have devastating consequences for local populations and the poultry industry. Kelly *et al.* (2008) provide a good review of HPAI pathogenesis, prevention, and control.

Clinical signs

- These vary widely depending on the virulence of the particular strain and can range from anorexia, depression, respiratory signs, diarrhea, and neurologic signs to sudden death.

Diagnosis

- Virus isolation or PCR from cloacal or choanal swabs.
- Serology.

Treatment

- Supportive but not recommended. Consult your local regulatory agencies for guidance.
- Antivirals such as Tamiflu® (Genentech, South San Francisco, CA, USA) can be considered but their use is controversial due to the potential for the development of resistance.
- Strict isolation. Euthanasia may be required by local health regulations.

Prevention

- Strict biosecurity and quarantine procedures should be followed. The virus is destroyed by sunlight and by most disinfectants and detergents.
- Avoid waterfowl and poultry.
- Vaccination in raptors has been described (Lierz *et al.*, 2007; Samour *et al.*, 2007).

Avian Vacuolar Myelinopathy (AVM)

Etiology: unknown

This is a neurologic disease that affects water birds as well as raptors, including the bald eagle. It is believed to be caused by a toxin produced by a cyanobacterium (a blue-green alga). This bacterium grows well on aquatic plants such as *Hydrilla verticillata*. Eagles become affected after consuming water birds, especially coots, which have fed on this plant. It has only been reported in the south-eastern USA and has a peak in November and December.

Clinical signs

- Incoordination, ataxia, weakness.

Diagnosis

- AVM must be differentiated from other causes of neurologic disease (see Raptor Tip for a list).
- Histopathology of the brain and spinal cord. There is no definitive ante-mortem diagnostic test.

Treatment

- Supportive care, but prognosis is very poor. Euthanasia is probably the best choice.

Prevention

- Not possible.

Blood Parasites

Etiology: *Hemoproteus* spp., *Leukocytozoon* spp., and *Plasmodium* spp.

These protozoans are obligate intracellular parasites. *Hemoproteus* (Fig. 6.6) is spread by the hippoboscid "flat fly" (Fig. 6.7); *Plasmodium* (the cause of malaria) by mosquitoes (Fig. 6.8); and *Leukocytozoon* (Fig. 6.9) by black flies or mosquitoes. Note that mixed infections are not uncommon.

Clinical signs

- *Hemoproteus* and *Leukocytozoon* are found relatively commonly but clinical disease is thought to be rare. If present, clinical signs may include weight loss and lethargy. Mixed infections are thought to be more pathogenic.
- *Plasmodium*, on the other hand, can produce serious disease ranging from mild depression and anemia to severe dyspnea and sudden death. Massive hemolysis is possible, resulting in jade-green urates.

Diagnosis

These parasites are easily detected on a blood smear. *Leukocytozoon* is unmistakable, but *Plasmodium* and *Hemoproteus* can be difficult to differentiate.

- In general, *Hemoproteus* gametocytes will wrap around the RBC nucleus without displacing it (Fig. 6.6).
- *Plasmodium* gametocytes, on the other hand, may displace the nucleus from the center of the cell (Fig. 6.8). In addition, *Plasmodium* can infect thrombocytes and WBCs,

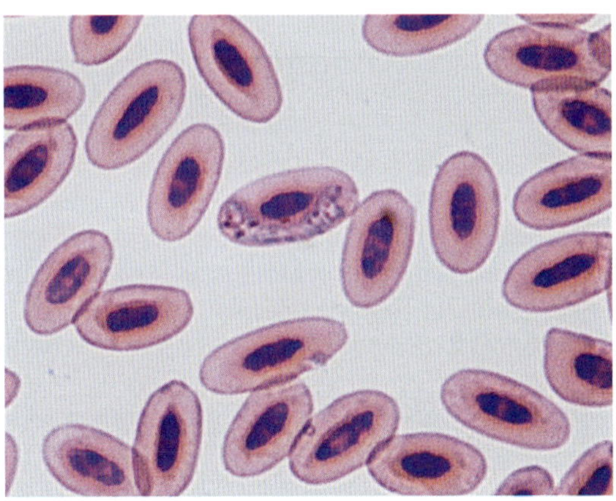

Fig. 6.6. *Hemoproteus.*

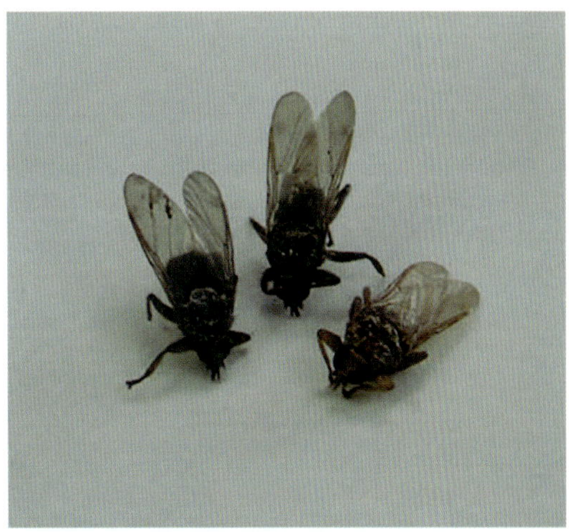

Fig. 6.7. Hippoboscid flies.

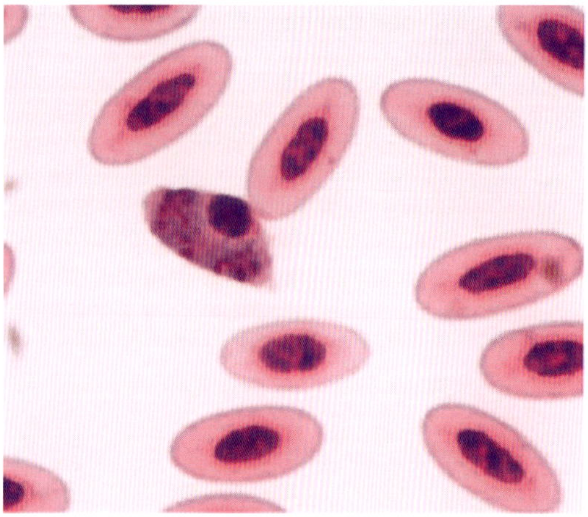

Fig. 6.8. *Plasmodium*.

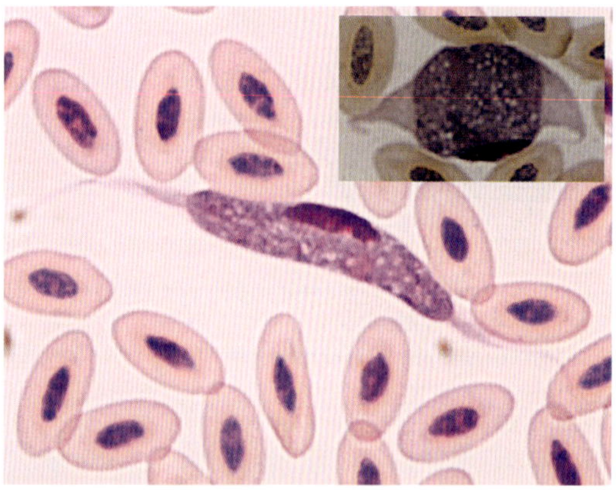

Fig. 6.9. *Leukocytozoon*. Different species can have a markedly different morphology and shape (inset).

and schizonts may also be present in peripheral blood.

- Splenomegaly with a black discoloration is strongly suggestive of a *Plasmodium* infection.

Treatment

- Supportive care. Treatment is generally not warranted or effective for *Hemoproteus* and *Leukocytozoon*.
- *Plasmodium* infections are treated with oxygen therapy or transfusions as needed, and mefloquine (the chloroquine/primaquine combination) no longer appears to be effective.

Prevention

- Insect control with mosquito netting is effective.
- Weekly prophylactic treatment for malaria during the high-risk season can also be helpful.

Candida

Etiology: *Candida albicans*

This organism may be found in low numbers in the crop and feces of a healthy bird. It is considered opportunistic and will cause disease when a predisposing factor such as immunosuppression is present, or when long-term antibiotics are in use.

Clinical signs

- Caseous lesions in the mouth and crop can form.
- *Candida* infections can cause pseudomembranous necrosis of the oral cavity and a marked thickening of the crop wall.
- Dysphagia and “food flicking”, along with secondary weight loss, are common. Systemic spread is also reported but is rare.
- This disease can be confused with lesions produced by *Capillaria*, *Trichomonas*, or possibly the wet (diphtheritic) form of avian pox.

Diagnosis

- Crop swab cytology. With a Gram stain, you will see budding yeast and possibly hyphae. It is important to see budding yeast, as an occasional non-budding yeast could be considered normal. The yeast generally measures 3–5 µm in diameter. For comparison, an avian RBC is 6 × 12 µm.

Treatment

- Nystatin works well. Note that it is not systemically absorbed and needs contact time with the organism to be effective. This makes it hard to treat lesions in the oral cavity. In these cases, a systemic antifungal such as fluconazole should be used. Itraconazole is not very effective against *Candida*.

Prevention

- Correct predisposing factors. Make sure that all tube-feeding utensils are properly cleaned and disinfected to prevent spread to other birds.

Capillaria

Etiology: *Capillaria* spp.

This is a nematode that inhabits the oral cavity, crop, and intestines (Figs 6.10 and 6.11). It is very common in birds of prey. Infection is from ingestion of fecal-contaminated material or food.

Clinical signs

- Clinical signs can be absent or can include dysphagia and "food flicking", anorexia, and weight loss secondary to necrotic lesions in the mouth and digestive tract.
- The oral lesions can look very similar to those produced by trichomoniasis, and mixed infections are not uncommon.

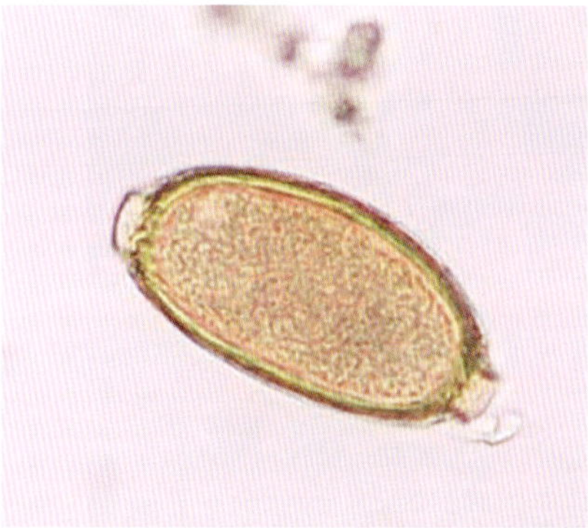

Fig. 6.10. A double-operculated *Capillaria* egg seen on fecal flotation.

Diagnosis

- Identify double-operculated eggs on fecal flotation or from a swab of oral lesions.

Treatment

- A 5-day course of fenbendazole is usually curative. Note: a single dose will not be effective.

Prevention

- Difficult or impossible.

Chlamydia/Chlamydophila

z c r

Etiology: *Chlamydia psittaci*

This is the etiologic agent of psittacosis in parrots. Studies (Hawkins, 2010) suggest that the prevalence of infection with this organism may be quite high in wild raptors. However, the clinical significance is not clear. The disease is spread by aerosolization of respiratory secretions and feces. This disease is zoonotic.

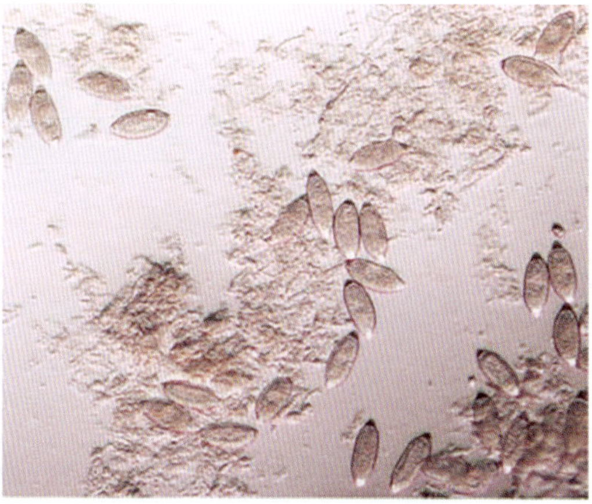

Fig. 6.11. *Capillaria* eggs seen in an oral swab.

Clinical signs

- Non-specific respiratory signs including conjunctivitis, rhinitis, and air sacculitis, as well as diarrhea.
- Splenomegaly (Fig. 6.12) and hepatomegaly are common findings on necropsy.
- Green urates due to biliverdinuria and hepatic disease are also common.

Diagnosis

- Severe leukocytosis with a toxic heterophilia and a monocytosis.
- Radiographs may show hepatomegaly or splenomegaly.
- PCR from choanal, cloacal, or conjunctival swab can be definitive.

Treatment

- Supportive care.
- Doxycycline for 45 days.

Prevention

- Quarantine and disinfection with bleach, as reinfection is possible after successful treatment.
- Treat all potentially exposed birds.

Coccidia

Etiology: *Eimeria* spp., *Isospora* spp., and *Caryospora* spp.

The coccidia protozoans are endocellular parasites of the intestinal mucosa.

Clinical signs

- These parasites generally do not cause disease in raptors.
- The exception is in young birds, when *Caryospora* spp. (Fig. 6.13) can cause lethargy, failure to thrive, abdominal pain, and bloody diarrhea.

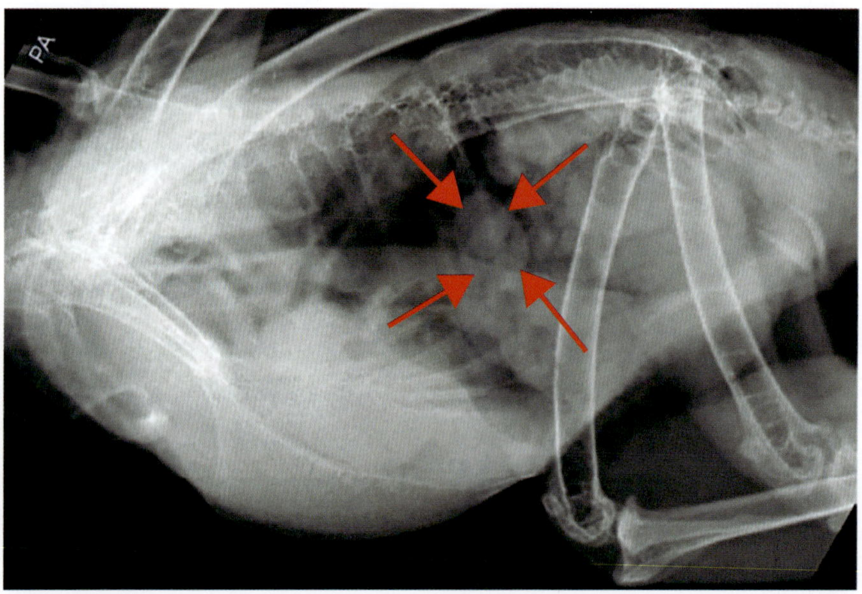

Fig. 6.12. Splenic enlargement in a red-tailed hawk.

Diagnosis

- Detection of oocysts on fecal flotation. *Caryospora* oocysts contain one sporocyst, *Isospora* contain two, and *Eimeria* contain four.

Treatment

- Toltrazuril seems to be the most effective treatment.

Prevention

- Routine fecal screenings and treatment.
- Probably not possible to clean an already contaminated environment.

Gapeworm

Etiology: *Syngamus trachea*

These worms live in the trachea, and sometimes in the air sacs, and can cause a marked inflammatory response. The males are 6 mm long and females can reach over 20 mm in length. Earthworms serve as an intermediate host.

Clinical signs

- Dyspnea and voice change; the neck may be stretched with the mouth gaping open (hence the name "gapeworm"), as well as death from complete blockage/asphyxia.
- The production of large amounts of mucus can lead to coughing and unusual URT sounds.

Diagnosis

- Identify eggs (Fig. 6.14) on fecal flotation or adults via endoscopic evaluation of trachea.

Treatment

- Fenbendazole or ivermectin are effective. However, dead worms can cause further respiratory damage, so physical removal (Fig. 6.15) should be attempted if possible.

Prevention

- Routine fecal screening and deworming.
- Prevent exposure to earthworms.

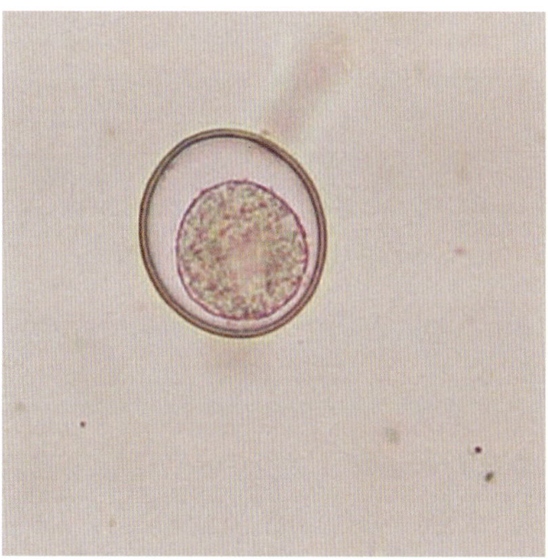

Fig. 6.13. *Caryospora* egg.

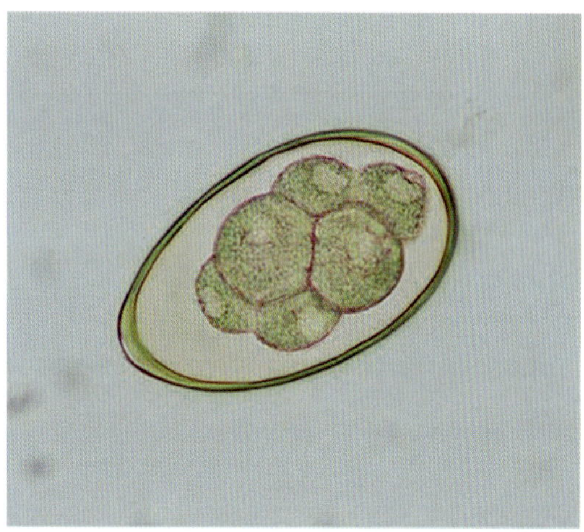

Fig. 6.14. *Syngamus trachea* egg.

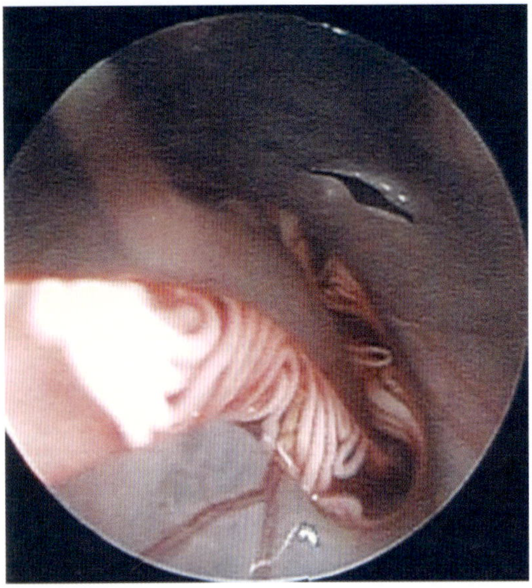

Fig. 6.15. A gapeworm is being removed endoscopically from the air sacs of a red-shouldered hawk.

> **Raptor Tip**
>
> Common causes of neurologic disease:
>
> - Lead intoxication—see Chapter 7.
> - Pesticide intoxication (organochlorines, organophosphates)—see Chapter 7.
> - Paramyxovirus (PMV-1).
> - West Nile virus (WNV).
> - Avian vacuolar myelinopathy (AVM).
> - Head trauma—see Chapter 7.
> - Avian influenza (AI).

Herpes Virus (C)

Etiology: various *Herpes* viruses

These viruses lead to lifelong, latent infections with intermittent shedding. Many avian species including all birds of prey are affected, but these infections seem particularly threatening to falcons. Other strains produce Marek's disease in chickens, a lymphoproliferative infiltration of the nerves, and can lead to paralysis, ataxia, and blindness. The route of infection is not clear, but may be from ingestion of infected pigeons or via the respiratory route.

Clinical signs

- Necrosis of liver and spleen.
- Depression and anorexia.
- Hepatomegaly and lime-green urates secondary to liver failure.
- Death within 48 h of onset of clinical signs.

Diagnosis

- Virus isolation or PCR on post-mortem tissues.
- On histopathology, eosinophilic intranuclear inclusions in liver, kidney, and spleen are pathognomonic for this disease.

Treatment

- Nothing is very effective.
- Can try supportive care and acyclovir.

Prevention

- Never feed pigeons and doves (even if frozen).
- This disease is contagious, so implement strict biosecurity measures in the face of an outbreak.

Mycobacterium avium Complex (MAC) (Z)

Etiology: *Mycobacterium avium* complex

MAC causes a chronic, granulomatous disease involving many organs. This organism is spread by the fecal–oral route and the spores can survive for years in the environment. This disease is potentially zoonotic, especially in immunocompromised individuals.

Clinical signs

- The intestinal tract is commonly affected. This leads to diarrhea and weight loss despite a good appetite.
- Granulomas and tubercles can form in other organs including the liver, spleen, and the respiratory tract.

Diagnosis

- Demonstration of acid-fast organisms on cytology or histology or in feces (examine fecal samples for a minimum of five consecutive days). The organism can also sometimes be seen as non-staining "ghosts" when a DipQuick stain is used.
- Histopathology of biopsy samples is considered the gold standard for diagnosis.
- PCR from affected tissues.

Treatment

- Not recommended due to the zoonotic nature of disease, although the risk is considered low in an immunocompetent individual. In addition, the treatment protocol is complicated, must be continued for 6–12 months minimum, and the prognosis is poor.

Prevention

- Decontamination of contaminated aviaries is difficult or impossible.
- Aviary substrate and furniture should be removed and destroyed.

Paramyxovirus-1 (PMV-1)

z c r

Etiology: Paramyxovirus PMV-1

The disease is known as Newcastle Disease in poultry. Raptors can be infected by consuming poultry that have been vaccinated for PMV. This disease can be zoonotic and causes a mild conjunctivitis in people.

Clinical signs

- Signs can be variable and vague but neurologic (torticollis (Fig. 6.16), tremors, ataxia) and respiratory (conjunctivitis) signs are common.
- GI signs including anorexia, diarrhea, and vomiting have also been reported.
- Many cases can be acutely fatal.

Diagnosis

- PMV-1 must be differentiated from other causes of neurologic disease (see Raptor Tip for a list).
- Can be difficult due to fast clinical course.
- PCR on cloacal swabs or post-mortem samples.
- Must be differentiated from trauma, lead toxicity, or other infections such as West Nile virus (WNV).

Treatment

- Supportive.

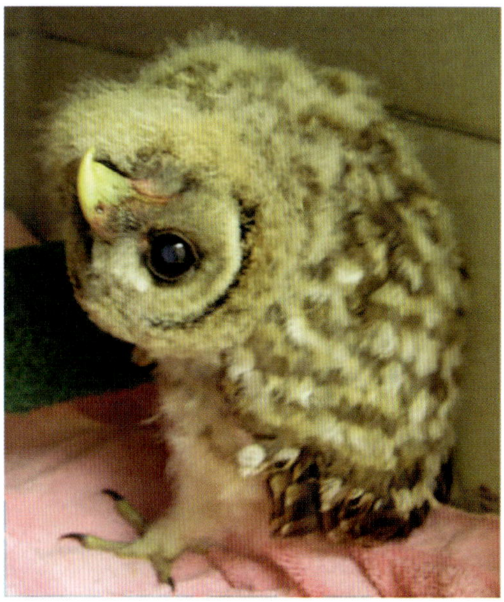

Fig. 6.16. Torticollis in a young barred owl could indicate PMV-1 infection.

Prevention

- Avoid close contact between raptors and poultry, since the disease is spread through respiratory secretions and feces.
- Inactivated vaccines may be useful.

Pox Virus

Etiology: Avipox virus

There are many different variants that are generally considered to be species-specific. The virus is distributed worldwide and is spread by biting insects such as mosquitoes and biting flies, but also directly by contaminated fomites (such as gloves). The virus can survive for years in dried scabs, so strict quarantine procedures and decontamination should be followed. The virus cannot pass through intact skin so there must be some sort of wound through which it gains entry. This virus is not considered a zoonotic risk.

Clinical signs

- The dry or cutaneous form affects the featherless areas on the feet, around the eyes, and mouth (Fig. 6.17). Nodular, ulcerated wounds with scabs form and will enlarge and worsen for 2 weeks. Most eventually regress and heal but secondary bacterial infection and substantial scarring around the eyes and eyelids can occur in the process. In addition, damage to the germinal layer of the beak can result in beak growth deformities.

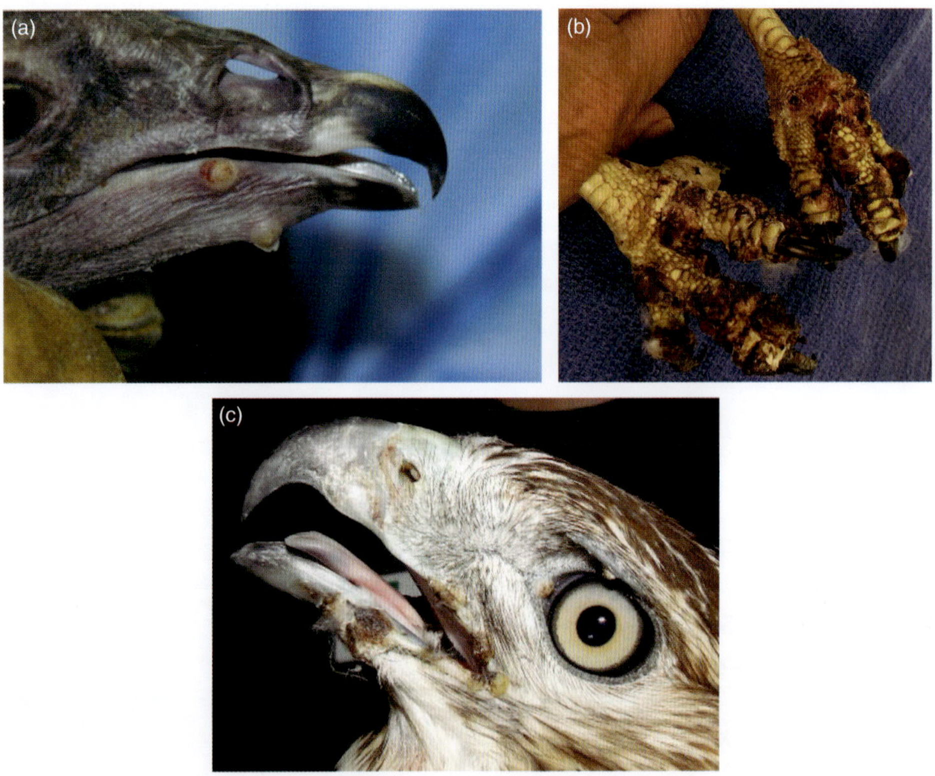

Fig. 6.17. Avian pox: the cutaneous form on the face of a turkey vulture (a), a very aggressive but resolving case on the feet of a red-tailed hawk (b), and a mild case around the mouth and eyes also on a red-tailed hawk (c).

- The wet or diphtheritic form affects the mucous membranes of the mouth, trachea, and esophagus. Caseous plaques develop and can lead to anorexia and sepsis. Prognosis for the wet form is poor. This form is very uncommon in raptors.

Diagnosis

- The lesions are characteristic, but diagnosis can be confirmed with histopathology. Large eosinophilic intracytoplasmic inclusion bodies ("Bollinger bodies") may be seen.

Treatment

- Systemic antibiotics are important to protect against secondary bacterial infections.
- The wounds should be cleaned topically and Vitamin A supplementation has shown to be helpful in some cases. There have been reports that surgical removal of larger lesions may speed the healing process and reduce scarring.

Prevention

- Vector control: make sure enclosures have netting small enough to prevent entry of the vectors.
- Prevent spread by fomites (e.g. gloves, shoes, perches, etc.) and use strict quarantine procedures.
- Pigeon pox and turkey pox vaccines have been used with variable success.

Trichomoniasis

Etiology: *Trichomonas gallinae*

This flagellated protozoan infects the oral cavity and upper GI tract (Figs 6.18 and 6.19). Pigeons and other columbiforms, as well as some passerines, commonly carry it, causing a disease known as "canker". Raptors are usually infected after eating fresh pigeons and the disease is known as "frounce".

Clinical signs

- Large caseous/cheesy lesions are commonly found in the mouth under the tongue and around the choana. The masses can get so large that eating and breathing can become difficult and it is not uncommon for birds to become emaciated as a result. In addition,

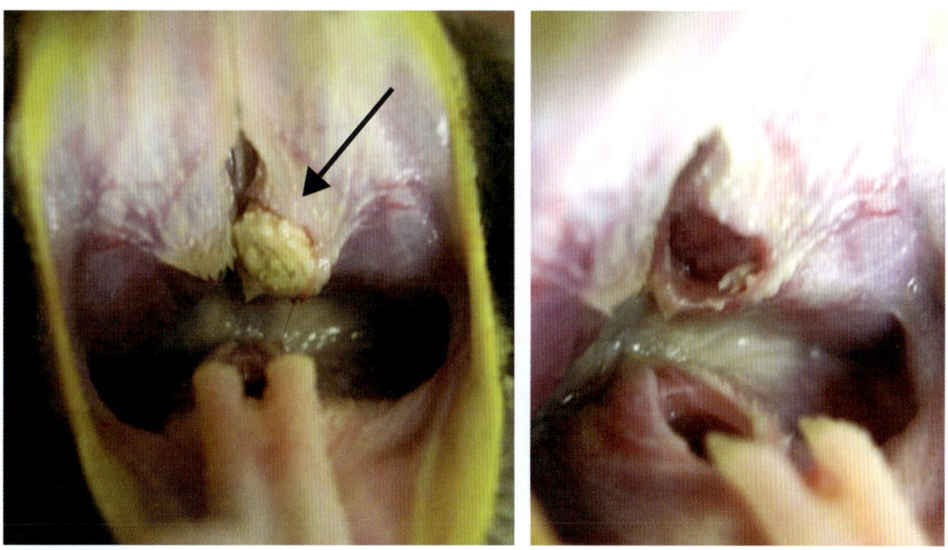

Fig. 6.18. A typical *Trichomonas* lesion in the oral cavity (arrow). Notice how cleanly they sometimes "shell out" as seen in the right-hand photo.

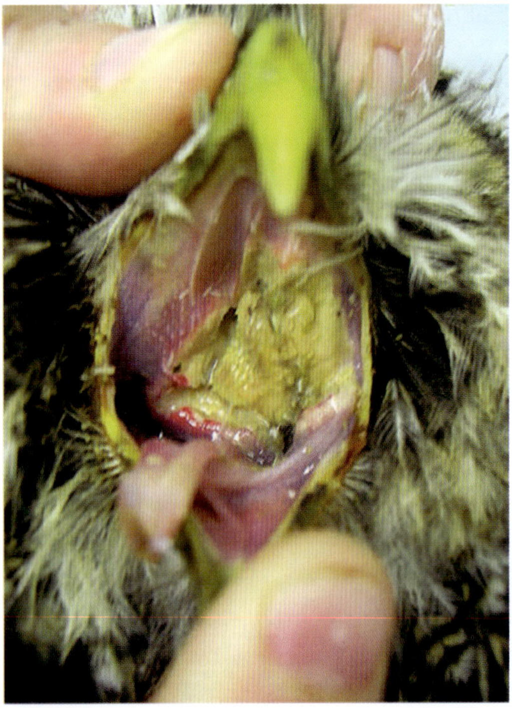

Fig. 6.19. Severe *Trichomonas* lesions like this are not uncommon.

lesions in the roof of the mouth can erode through the hard palate and into the sinuses.

- Dysphagia and "food flicking" are also common.
- May only see stringy mucus and not actually have a caseous lesion (Redig and Ponder, 2010).

Diagnosis

- Lesions and clinical signs can be mistaken for *Capillaria* and possibly *Candida*.
- Cytology of warm saline wet mount. The organisms are fragile so the slide must be viewed quickly. Motile flagellated protozoa will be seen.
- Very common in barred owls.

Treatment

- Treatment with carnidazole (see Appendix B, Formulary) is usually effective.
- A few days after treating, the lesions should become loose and can be debrided away, often leaving very large, but generally clean, defects (Fig. 6.18).
- Disinfection of the resulting cavity with a topical agent such as F10® is helpful, in addition to systemic antibiotics, to prevent secondary infections.

Prevention

- Do not feed pigeons to raptors (even if frozen).

> **Raptor Tip**
>
> Do not forget to rule out *Capillaria*.

West Nile Virus (WNV) Z

Etiology: Flavivirus

This virus primarily causes an encephalitis and it is spread by mosquitoes, but consumption of infected animals can also lead to infection. Birds may act as a reservoir but can also become ill from the virus. It was first seen in the western hemisphere in 1999 and has now been reported in all 50 US states, and across Europe, much of Africa, the Middle East, and South-east Asia. It affects many species of birds. Corvids seem to be highly susceptible but most species of raptors have also been seriously affected. This disease is zoonotic but is not transmitted directly from birds to humans.

Clinical signs

Clinical signs develop 10–12 days post-infection and can include:

- Any type of neurologic signs including ataxia and seizures.
- Vision loss from retinal pathology.
- Sudden death.

- Feather growth abnormalities including a "pinched off" or hemorrhagic calamus (Fig. 6.20; see Chapter 13).
- Many cases are terminal but some birds with milder clinical signs may recover.

Diagnosis

- WNV must be differentiated from other causes of neurologic disease (see Raptor Tip for a list).
- PCR of combined cloacal/choanal swabs may not be helpful due to a potentially short period of shedding (2–7 days) (Redig and Ponder, 2010).
- PCR on whole blood or paired serology samples may be helpful.
- Diagnostic testing is complicated by the fact that many of the tests will only be positive at various points in the infection.
- An elevated white count may be seen.
- The gold standard is to do histopathology with immunohistochemical stains on brain tissue (Fig. 6.21).
- Fundic exam may show a chorioretinitis.
- Splenomegaly may be present, but a typical gross necropsy may be completely normal.
- Must be differentiated from lead toxicity, insecticides, AI, and PMV-1.

Treatment

- Purely supportive.
- Meloxicam at a high dose of 1 mg/kg SID or BID × 7 days has been effective in some cases (Redig and Ponder, 2010).
- Note: birds can recover neurologically but may still have serious retinal damage that would prohibit release, so repeated fundic exams are important.

Prevention

- Mosquito control.
- Annual vaccination may be helpful. Fort Dodge (Fort Dodge, IA, USA) and Merial (Duluth, GA, USA) both have commercial equine WNV vaccines that have been used successfully in raptors.

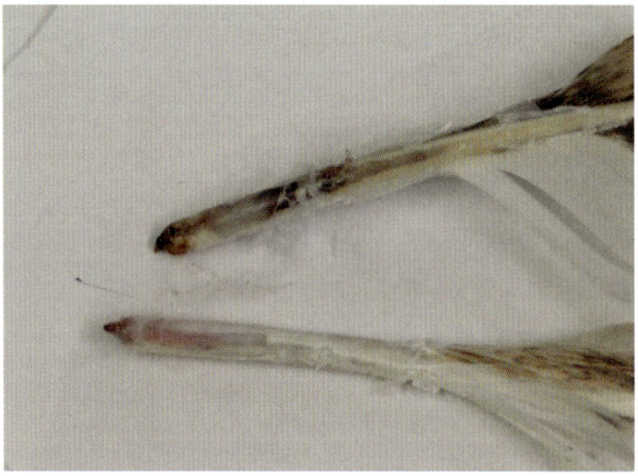

Fig. 6.20. Feathers affected by WNV.

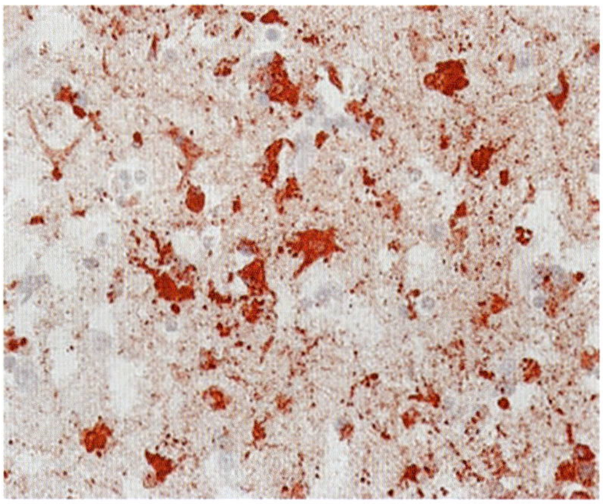

Fig. 6.21. Positive immunohistochemical stain for WNV in brain tissue in a red-shouldered hawk.

Summary

Table 6.1. Summary of diseases.

Agent	Clinical signs	Diagnosis
Aspergillosis	Emaciation, respiratory signs, voice change	Endoscopy, CBC, history, species
Avian influenza (AI)	**Zoonotic** (some strains) Anorexia, depression, respiratory signs, neurologic signs, sudden death	Virus isolation from cloacal swabs or post-mortem tissues, PCR
Avian vacuolar myelinopathy (AVM)	Incoordination, ataxia, weakness	Histopathology
Blood parasites (*Hemoproteus*, *Leukocytozoon*, *Plasmodium*)	Malaria: Depression, anemia, dyspnea, hemolysis, jade-green urates, sudden death	Blood smear
Candida	Caseous lesions in the mouth and crop, thickening of the crop wall, dysphagia, "food flicking"	Cytology
Capillaria	Dysphagia and "food flicking", necrotic lesions in the mouth and digestive tract	Cytology, fecal exam
Chlamydia	**Zoonotic** Conjunctivitis, rhinitis, air sacculitis, splenomegaly and hepatomegaly, green urates	Severe leukocytosis, PCR from choanal, cloacal swab
Coccidia	Lethargy, failure to thrive, abdominal pain, bloody diarrhea in young animals	Fecal exam
Gapeworm	Dyspnea, voice change, the neck may be stretched with the mouth gaping open	Fecal exam, endoscopy
Herpes virus	Depression and anorexia. Hepatomegaly and lime-green urates. High mortality rate	Virus isolation and PCR on post-mortem tissues
Mycobacterium avium complex (MAC)	Potentially **zoonotic** Chronic wasting despite good appetite	Demonstration of acid-fast organisms on cytology or from feces. Histopathology of intestinal biopsy is the gold standard
Paramyxovirus-1 (PMV-1)	**Zoonotic** Neurologic (torticollis, tremors, ataxia) and respiratory (conjunctivitis) signs are common, sudden death	PCR on cloacal swabs or post-mortem samples
Pox virus	Proliferative or ulcerative lesions on featherless areas on feet, around mouth and eyes, or in oral cavity	Clinical signs, histopathology
Trichomonas	Large caseous lesions in the mouth. Dysphagia and "food flicking"	Cytology, clinical appearance
West Nile virus (WNV)	**Zoonotic** Sudden death, central nervous system signs, blindness	PCR from choanal/cloacal swabs or blood. Histopathology on brain tissue (with special stains)

Bibliography

Cray, C., Reavill, D., Romagnano, A., Van Sant, F., Champagne, D., Stevenson, R., *et al.* (2009) Galactomannan assay and plasma protein electrophoresis findings in psittacine birds with aspergillosis. *Journal of Avian Medicine and Surgery* 23(2), 125–135.

Fischer, D., Van Waeyenberghe, L., Cray, C., Gross, M., Usleber, E., Pasmans, F., *et al.* (2014) Comparison of diagnostic tools for the detection of aspergillosis in blood samples of experimentally infected falcons. *Avian Diseases* 58(4), 587–598.

Hawkins, M. (2010) *Chlamydophila psittaci* in wild raptors in northern California: 2000–2009. *Proceedings of the 31st Conference of the Association of Avian Veterinarians, San Diego, CA, USA*. Association of Avian Veterinarians, Teaneck, NJ, USA, p. 349.

Kelly, T.R., Hawkins, M.G., Sandrock, C.E. and Boyce, W.M. (2008) A review of highly pathogenic avian influenza in birds, with an emphasis on Asian H5N1 and recommendations for prevention and control. *Journal of Avian Medicine and Surgery* 22(1), 1–16.

Krautwald-Junghanns, M.-E., Cramer, K. and DellaVolpe, A. (2008) Avian influenza in wild, zoo, and pet birds: 2006 and 2007 in review. *Proceedings of the 29th Conference of the Association of Avian Veterinarians, Savannah, GA, USA*. Association of Avian Veterinarians, Teaneck, NJ, USA, pp. 379–384.

Kummrow, M., Silvanose, C., Di Somma, A., Bailey, T.A. and Vorbrüggen, S. (2012) Serum protein electrophoresis by using high-resolution agarose gel in clinically healthy and Aspergillus species-infected falcons. *Journal of Avian Medicine and Surgery* 26(4), 213–220.

Lierz, M., *et al.* (2007) Highly pathogenic avian influenza (H5N1) in falcons – susceptibility and vaccination. *Proceedings of the 9th Conference of the European Association of Avian Veterinarians*. European Association of Avian Veterinarians, pp. 149–154. Available at: www.eaavonline.org (accessed February 2016).

Nemeth, N.M., Kratz, G.E., Bates, R., Scherpelz, J.A., Bowen, R.A. and Komar, N. (2009) Clinical evaluation and outcomes of naturally acquired West Nile Virus infection in raptors. *Journal of Zoo and Wildlife Medicine* 40(1), 51–63.

Raghav, R. and Samour, J. (2019) Inclusion body herpesvirus hepatitis in captive falcons in the Middle East: a review of clinical and pathologic findings. *Journal of Avian Medicine and Surgery* 33(1), 1–6.

Redig, P. and Ponder, J. (2010) Raptors: practical information every avian practitioner can use. *Proceedings of the 31st Conference of the Association of Avian Veterinarians, San Diego, CA, USA*. Association of Avian Veterinarians, Teaneck, NJ, USA, pp. 171–180.

Samour, J., *et al.* (2007) Humoral response in saker (*Falco cherrug*) and peregrine (*Falco peregrinnus*) falcons to an inactivated H5N1 avian influenza vaccine. *Proceedings of the 9th Conference of the Association of Avian Veterinarians*. Association of Avian Veterinarians, Teaneck, NJ, USA, pp. 5–6. Available at: www.eaavonline.org (accessed February 2016).

7 Miscellaneous Conditions

There are many conditions affecting raptors that are not directly infectious in nature. Some are secondary to trauma or poor husbandry or due to exposure to toxic chemicals and substances in the environment.

Learning Objectives

1. Diagnosis and treatment of lead poisoning.
2. Dealing with bumblefoot.
3. The emaciated bird.
4. Treatment of spinal trauma.

Air Sac Rupture/ Subcutaneous Air

Etiology

Air sac ruptures and subcutaneous air can occur for many reasons. The most common cause is trauma such as hit-by-car, window-strike, or gunshot. It can also be caused accidentally, secondary to a lacerated trachea during intubation, or if the oxygen flow rate is too high during anesthesia. Mild cases can also result after endoscopic examination of the coelomic cavity.

Clinical signs

- Subcutaneous air accumulation may be substantial and can cover many parts of the body. It usually does not represent a serious danger but needs to be managed and treated.

Treatment

- Aspirate air from the pockets with an 18-gauge needle. Make a small nick with the needle as you are withdrawing to make a larger hole. This should be repeated as necessary. Anesthesia is not required.
- Pressure bandages are helpful if the location allows a bandage to be placed.
- Do not give SQ fluids.
- Attempt to correct the underlying cause.

Anticoagulant Toxicity

Etiology

Exposure to the anticoagulant rodenticides is likely quite common but this toxicity is difficult to diagnose definitively. Exposure is usually from contaminated prey. Warfarin is a first-generation anticoagulant. It has a short half-life and usually requires multiple exposures to reach toxic levels. Brodifacoum has a much longer half-life and can be toxic after a single exposure. Another potential source of toxicity is iatrogenic over-heparinization of catheters.

Clinical signs

- Bleeding into body cavities (joints, abdomen, pulmonary space) is less common in birds than it is in mammals. Instead, excessive bleeding from superficial wounds is much more likely.

Diagnosis

- Based on clinical signs and response to treatment.
- Coagulation panels are not useful in birds.

Treatment

- Control the bleeding with pressure bandages.
- Supportive care including fluid therapy.
- Vitamin K_1 (see Appendix B, Formulary). Continue to treat and monitor for 2 weeks beyond resolution of clinical signs.
- Fluid therapy and blood transfusions as needed.

Prevention

- For cases due to over-heparinization of catheters, it is important to minimize the amount of heparin used. Try flushing with saline instead and use heparin only once per day in a very dilute concentration (see Appendix B, Formulary).

Bumblefoot

Etiology

Bumblefoot, or pododermatitis, refers to any injury, lesion, or inflammatory process on the pads of the feet and toes. It is primarily caused by pressure necrosis. It is rare in wild birds but can be commonplace in captive raptors. Bumblefoot will develop for any reason when weight cannot be borne on the contralateral leg. Therefore, it is common to see bumblefoot on the "good" foot when a bird is recovering from a fracture or other non-weight-bearing injury in the opposite leg.

Some husbandry-related causes in captive populations include:

- Improper perch size, type, or covering (see Chapter 15).
- Too little perch variability.
- Sharp or jagged ground substrate.
- Obesity.
- Punctures caused by overgrown talons.

Clinical signs

Severity is graded as described in Table 7.1. Initially, bumblefoot may simply present as a pink area that is smooth and has lost the normal texture, but it can rapidly progress to a deep, painful abscess (Figs 7.1–7.3). *Staphylococcus* spp. and *Escherichia coli* are often cultured from these wounds. In general, perches that are too small result in lesions in the center of the foot, while perches that are too large result in lesions on the distal toes (Fig. 15.7).

> **Raptor Tip**
>
> Large falcons are very susceptible to bumblefoot.

Treatment

In all cases, the underlying cause must be identified and corrected.

In minor cases, simple padded bandages and topical or systemic anti-inflammatories (Preparation H®, Pfizer, Kings Mountain, NC, USA; or hydrocortisone, meloxicam, for example) can be effective. If there is an open wound, systemic antibiotics are required (enrofloxacin and amoxicillin with clavulanic acid work well in combination). Bacterial culture and sensitivity are recommended, and treatment may be long term.

Soaking affected feet in dilute chlorhexidine can be helpful and can be achieved by removing the perch from the bird's kennel, thereby forcing it to stand in the soaking solution.

Once abscessation has occurred, aggressive surgical debridement is required. These wounds can be very bloody and a tourniquet is often necessary to control bleeding during surgery. It is usually not possible to close the resulting wound without tension; therefore, they must be allowed to granulate and heal slowly over time.

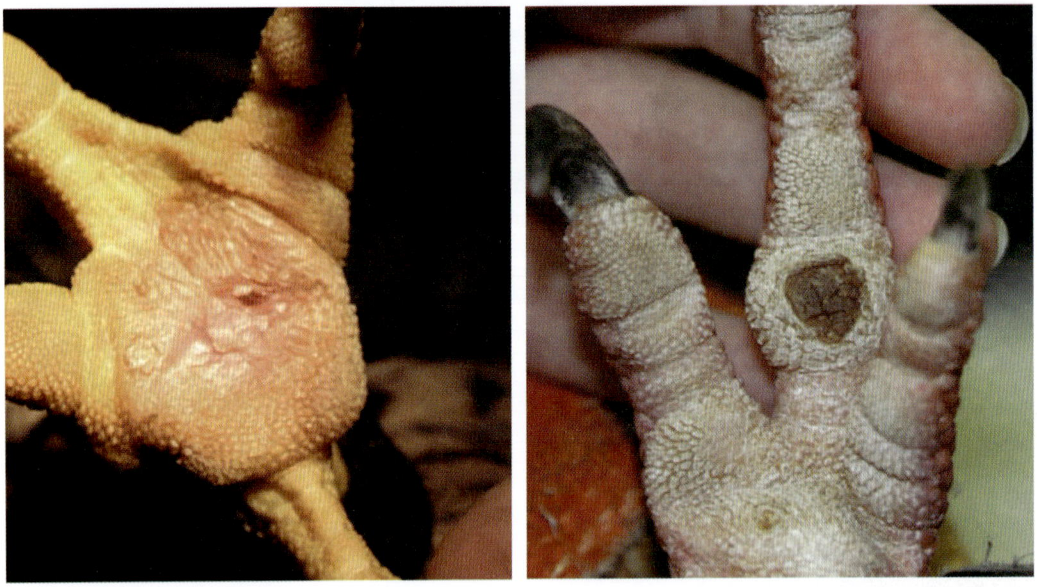

Fig. 7.1. Early bumblefoot. Grade I on the left has smooth, slightly pink skin. Grade II–III on the right has subcutaneous involvement and some swelling.

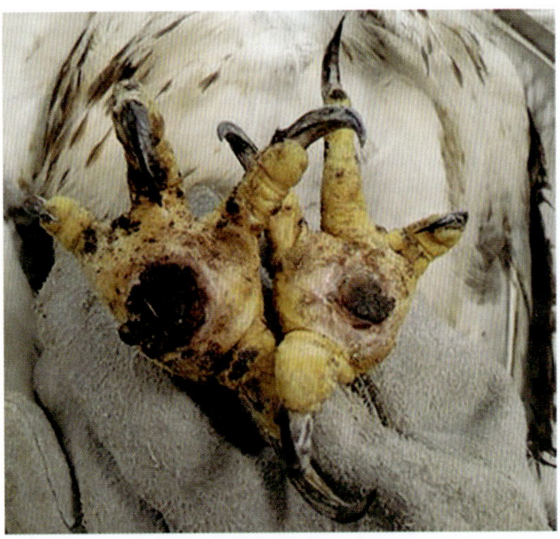

Fig. 7.2. End-stage Grade V bumblefoot in a wild red-tailed hawk. This is very unusual in a wild bird and the underlying cause was not identified.

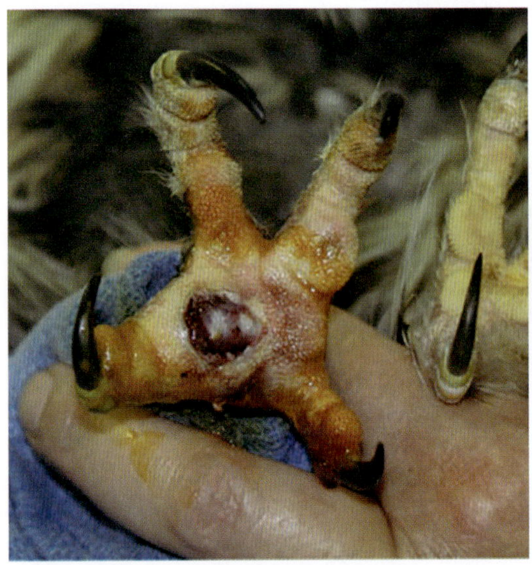

Fig. 7.3. Grade IV bumblefoot in a barred owl recovering from a fractured tibiotarsus in the opposite leg.

Raptor Tip

Try to catch bumblefoot early. Always look at the bottom of the feet whenever a bird is handled.

Be patient, since these cases often take 6–8 weeks (or longer) to heal.

Frequent bandage changes (every 2–3 days) and cleansing/debriding are critical. Many different bandaging methods, including the use of small

Table 7.1. Bumblefoot grades.

Grade	Clinical signs
I	Smooth, shiny epithelium. May be pink
II	Infection of subcutaneous tissue but no gross swelling
III	Infected, warm, and swollen but without involvement of deeper tissues
IV	Involvement of tendon and bone
V	End stage with loss of function

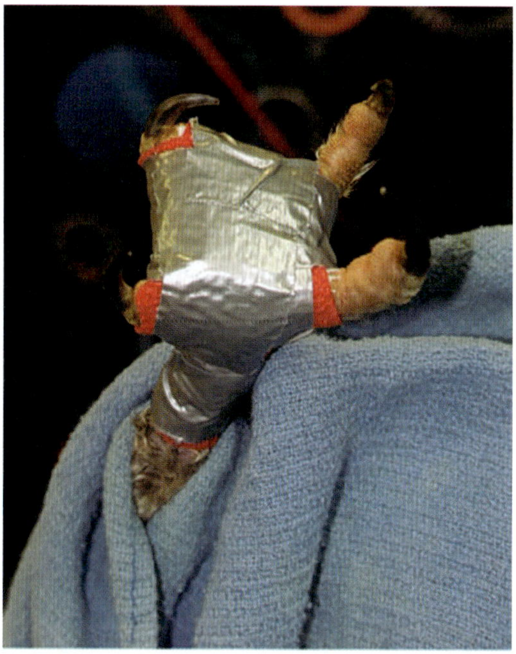

Fig. 7.4. Typical bumblefoot bandage.

"donuts" or foam shoes, can be used to relieve pressure on the wound (Figs 7.4–7.6).

The use of composite, form-fitting silicone shoes (Fig. 7.7a–g) is very useful in relieving pressure on a bumblefoot lesion. The shoes are created from an equine silicone composite material, Advanced Cushion Support™ (Nanric, Lawrenceburg, KY, USA). The procedures described in Fig. 7.7 are adapted from Remple (2006).

Duct tape can be useful to help protect and waterproof the bandage. Remove water dishes from the enclosure of any bird with a foot bandage. Always monitor for development of bumblefoot

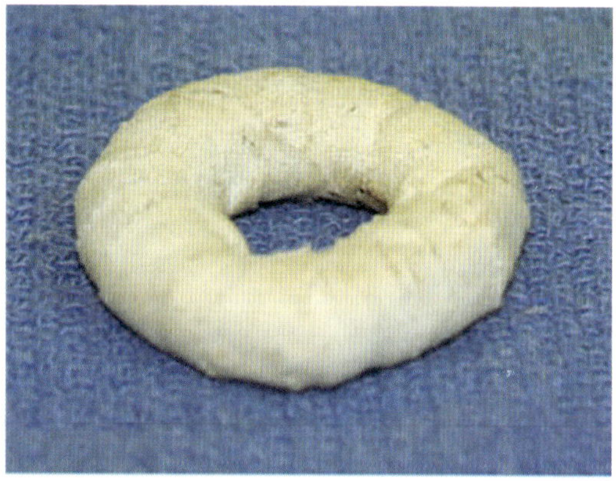

Fig. 7.5. Foot bandage donut.

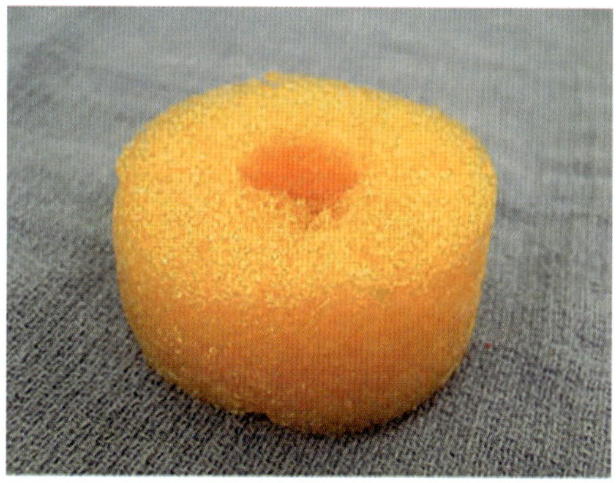

Fig. 7.6. Foam "water noodles" are great for creating pressure-relieving foam shoes.

in the opposite foot as weight bearing will not be shared equally during the healing process.

While systemic antibiotics are often useful, chronically abscessed lesions often require a different approach. The use of antibiotic-impregnated polymethyl methylmethacrylate (AIPMMA) beads (Table 7.2) is very helpful in these cases as it allows for high local concentrations without any toxic side effects. These instructions are adapted from Remple (2006). You will need polymethyl methylmethacrylate (PMMA) bone cement (Simplex™ P, Stryker Corporation, Kalamazoo, MI, USA) and an appropriate antibiotic (ideally based on culture and sensitivity). The antibiotic must come in powder form, it must be water soluble, and it must be heat stable to withstand the heat generated when the bone cement polymerizes.

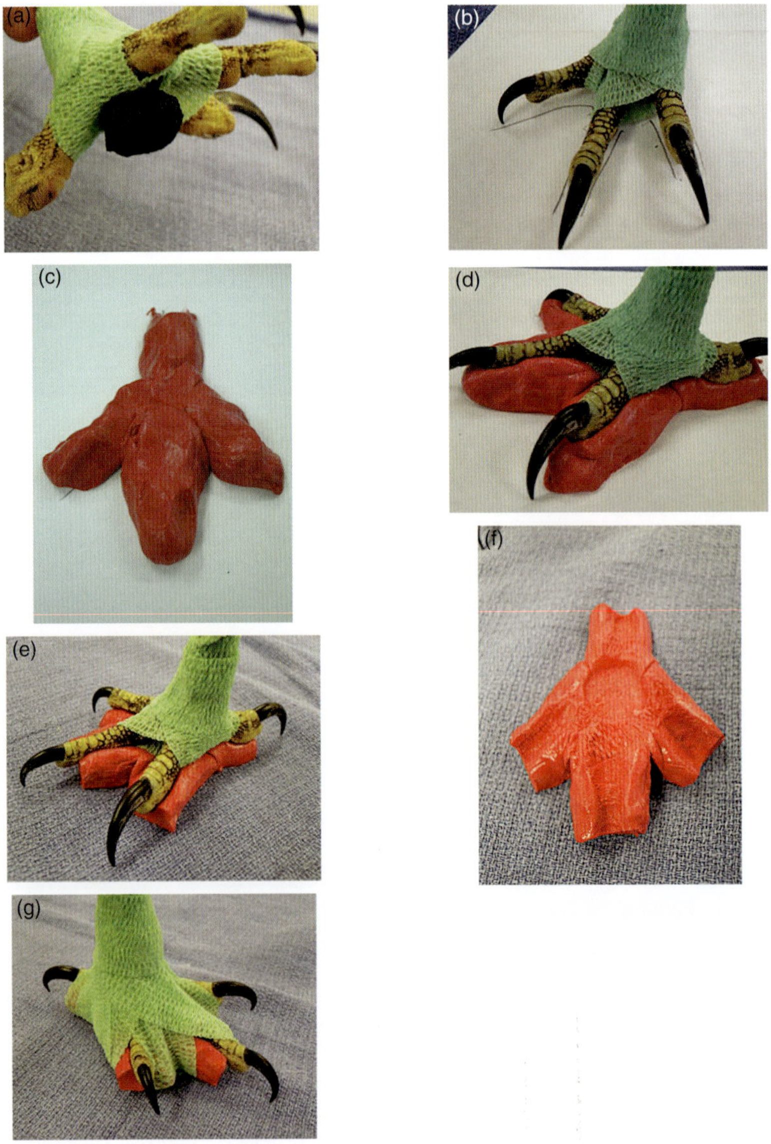

Fig. 7.7. Silicone shoe. (a) The wound is cleaned, debrided, and dressed with a sterile bandage. A piece of thick foam spacer is placed over the wound. (b) The foot and toes are outlined on a piece of paper. (c) The composite material is mixed and formed into a rough approximation of the foot. (d) The foot (with the foam spacer in place) is pressed into the composite material and the material is worked into a tight fit around the toes. (e) The composite material is allowed to harden and it is trimmed so that the distal phalanges can be flexed easily. (f) This is the shoe after it has been trimmed. The gap or cavity created by the foam spacer is clearly visible. (g) The foam spacer is removed and the shoe is firmly attached to the foot with elastic wrap. Duct tape can be used as an outer layer to protect the shoe.

Table 7.2. Antibiotics to mix with PMMA powder.

Antibiotic	Ratio	Antibiotic (g) per 40 g packet of bone cement
Gentocin or tobramycin	1:14	3
Penicillin	1:5	8
Fluoroquinolone	1:6	7
Clindamycin	1:1.7	6
Cefotaxime	1:10	4
Ceftazidime	1:10	4
Ceftiofur	1:10	4

To create the beads:

- Grind the appropriate amount of antibiotic powder to a very fine consistency. Refer to Table 7.2.
- Mix it with the PMMA powder.
- Divide the mixture into 1 g portions.
- Chill the PMMA liquid monomer in the freezer at 0°C.
- Mix 0.7 ml of the liquid monomer with 1 g of the combined powder.
- Load the mixed "batter" into a syringe and expel the dough in a line on a sterile surface.
- Create 2–3 mm beads from the dough by rolling them in the palm of your gloved hand. Make sure they are smooth with no sharp points or edges.
- Sterilize the beads using ethylene oxide and allow them to aerate for 24 h before using them. You *cannot* use steam sterilization. If gas sterilization is not available, then you may still use the beads if you are very careful and clean while making them.

The beads are inserted into a freshly debrided wound. The skin should be closed over the beads if possible. Avoid placing the beads in areas that are likely to cause ulceration of the skin. The beads often work themselves out of the wound, so they rarely need to be removed.

Prevention

- Address all potential causes listed above (see Chapter 15).
- Routinely check feet whenever a bird is handled.
- Treat early and aggressively.
- Repair leg fractures quickly so that weight bearing on both legs can be restored as soon as possible.

Cloacal Prolapse

Etiology

Cloacal prolapse (Fig. 7.8) can occur for many reasons including:

- Straining due to obstruction, egg binding, parasitism.
- Intussusception, foreign body, ureteroliths.
- Diarrhea/colitis.
- Trauma.

Prolapses are not common in wild raptors but may be seen in a large captive population. Note: a cloacal papilloma must be differentiated from a prolapse. Papillomas are common in parrots but not in raptors. They have a rough, cobblestone appearance, protrude from the cloacal mucosa, and will turn white when dabbed with vinegar.

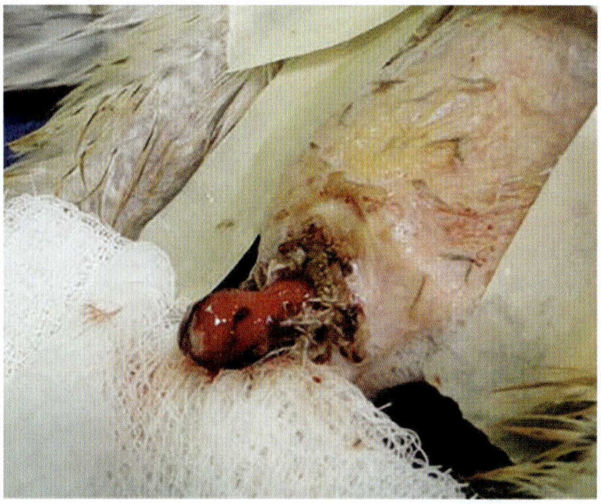

Fig. 7.8. A colonic intussusception prolapsed from the cloaca in a juvenile red-shouldered hawk.

Clinical signs

Many tissues/organs can be involved in the prolapse.

- In simple cases, the cloaca itself is prolapsed and it will appear as a smooth (or somewhat rough if more chronic) red ball. You may be able to see the openings to the colon, ureters, and oviducts.
- The colon may be prolapsed.
- The oviduct may be prolapsed and can be identified by longitudinal mucosal folds.
- Refer to Fig. 2.12.

In addition to the prolapse, the bird may be systemically ill, may be dehydrated, lethargic, and in shock.

Treatment

- Stabilize patient with fluids, analgesics, antibiotics, and anti-inflammatories, as indicated.
- Radiographs can be used to identify an egg in dystocia cases. Oral barium can be used to outline the GI tract in cases of rectal prolapse.
- Lavage and lubricate tissues with lidocaine jelly and gently replace the tissue with a lubricated cotton-tipped applicator, if possible. Necrotic tissue will need to be resected.
- The cloaca can be partially closed temporarily with a simple interrupted or horizontal mattress suture on each side. A non-absorbable monofilament suture such as nylon is a good choice. Do not use a purse-string pattern as that can cause damage to the cloacal sphincter.
- Monitor for defecation and straining.
- Remove the sutures in 7 days.

Prolapses of the colon and oviduct are often due to an intussusception and cannot be treated as described above. These cases require a laparotomy in order to reduce the intussusception and remove any devitalized tissue.

Recurrent or chronic cases of cloacal prolapse should be surgically repaired. See Chapter 9.

Ectoparasites

Etiology

Ticks, Mallophaga chewing lice, hippoboscid (flat) flies, mites, maggots, and warbles are common ectoparasites affecting raptors.

Clinical signs

Ticks tend to attach themselves on the head, around the eyes, and on the eyelids (Fig. 7.9). Oftentimes, the only thing noticeable is a feather sticking up after being displaced by an engorged tick. Some infestations can lead to severe blepharitis and conjunctivitis.

Feather lice are dorsal–ventrally flattened and are typically around 2 mm in length. They are relatively common in apparently healthy birds, but an ill bird may develop a severe infestation. Louse eggs may also be present on or near the feather shafts (Fig. 7.10).

Hippoboscid flies (Fig. 6.7) are often seen in ill birds and become very apparent during the intake exam. These flies transmit the *Hemoproteus* protozoal parasite.

Maggot infestations should be treated as an emergency since maggots can produce a staggering amount of damage in a very short period of time (Fig. 7.11). Contrary to popular belief, these maggots do consume healthy tissue. In addition to

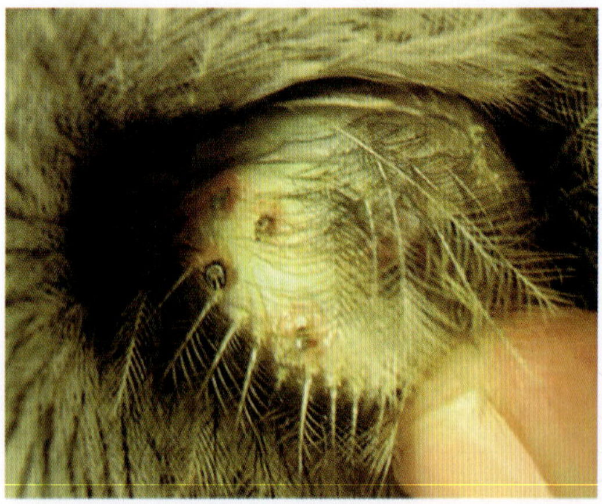

Fig. 7.9. Ticks attached to the eyelid.

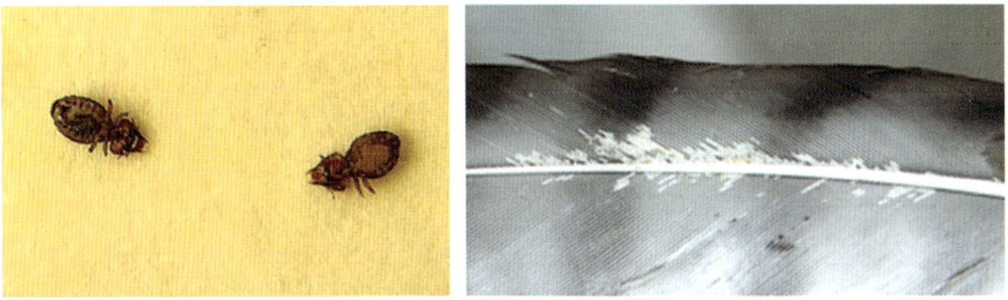

Fig. 7.10. Lice and their eggs on a feather shaft.

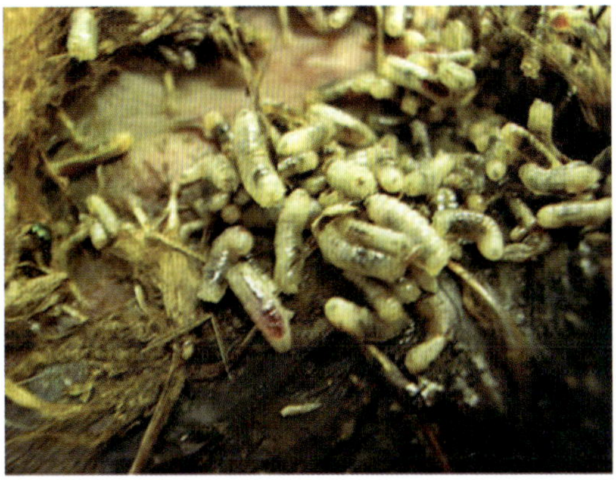

Fig. 7.11. Maggot infestations can be devastating.

actual maggots, there may be clumps of fly eggs attached to the feathers. All wounds and blood feathers should be carefully inspected for maggots or fly eggs. In addition, areas such as the vent and the elbows seem to be preferred locations for maggots.

Warbles are large insect larvae (species variable) that often are located in the ear canals of young raptors, especially hawks. A dried, brown exudate on the feathers overlying the ear canals is a common indicator of their presence. They are large (5–6 mm in length) but it is not uncommon for a half dozen larvae to be in each ear canal.

Treatment

Ticks should be carefully removed. Inflammation around the eye can be treated with topical prednisone and an injection of dexamethasone. Fipronil (Frontline®, Merial, Duluth, GA, USA) can be used as a preventative. The spray-on formulation is applied to cotton balls and then wiped on the featherless areas in the leg webs, axillas, along the keel, and between the shoulder blades.

> **Raptor Tip**
>
> Recheck wounds repeatedly to make sure that all maggots were removed.

Flat flies and lice can be treated with water-based pyrethrin or permethrin sprays. Products with pyrethrin, piperonyl, and permethrin (Bronco Equine Fly Spray, for example) are safe and effective. Mites can be treated with selamectin (Sadar *et al.*, 2015).

Maggots and fly eggs must be removed physically. Removal can sometimes take a great deal of time and anesthesia is helpful. The infestation can be very severe and require that feathers be plucked. Any wounds should be thoroughly flushed and dressed as indicated. Application of topical nitenpyram (Capstar—tablets can be crushed and mixed with water; see Appendix B, Formulary) is very effective in killing the maggots quickly and will help greatly in their removal. In addition, nitenpyram should be given orally to infested birds.

Warbles should be carefully removed from the ear canal. Topical nitenpyram is helpful in killing them prior to their removal and the ear canal should then be gently flushed with warm saline. The ears should be checked for the next few days to ensure that all warbles have been removed.

Egg Binding

Etiology

Egg binding is defined as the inability to lay an egg and may or may not include dystocia. The egg can be located in any part of the reproductive tract from the oviduct to the cloaca. It can occur for a variety of reasons including:

- Inflammation or other disease of the oviduct.
- Hypocalcemia.
- Systemic illness, hypothermia.
- Pelvic malformation/trauma.
- Over-sized or oddly shaped eggs.
- Lead toxicity.

As with cloacal prolapses, egg binding is not common in wild raptors, but may be seen in a large captive population.

Clinical signs

- The egg may be visible in or palpable inside the vent and the abdomen may be distended.
- The bird may be visibly straining or may be very lethargic.
- The bird may be systemically ill and in shock if the condition has persisted for any length of time.
- Paresis of one or both legs is possible due to compression of the sciatic nerve.

Treatment

- Since there are limited data regarding the length of time it takes various species to lay an egg, it is difficult to know when an egg is overdue. It can therefore be unclear when it is time to intervene. In general, the process should not take longer than 24 h.
- Stabilize the patient with fluids, analgesics, and anti-inflammatories as indicated. Provide heat and increased humidity.
- Supplementation with IM calcium (see Appendix B, Formulary). Note that use of oxytocin is contraindicated in birds.
- Radiographs are useful to determine the exact location and size of an egg. Additional radiographs allow evaluation of the long bones for medullary bone deposition. In a healthy hen, the long bones (such as the tibiotarsus) should demonstrate a massive deposition of calcified bone in the medullary canal of the diaphysial regions. Hypocalcemia is more likely if this deposition of bone is reduced or absent and can then be confirmed with a serum chemistry panel.
- Lubrication with warm KY jelly and manual expression/removal of the egg can be accomplished if the egg is present in the cloaca.
- If the egg cannot be removed whole, cloacal ovocentisis should be attempted. Use an 18-gauge needle to aspirate contents of the egg. The shell can then be collapsed and removed in pieces.
- If the egg cannot be visualized in the cloaca, percutaneous ovocentisis can be attempted. Surgically prep the *left* side of the abdomen and press the egg towards the body wall. This displaces the intestines out of the way. The contents of the egg can then be aspirated, the egg is collapsed, and the pieces of shell should eventually be expelled.
- If all else fails, a salpingohysterectomy is required.

Electrocution

Etiology

Electrocution occurs after contact with a power source. The contact point is usually on a wing and the current will travel through the body to ground, usually exiting through a foot. The current can cause cardiovascular anomalies and physiologic changes. The blood supply to affected limbs is often compromised, leading to massive necrosis and sloughing of tissue.

Clinical signs

- In cases that survive the electrocution, there can be evidence of singed feathers and/or burned flesh.
- In less severe cases, there may be minor tissue damage or areas that are damp or where the skin tears easily with no bleeding. The affected areas may be cold to the touch and swollen. These cases often progress to the point where all the tissue of an affected area can die and slough (Fig. 7.12).

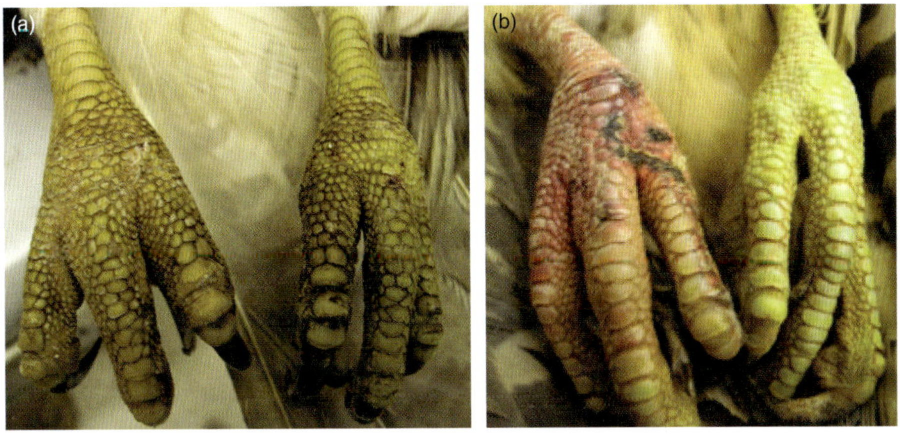

Fig. 7.12. The feet of a red-tailed hawk after electrocution. On admission (a), the right foot is cool and swollen and, after a few days (b), the tissue has begun to slough.

Diagnosis

- History and physical examination. The classic appearance of electrocution is unmistakable but may not be obvious for several days after the exposure.

Treatment

- None. Prognosis is very poor. Humane euthanasia is often the only option.

Emaciation

Etiology

Emaciation is not a disease but the result of some other underlying problem such as:

- Systemic disease.
- Poor hunting ability in a young bird.
- Traumatic injury (e.g. fracture, eye damage).

Severely emaciated birds are in a hypometabolic state and they need to be slowly and gradually returned to a normal physiologic state. These birds are very much at risk of "refeeding syndrome". Patience is required when treating these birds.

> **Raptor Tip**
>
> Keel score < 2.0, PCV < 15%, and TS < 1.0 g/dl indicates a poor prognosis.

Clinical signs

It is not uncommon to admit birds with a keel score of 1 or 1.5 that have lost 40% of their BW (Fig. 7.13). Emaciation is commonly accompanied by severe anemia and hypoproteinemia, lethargy, and hypothermia. Refer to Fig. 1.2 for a diagram of keel scores.

Treatment

- As much as you may feel compelled to, *do not feed these birds immediately*. It is critical that they be rehydrated first before introducing food. The one exception is with young orphans. These birds are generally not in a chronically emaciated state since their condition is likely the result of a very short period of malnutrition. As such, young birds/hatchlings should be quickly rehydrated and provided with food almost immediately.

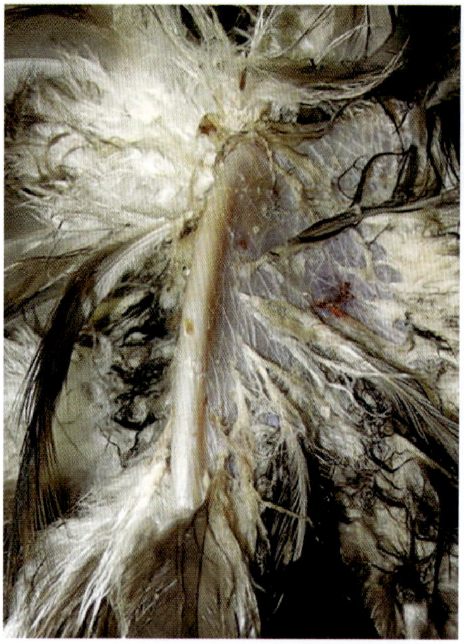

Fig. 7.13. Keel score of 1.5. There is not much muscle mass and both sides of the keel bone can be palpated easily.

- A baseline PCV and TS is a helpful guide to treatment and is a good prognostic indicator. Birds with a keel score < 1.5, PCV < 15%, and/or TS < 1.0 g/dl generally do not survive.
- Rehydration can be difficult: fluids are clearly needed but the danger of hemodilution is a serious consideration. This author prefers to rehydrate slowly via the SQ route.
- Typical protocol:
  - Provide supplemental heat and minimize stress.
  - Injection of iron dextran.
  - Fluid therapy with LRS at 2 × maintenance via the SQ or IO/IV route. Hetastarch can be helpful and Vitamin B supplementation (0.5 ml Vitamin B per 30 ml fluids) in the fluids is also indicated.
  - Whole blood transfusions are indicated if the PCV is less than 20%.
  - A single dose of fenbendazole should be given once the bird is rehydrated.
  - Broad-spectrum antibiotics may be indicated as the bird's immune system may be compromised.
  - An antifungal such as itraconazole or terbinafine should be started immediately, especially for juvenile red-tailed hawks.
  - After 18–24 h, begin providing food. Start with furless whole mice at a rate of 10–15 g/kg BW TID. This can be slowly increased by 10–20% per day over the next few days as long as the bird is not regurgitating or developing crop stasis.
  - Formula diets such as Carnivore Care™ (Oxbow Animal Health, Murdock, ME, USA) may also be helpful, especially in cases that are regurgitating. Anti-emetics such as metoclopramide can be tried but may not be effective in birds.
  - Monitor the weight daily.
  - Gradually move the bird to a whole-prey diet over a 7–10-day period.

Raptor Tip

Rehydrate first. Introduce food very slowly.

Many cases can be saved but it is important to remember that there was an underlying cause that must be addressed.

Raptor Tip

Be aware that many birds will improve dramatically for the first 3 or 4 days and then die unexpectedly.

Head Trauma

Etiology

Blunt force trauma from moving vehicles or window-strikes is very common. This can result in massive intraocular damage as well as intracranial hemorrhages (Figs 7.14 and 7.15) and compression on the brain.

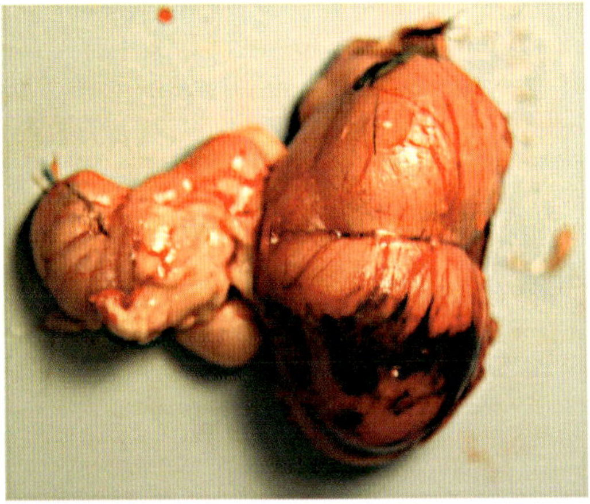

Fig. 7.14. Intracranial hemorrhage.

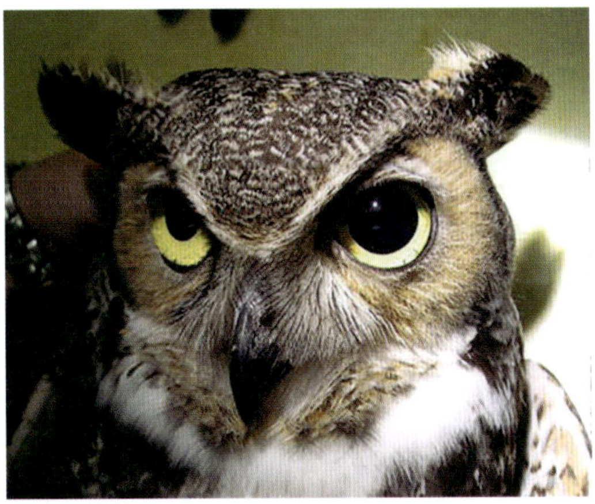

Fig. 7.15. Pronounced anisocoria in a great-horned owl with head trauma.

Clinical signs

- Extreme lethargy, head tilt, head tremors, nystagmus, and anisocoria (unequal pupil size) are common findings.
- Severe damage to one or both eyes as well as fresh blood in the ears and oral cavity are also common.

Diagnosis

- Signs of trauma are usually clear, but it is important to rule out lead toxicity and infectious disease (PMV-1, WNV, etc.) as the cause.

Treatment

- Provide oxygen by mask or in an oxygen cage.
- Butorphanol for analgesia and sedation.
- A single dose of dexamethasone (2 mg/kg) may be helpful although the data are inconclusive and use of corticosteroids in these cases is controversial.
- Meloxicam.
- Mannitol or hypertonic saline with crystalloids can be effective if given within 24 h of the trauma (see Appendix B, Formulary).
- Do *not* provide supplemental heat.
- Supportive care including fluids and midazolam for seizures.
- Resolution of clinical signs, if they are going to resolve, is usually relatively quick and can occur within 7 days. However, some cases can have a more prolonged recovery, so it is hard to know when to "give up". The rule of thumb is to continue as long as you are seeing any signs of improvement.

Lead Toxicosis

Etiology

Lead toxicosis is most commonly caused by the ingestion of prey containing lead shot (Hunt *et al.*, 2009; Redig, 2009), fragments from bullets, or fishing sinkers. It is usually seen in bald eagles which often scavenge deer carcasses but can also be seen in osprey (Slabe, 2019) and vultures due to their eating habits. The disease causes physical damage to nervous tissue which it is thought to be secondary to a vasculitis and resulting hemorrhage/necrosis (Redig, 2010).

Clinical signs

Lead poisoning may present in an acute or chronic form.

- In the acute form, seizures, ataxia, and blindness are common.
- In the chronic form emaciation and generalized weakness are common, as well as hind limb paresis/paralysis.

- In addition, any presentation between these two extremes is possible.
- Anemia and hemoglobinuria can also be present.

> **Raptor Tip**
>
> Check blood lead on all neurologic birds that do not have obvious evidence of trauma and on all scavengers (bald eagles and vultures).

Diagnosis

Diagnosis is based on the blood lead level. Most references consider *concentrations greater than 20 μg/dl to be diagnostic*. However, some species can be either more or less resistant to the effects of lead and concentrations less than 50 μg/dl may be sub-clinical (Stauber *et al.*, 2010). Therefore, the concentration should be interpreted on a case-by-case basis. The LeadCare® (Magellan Diagnostics, North Billerica, MA, USA) (Fig. 7.16) in-house system is an excellent device for testing lead levels. It requires a few drops of whole blood and provides results in 90 s. Note that it is not uncommon for healthy birds to have a background lead level of from 0.5 to 4.0 μg/dl.

Radiographs should also be taken to look for metallic fragments. It is important to realize that lead fragments embedded in muscle tissue (i.e. from a gunshot wound) generally will not cause lead toxicosis (LaDouceur *et al.*, 2015). Removing these fragments is generally not warranted as it can be very difficult to find the fragments and even careful dissection can result in additional tissue trauma. However, lead fragments embedded in fracture sites can lead to toxic levels of absorption (LaDouceur *et al.*, 2015) and should be removed if possible. Lead fragments in the GI tract should also be removed (see below). Note, however, that lead cannot be differentiated from other metals based on radiography.

Treatment

- Prognosis is poor if clinical signs are severe or if the blood lead level on admission is greater than 120 μg/dl (Redig and Ponder, 2010) although birds have been successfully treated with levels as high as 600 μg/dl (L. Degernes, personal communication, 2014). Euthanasia should be considered in these cases.
- Supportive care, including fluid therapy and nutritional support, should be given as many

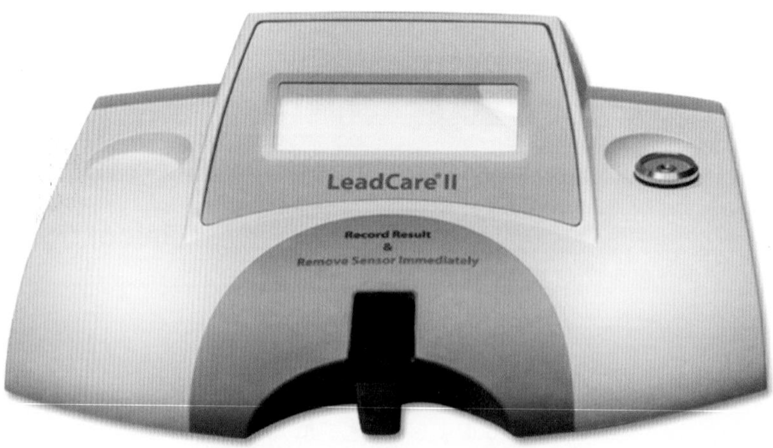

Fig. 7.16. LeadCare® II tester (www.magellandx.com (accessed May 2020)).

of these birds are extremely emaciated and weak.

- Midazolam, as needed, for seizures.
- Treat the anemia if present.
  - Iron dextran for anemia. Repeat in 10 days.
  - Blood transfusions if necessary.
  - Chelation of lead. This step is critical and can be very effective.
  - CaEDTA is considered the treatment of choice. The "name brand" calcium disodium versenate product is expensive; however, compounded products are effective and much more affordable. This is given by injection only (either SQ or IM). CaEDTA tends to chelate heavy metals from the bone.
  - Dimercaptosuccinic acid (DMSA, Succimer) is an oral chelator that preferentially chelates from soft tissues. It can be used alone or in combination with CaEDTA.
  - Duration of chelation therapy is variable and depends on blood lead levels as well as on continued exposure from lead still in the GI tract. In general, plan to chelate for 2–4 weeks but it should be continued until blood lead concentrations have returned to a normal level. There is a chance of a "rebound" toxicity after chelation therapy has ended due to lead leaching back out of the bones (Fig. 7.17). Because of this, the lead level should be checked 1–2 weeks after the cessation of chelation therapy.
- Remove lead in the GI tract.
  - Stomach gavage: the bird is anesthetized on a board with head down at 45° angle. The airway is protected with an ET tube. Gavage with warm water. Measure the tube so it is placed into proventriculus or ventriculus. Repeat the gavage several times and catch all exiting fluid to see if pieces of lead are removed.
  - Raptors produce a pellet in the ventriculus and eject the pellet orally. This process may help in the removal of any lead fragments still in the stomach, so

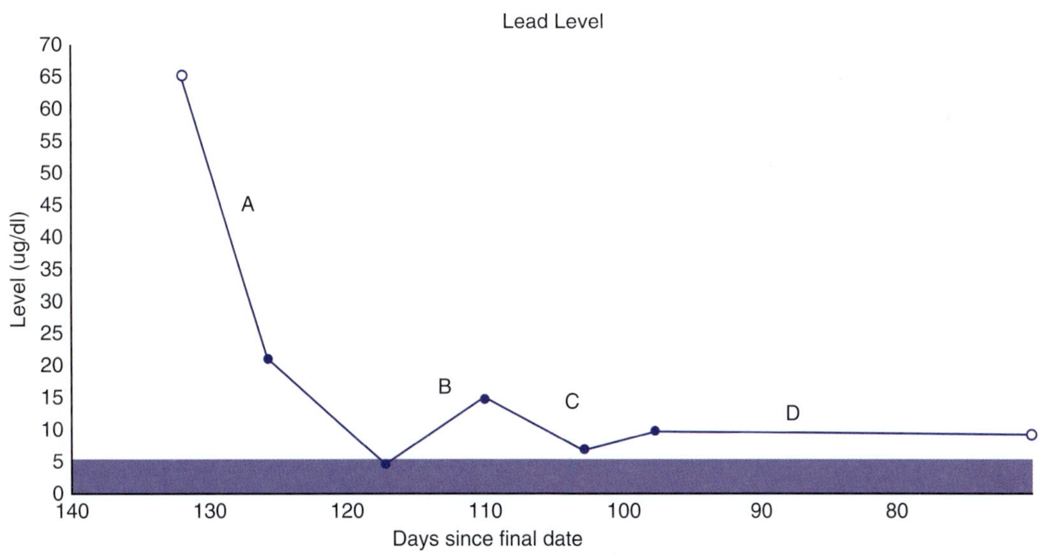

Fig. 7.17. A typical lead chelation curve. A: the lead level can drop quickly during the initial treatment. B: once chelation is stopped, the lead level may rebound. C: the second chelation cycle. D: the second rebound was not very severe so a third chelation was not needed and the level slowly returned to normal without further treatment. Note: the blue band near the bottom represents the target lead level of 5 μg/dl. As displayed in the RaptorMed™ medical records software.

providing casting material such as mouse or rat skin/fur may be beneficial.

- Various cathartics and bulk laxatives can also be tried to attempt to move the fragments out of the GI tract.
- MgSulfate (Epsom salts): 0.5–1 g/kg SID for 1–3 days. Can mix with honey or 50% dextrose.
- Psyllium (Metamucil®, Procter & Gamble, Cincinnati, OH, USA) mixed in a slurry via tube.
- Endoscopic or surgical removal may be required in some cases. Note that surgical removal is not without risk and should only be attempted if all other options have failed.
- Repeat radiographs to monitor removal and movement of the fragments.

Raptor Tip

Recheck blood lead level 2 weeks after stopping chelation therapy.

Metabolic and Nutritional Disorders

Etiology

Deficiencies in the diet can lead to various pathological conditions which can be difficult to prove unless a very complete history is available. Response to treatment leads to a presumptive diagnosis.

Clinical signs

Metabolic bone disease (MBD) results in multiple fractures or curvatures of the long bones (Fig. 7.18), especially in young, growing birds. This is generally due to a diet with an inappropriate calcium:phosphorus ratio and/or a deficiency in calcium such as one composed entirely of boneless meat (i.e. "pinkies"). Clinical disease can progress quickly after an inappropriate diet is begun. Note that this is typically a problem that results from poor husbandry but is also seen in the wild birds (Fig. 7.18). MBD can also be caused by Vitamin D deficiencies due to inadequate access to UVB/sunlight.

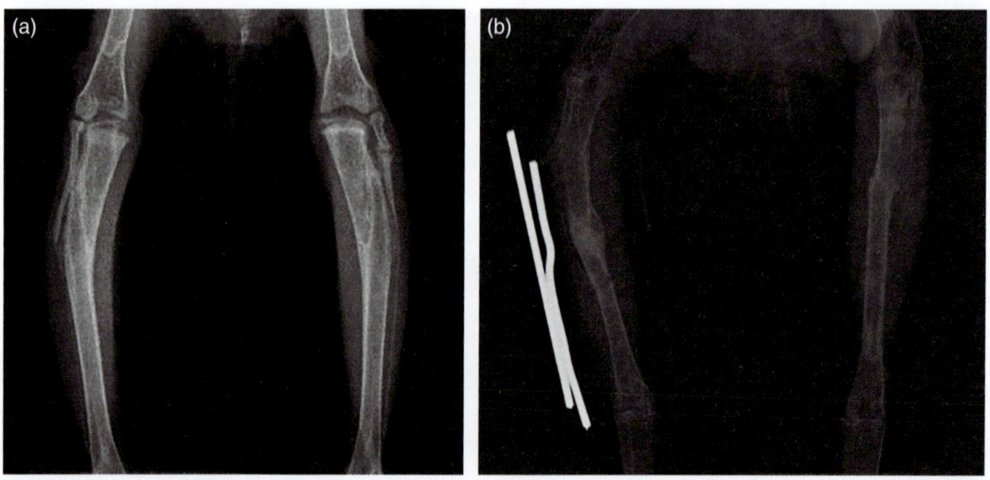

Fig. 7.18. MBD can affect any long bone but is often seen in the legs in young birds. A young barred owl (a) with bilateral curvatures and healing fractures of both tibiotarsus bones and also in a young red-shouldered hawk (b) with five fractures in both legs. Note the perpendicular pin tracts in the left leg after an external fixation device had been removed.

Hypovitaminosis A is rare in wild birds that eat whole prey. When present, it can cause hyperkeratosis, squamous metaplasia of mucous membranes, blunted choanal papillae, blocked nasolacrimal ducts, and/or a reduced mucosal immunity resulting in URT infections.

Hypocalcemia can cause extreme lethargy and neurologic signs such as tremors and seizures. Diagnose with a serum chemistry panel.

Hypovitaminosis E is also rare. Neurologic signs are seen due to encephalomalacia and myopathy.

Thiamine (Vitamin B_1) deficiency can result in a range of neurologic signs such as "star gazing" and ataxia. It is more of a problem in fish-eating birds due to a thiaminase enzyme found in many fish. This is of particular concern in birds whose diet consists of frozen fish.

Treatment

Supplementation of the deficient nutrient can be very helpful and/or curative. Correction of the underlying cause of deficiency is obviously crucial and all fish should be supplemented with vitamins such as Vitahawk (DB Scientific, Oakley, CA, USA). Juvenile raptors with fractures and bone deformities due to MBD may never return to normal and these birds are often non-releasable. Refer to the Feeding Guide in Appendix A.

Paraparesis and Spinal Trauma

Etiology

Blunt force trauma secondary to moving vehicles or window-strikes is very common. The trauma can lead to spinal cord damage and this usually occurs at the junction of the notarium and synsacrum, although confirmation via radiography ± myelogram is difficult.

Clinical signs

- Flaccid paralysis of both legs.
- The vent may be soiled with little or no sphincter tone.
- There may be bruising or instability over the dorsal spine.
- These birds are unable to empty the cloaca normally so their feces often become very gritty and foul smelling, mostly due to fecal stasis and bacterial overgrowth. In addition, the urates may precipitate to form large, rough cloacoliths.
- There may be evidence of keel and feather damage depending on how long the bird has been down.

Diagnosis

- Based on clinical signs.
- A fracture is rarely seen on radiographs.
- Measure the blood lead concentration to rule out lead toxicosis, especially in cases where trauma is not obvious.

Treatment

Treatment and prognosis very much depend on the extent of the clinical signs on admission. Birds can be categorized (Scott, 2015) as shown in Table 7.3. As can be seen, the prognosis is very poor for all except category 1 birds, and many should be euthanized.

> **Raptor Tip**
>
> When a bird appears to have recovered, keep a watch for residual ataxia. This may only be apparent when the bird attempts to turn on a perch, for example.

For birds that will be rehabilitated, the following guidelines are helpful:

- Supportive care. Keep well hydrated via SQ fluid administration and maintain BW. Use furless whole food to decrease the need to produce a pellet. Force-feed as necessary. Note that a formula diet is *not* recommended if the bird is not able to stand since regurgitation and aspiration can occur.

Table 7.3. Spinal trauma categories.

Severity score	Release rate (%)	Clinical signs
1	58	Mild paresis, ataxia. Kicking and grasping strongly
2	7	Severe paresis, paralysis. Deep pain present
3	0	No deep pain, flaccid paralysis. No vent tone

- The use of corticosteroids in these cases is very controversial. A single dose of dexamethasone or Solu-Medrol may or may not be helpful.
- Anti-inflammatories: meloxicam 0.5 mg/kg BID.
- Protect the tail with a tail wrap.
- Keep the bird evacuated and the vent clean.
- Keep on thick padding with head elevated.
- A broad-spectrum antibiotic such as trimethoprim-sulfa seems to help minimize colonic overgrowth. It is crucial to keep these birds well hydrated as this drug can be nephrotoxic.

Birds should be euthanized if there is no improvement in 10 days, if the bird is not self-feeding or is unable to evacuate itself, or if there is radiographic evidence of a spinal fracture.

Pesticide/Insecticide Toxicities

Etiology

Many pesticides and insecticides are in use and toxicity after exposure is likely very common. However, they are usually unrecognized since definitive diagnosis is difficult. There are several categories of chemicals to consider:

- 4-Aminopyridine (Avitrol) affects K^+ channels and induces seizures/convulsions.
- Organophosphates (Diazinon, Malathion, Parathion, Dichlorvos) are irreversible acetylcholinesterase (ACHE) inhibitors. May respond to treatment with atropine.
- Carbamates (Methomyl) reversibly inhibit ACHE. May respond to treatment with atropine.
- Metaldehyde is used in snail bait.
- Organochlorines (Aldrin, Heptachlor) are DDT-like and affect the Na^+ channels in the peripheral nervous system.

Clinical signs

- Diarrhea, vomiting, salivation, and lacrimation may be seen.
- Generalized neurologic signs such as depression, tremors, or seizures may be observed.
- Bradycardia.

Diagnosis

- Measurement of plasma cholinesterase levels is possible but not practical.
- Response to treatment with atropine may indicate an organophosphate.
- Toxin screens of liver, brain, or stomach contents are possible but expensive and are really only available post-mortem.

Treatment

- Supportive care (fluids, etc.).
- Treatment is often difficult as the type of pesticide is rarely known.
- High doses of atropine (see Appendix B, Formulary) and/or 2-PAM/Pralidoxime for organophosphates.
- Midazolam as needed for seizures.
- No treatment for organochlorine intoxications. In this author's experience, there is 100% mortality within 12–24 h.

Soiled Feathers

Etiology

Feathers can be soiled by many different sources and chemicals. The most common are chimney soot, rodent glue traps, and petroleum products including various types of crude oil (Fig. 7.19). Other more unusual sources include sewage at water treatment plants.

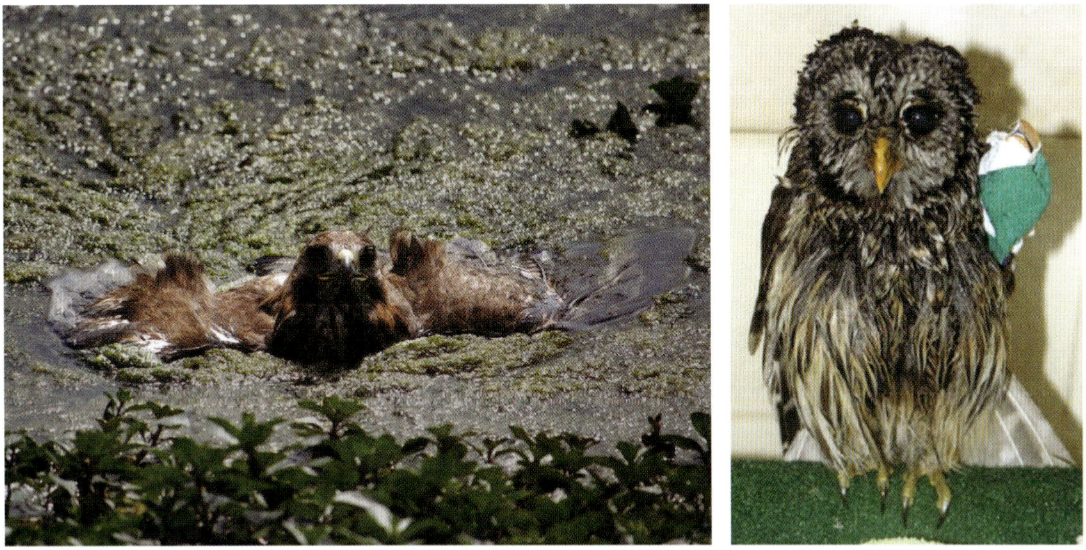

Fig. 7.19. A red-tailed hawk trapped in algae in a pond (left) and a barred owl soiled in cooking oil (right).

Clinical signs

- Besides the obvious damage to the feathers, systemic clinical signs may be present depending on the offending agent.
- Various chemicals and oils may be toxic.
- The feathers may have lost their insulating properties, resulting in hypothermia.
- Depending on the chronicity, the patient may be dehydrated and emaciated if feather damage is severe enough to prevent flight and the ability to hunt.

Treatment

- Supportive care as needed.
- Activated charcoal to reduce systemic absorption.
- Decontamination of feathers must be accomplished but will need to be staged and may need to wait until the bird is stabilized. The feathers may require one or more warm-water baths under general anesthesia (Fig. 7.20). The bird should be placed on an inclined tray with the head elevated. The airway should be protected carefully with an ET tube and gauze packed around the glottis. The eyes should be lubricated. Dawn® dish soap (Procter & Gamble, Cincinnati, OH, USA) works well in many cases and should be mixed as shown in Table 7.4. Do not exceed a concentration of 5%. Blow dry with hair dryer after blotting with a towel. Several baths may be required over 5–10 days. Do not try to do too much in a single bath.
- Thick oils or tarry/sticky substances can be dissolved with canola cooking oil prior to bathing with Dawn®.
- The feathers are clean if they are fluffy and airy when dry. Water should run off the feathers and be deflected when sprayed on them. Feathers that are still oily or soiled form small beads of water when sprayed but will quickly become wet and heavy. Repeated baths will be required until the plumage is completely clean and waterproof.

Table 7.4. Mixing Dawn® dish soap.

%	Dawn® (ml) in 12 US ounces (355 ml) water
1	3.5
2	7
3	10
4	14
5	18

Sour Crop

Etiology

Bacterial or yeast overgrowth due to crop stasis. Crop stasis can be caused by systemic illness and dehydration and it is more common in severely emaciated and debilitated birds.

Clinical signs

- The crop may be full of undigested, spoiled food.
- The bird's breath can be quite malodorous.
- The bird may be depressed and lethargic.

Treatment

- Supportive care including fluid therapy.
- Physically remove all spoiled food with forceps. Be careful not to grab the mucosa inadvertently.
- Repeatedly flush the crop with warm saline until the returned fluid becomes clear. This is done under general anesthesia with the trachea well protected and the bird on a slanted board or table with the head pointing downward. The crop can be filled via a red-rubber feeding tube while the esophagus is manually compressed. The crop is gently massaged and the fluid is then aspirated back out. The crop can also be flushed with dilute chlorhexidine solution.
- Prokinetic drugs such as metoclopramide may be tried.
- Systemic antibiotics or antifungals may be necessary based on cytology of the crop fluid.

Talon Trauma

Etiology

Damage to talons can occur from any type of trauma. Remember that the talon in a raptor is a thin layer of keratin tightly adhered to the distal phalanx. The underlying bone will extend to within 1 or 2 mm from the talon tip. Any significant trauma will likely affect the underlying bone (Fig. 7.21).

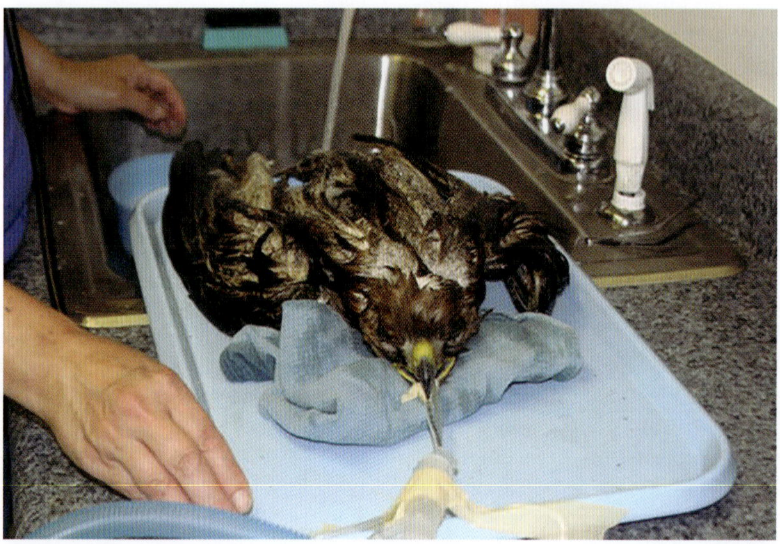

Fig. 7.20. Anesthetized hawk having Dawn® bath.

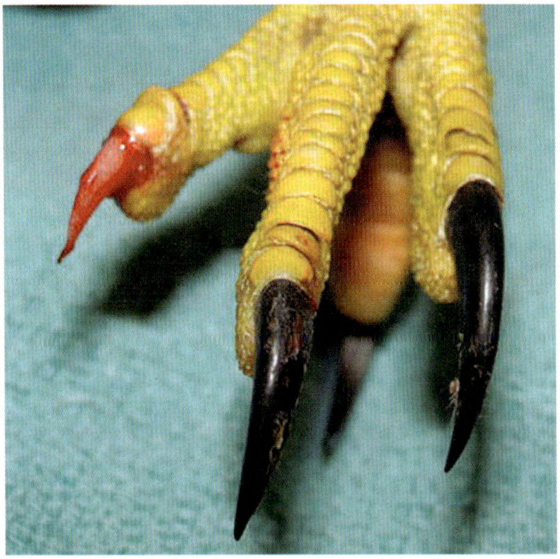

Fig. 7.21. A degloved talon.

Clinical signs

- Broken talon tips with or without bone exposure. Blood loss can be significant.
- In some cases, the entire keratin sheath can loosen and slide off exposing the sensitive phalange bone. This is obviously painful and the exposed bone is at significant risk of desiccation.

Treatment

- Under general anesthesia, gently clean and flush the affected digit. Application of a topical lidocaine gel can be helpful.
- Protect the exposed bone from desiccation with a hydrocolloid dressing such as Duoderm® (ConvaTec, Mulgrave, VIC, Australia). The affected toe and dressing are then protected with a typical foot bandage.
- Alternatively, the damaged talon can be "repaired" by the application of a beak repair product (Fig. 10.44). This has the advantage that a foot bandage is not always required and the bird can still use the foot and toes with minimal pain or discomfort. In addition to the typical beak repair products, multiple layers of cyanoacrylate glue ("Super glue") can be applied to build up a protective layer over the exposed bone. This can work well but reapplication will be necessary as the glue slowly wears off.
- Systemic antibiotics such as clindamycin as well as meloxicam and other analgesics (tramadol, butorphanol) are recommended.
- Note that talon regrowth is a very slow process. If the keratin germinal bed was traumatized, the keratin may not grow back completely or may grow abnormally. In some cases, amputation of the distal phalanx may be necessary (Chapter 9).

Wrist/Carpal Wounds

Etiology

The distal radius, the radial carpal bone, and the alular metacarpal bone all project out from the cranial edge of the carpus. These bones are covered by a thin layer of skin and are therefore at risk of injury when a bird is placed in an inappropriate enclosure.

Clinical signs

An open wound on the leading edge of the carpus accompanied by soiled feathers adjacent to the wound. The joint space is typically exposed (Fig. 7.22).

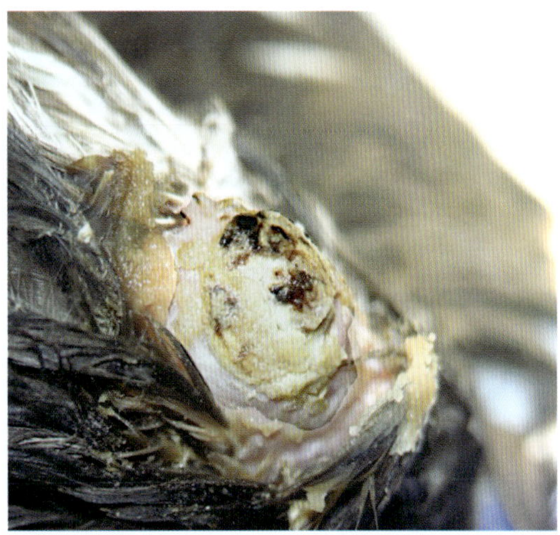

Fig. 7.22. Typical wrist wound.

Treatment

- Surgical debridement under general anesthesia.
- These wounds are typically too large to close with sutures and the high level of motion in the area makes early closure challenging. Fortunately, a granulation bed usually forms rapidly.
- Frequent (every other day) wound flushes and bandage changes. Silver sulfadiazine (SSD) ointment, a non-adherent pad/gauze for padding, and Tegaderm™ (3M, St Paul, MN, USA) work well. If the wound is flushed carefully so that the surrounding feathers stay dry, the Tegaderm™ will stick well. It is important that the Tegaderm™ be placed with the carpus extended (Fig. 7.23). If not, it will tear off as soon as the bird folds up the wing.
- Systemic antibiotics are usually not required but topical triple-antibiotic ointment is useful. An ointment that contains a steroid such as dexamethasone can be helpful to avoid excessive formation of granulation tissue.

Prevention

Place bandages on carpi pre-emptively, as described above, in species more prone to injury such as bald eagles and osprey. Additional layers of gauze or thin foam can be added under the Tegaderm™ to provide more padding. If placed correctly, the carpus maintains its full ROM and flight is not impeded.

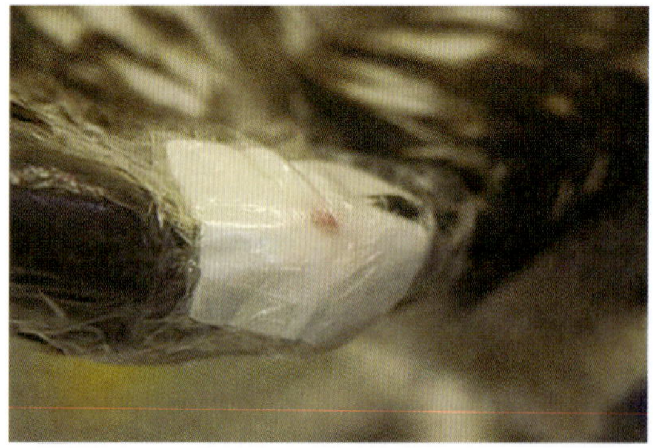

Fig. 7.23. Wrist bandage secured with Tegaderm™.

Bibliography

Ford, S., Chitty, J. and Jones, M. (2010) Surgical aspects of raptor feet. Handout. *31st Conference of the Association of Avian Veterinarians, San Diego, CA, USA*. Association of Avian Veterinarians, Teaneck, NJ, USA.

Hunt, W.G., Parish, C.N., Orr, K. and Aguilar, R.F. (2009) Lead poisoning and the reintroduction of the California condor in northern Arizona. *Journal of Avian Medicine and Surgery* 23(2), 145–150.

LaDouceur, E.E., Kagan, R., Scanlan, M. and Viner, T. (2015) Chronically embedded lead projectiles in wildlife: a case series investigating the potential for lead toxicosis. *Journal of Zoo and Wildlife Disease* 46, 438–442.

Redig, P. (2009) Lead from spent ammunition: a source of poisoning in bald eagles. *Proceedings of the 30th Conference of the Association of Avian Veterinarians, Milwaukee, WI, USA*. Association of Avian Veterinarians, Teaneck, NJ, USA, pp. 427–428.

Redig, P. (2010) Use of MRI and histological methods for detection of lead-induced lesions in the CNS of bald eagles. *Proceedings of the 31st Conference of the Association of Avian Veterinarians, San Diego, CA, USA*. Association of Avian Veterinarians, Teaneck, NJ, USA, pp. 33–34.

Redig, P. and Ponder, J. (2010) Raptors: practical information every avian practitioner can use. *Proceedings of the 31st Conference of the Association of Avian Veterinarians, San Diego, CA, USA*. Association of Avian Veterinarians, Teaneck, NJ, USA, pp. 171–180.

Remple, J.D. (2006) A multifaceted approach to the treatment of bumblefoot in raptors. *Journal of Exotic Pet Medicine* 15(1), 49–55.

Sadar, M.J., Guzman, D.S.-M., Mete, A., Foley, J., Stephenson, N., Rogers, K.H., *et al.* (2015) Mange caused by a novel *Micnemidocoptes* mite in a golden eagle (*Aquila chyrsaetos*). *Journal of Avian Medicine and Surgery* 29(3), 231–237.

Scott, D. (2015) A retrospective look at outcomes of raptors with spinal trauma. *Proceedings of the 2nd International Conference on Avian, Herpetological, and Exotic Mammal Medicine, Paris, France*. European Association of Avian Veterinarians, p. 391. Available at: www.eaavonline.org (accessed February 2016).

Slabe, V.A., Anderson, J.T., Cooper, J., Brown, B., Ortiz, P., Buchweitz, J., *et al.* (2019) Lead in piscivorous raptors during breeding season in the Chesapeake Bay Region of Maryland and Virginia, USA. *Environmental Toxicology and Chemistry* 38(4), 862–871.

Stauber, E.I., Finch, N., Talcott, P.A. and Gay, J.M. (2010) Lead poisoning of bald (*Haliaeetus leucocephalus*) and golden (*Aquila chrysaetos*) eagles in the U.S. inland Pacific northwest region—an 18-year retrospective study: 1991–2008. *Journal of Avian Medicine and Surgery* 24(4), 279–287.

8 Anesthesia

Learning Objectives

1. Basic anesthetic protocols.
2. Proper oxygen flow rates and endotracheal tube placement.
3. Safe monitoring of vital signs.

Induction and maintenance of anesthesia in raptors is relatively easy but, as with all species, careful monitoring is always necessary. Gas anesthesia is usually the safest and most convenient method. A non-rebreathing system such as an Ayers T-piece configuration with a high flow rate (Fig. 8.1) should be used. Isoflurane works very well, is safe, and has a fast duration of onset and recovery. Newer gases such as sevoflurane are also becoming popular and may be advantageous in patients with cardiac arrhythmias. However, they can be quite a bit more expensive.

Induction is carried out by masking the bird down with 3–4% isoflurane in oxygen at a flow rate of at least *1 liter/min/kg*.

Pre-oxygenation and premedication/pre-emptive analgesia with butorphanol are very useful and are highly recommended. Birds appear to have a predominance of kappa opioid receptors so butorphanol, which has primarily kappa agonist action, is currently the opioid of choice in birds.

Midazolam can also be a beneficial premedication and can be used in combination with butorphanol. The use of NSAIDs such as meloxicam is not recommended prior to anesthesia due to the chance for renal toxicity during potentially hypotensive periods while under anesthesia. Parasympatholytics such as atropine are not recommended as a pre-anesthetic since they tend to thicken respiratory secretions and can potentially cause a clogged ET tube. Atropine, however, can be used to combat bradycardia during anesthesia.

Premedications

Butorphanol: 10 mg/ml
Dosage: 2 mg/kg = 0.2 ml/kg IM
Midazolam:
Dosage: 1.25 mg/kg (volume depends on concentration)

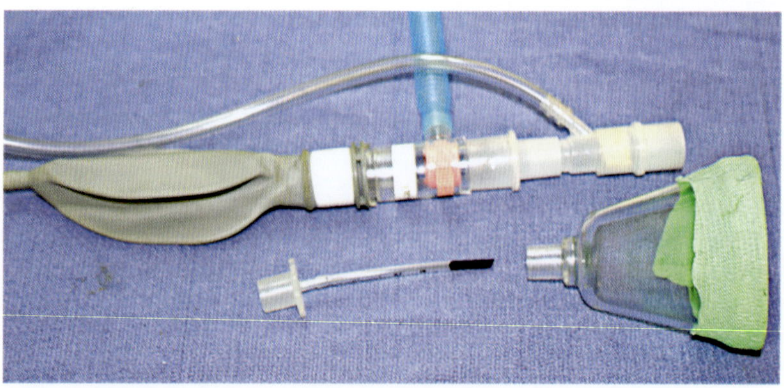

Fig. 8.1. Non-rebreathing system with a small mask and an uncuffed ET tube.

Raptor Tip

It may be wise to wait a few days before anesthetizing a patient with recent head trauma.

Table 8.1. ET tube sizes.

Species	ET tube size (outer diameter in mm)
Eastern screech owl	<2
Cooper's hawk	2.0–2.5
Red-shouldered hawk	2.5–3.0
Barred owl	3.0
Red-tailed hawk	3.0–4.0
Great-horned owl	3.5–4.5
Bald eagle	5.0–5.5

Intubation is recommended for any procedure lasting more than 10–15 min or if the risk of regurgitation and subsequent aspiration is high. The glottis is generally quite large and is easily accessible at the base of the tongue. Birds have complete tracheal rings, so ET tubes with inflatable cuffs should never be used since inflation can result in mucosal necrosis. Only non-cuffed tubes should be used (Table 8.1).

Small birds can be intubated with a tube fashioned from a urinary cannula or an oral suction catheter (Fig. 8.2). These tubes are 1–2 mm in diameter so the risk of clogging is significant. In these cases, using positive pressure ventilation helps keep the tube clear.

Once placed, the tube is secured to the lower beak with tape and usually fits nicely into the groove formed by the lower beak when the tongue is pushed to the side (Fig. 8.3).

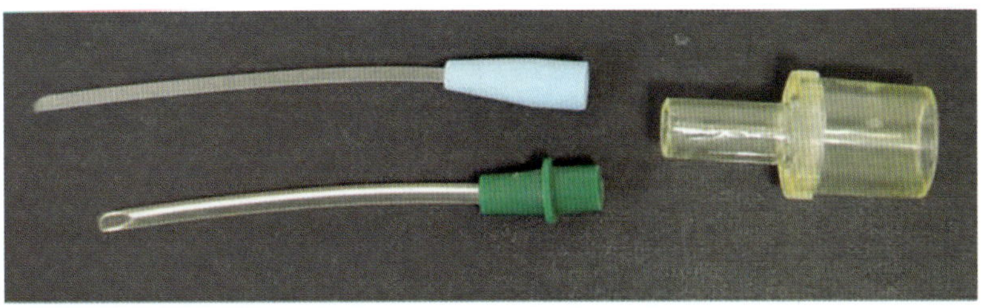

Fig. 8.2. Small ET tube made from a human oral suction catheter (Kimberly Clark, Irving, TX, USA). The tube can be attached to a common anesthesia tubing adapter with white cloth tape.

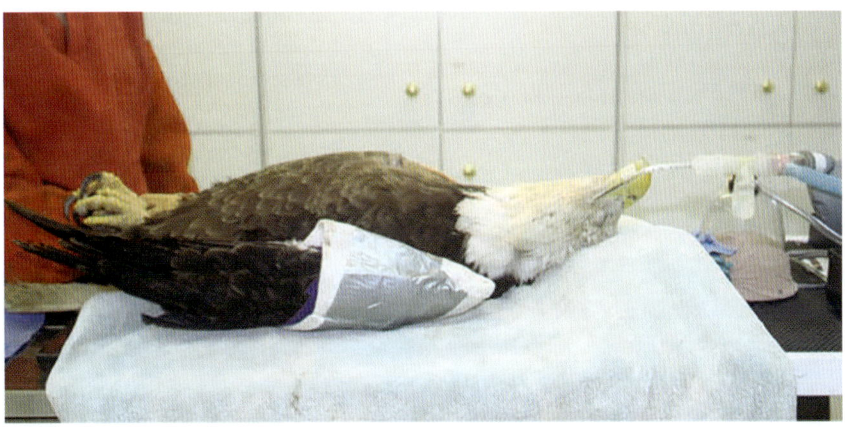

Fig. 8.3. Bald eagle under gas anesthesia.

> **Raptor Tip**
>
> To prevent the ET tube from getting loose, be sure to loop the tape around the tube completely before securing it to the beak.

Ideally, raptors should be fasted at least 12 h before induction of anesthesia. However, this may not always be possible, for example in a young bird or in one of the smaller species such as a sharp-shinned hawk. Always check for a full crop before inducing anesthesia. If the crop is full and anesthesia must be performed:

- Manually empty the crop with forceps if possible.
- Place a loop of elastic wrap around the neck to provide some pressure on the cranial esophagus.
- Keep the head elevated.
- Pack the throat with gauze.

> **Raptor Tip**
>
> For safety, wrap the talons with tape or elastic wrap while the bird is under anesthesia.

Monitoring

Depth of anesthesia can be determined by many factors. When a bird is too light:

- The wings will pull up to the sides and may begin to flutter.
- The talons will clench.
- The legs will be drawn upward towards the body.
- The respiratory rate will increase.

When a bird is at a good surgical plane of anesthesia:

- The respiratory rate is slow (15–20 breaths per min), deep, and regular.
- The palpebral reflex is gone and the eyelids are closed.
- The pupils may dilate.

When a bird is deep:

- The heart rate will decrease.
- The respiration rate will decrease and the breaths will be shallow.
- The corneal reflex is gone.

Note that birds have a tendency to appear deep, and then suddenly to become reactive with little or no warning regarding changes in heart and respiration rate. Paradoxically, it is not uncommon for the heart rate to drop in response to painful stimuli.

Heart Rate

Monitoring of any avian patient should include the heart rate via stethoscope. The Littman Infant Model® (3M, St. Paul, MN, USA) with a 2.5 cm head is ideal for most avian patients. In addition, an esophageal stethoscope is very helpful since it frees up both hands.

Heart rate can also be monitored with a Doppler flow probe (Fig. 8.4). The transducer may be placed in a few places:

- The superficial radial artery on the ventral side of the elbow joint near the basilic vein (see Figs 4.10 and 8.4).
- The deep radial artery on the ventral carpal joint.
- The cranial tibial artery on the cranial surface of the hock joint.
- The roof of the mouth. This is very useful in larger birds.

An electrocardiogram is helpful but can be frustrating at times since it is difficult to maintain a steady baseline, especially when the bird is being manipulated during an orthopedic procedure.

Respiratory Rate

The respiratory rate should always be monitored carefully. This is best done by visualizing the chest rise and fall, or by seeing the anesthetic bag inflate and deflate. Using clear drapes during a surgical procedure can aid in visualizing.

Shallow breathing is not uncommon and this can lead to hypercapnia and respiratory acidosis. An end tidal CO_2 ($ETCO_2$) monitor is useful to maintain the $ETCO_2$ around 30–45 mmHg and is especially important for procedures lasting longer than 45 min. Manual breaths (at least 2 per min) or use of a ventilator is helpful in preventing hypercapnia.

Raptor Tip

Under isoflurane anesthesia:

Great-horned owl: pupils often become fixed and maximally dilated.

Barred owl: the unfeathered areas around the beak can become bright pink.

Osprey: produces a large amount of mucus so be sure to swab the oral cavity.

Many falcons may not close their eyes so be sure to lubricate them.

Temperature

Body temperature can be monitored, but it is more important to provide supplemental heat. The high oxygen flow rates used in avian anesthesia, fluid flushed into wounds, and the surgical prep can have a significant cooling effect. A warm water (not electric) table-top heating pad is ideal, since there is no chance of inadvertent burns or fires. All fluids used for flushing wounds should be warmed.

Blood Pressure

Systolic blood pressure (BP) can and should be measured whenever possible. A sphygmomanometer (Fig. 8.5) is used in conjunction with the Doppler flow probe to indirectly measure BP. This can be difficult in smaller birds but works well in most species. The transducer is placed as

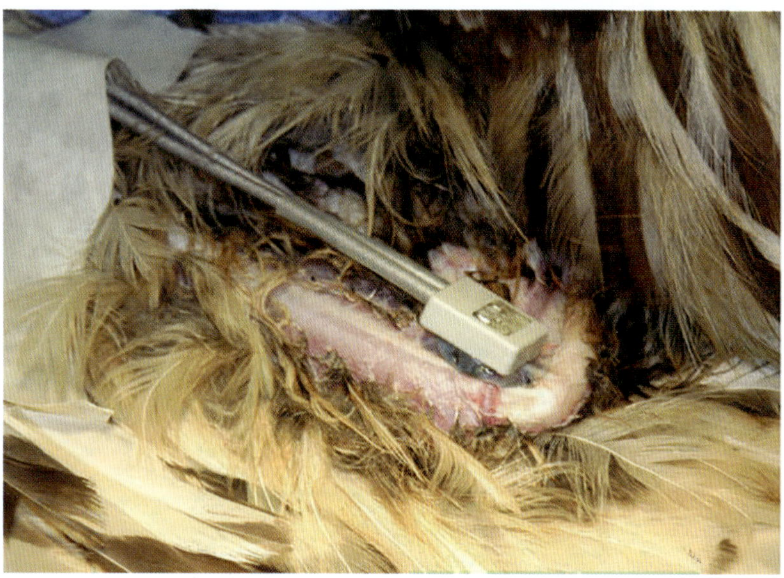

Fig. 8.4. A Doppler probe placed over the superficial radial artery on the ventral side of the elbow.

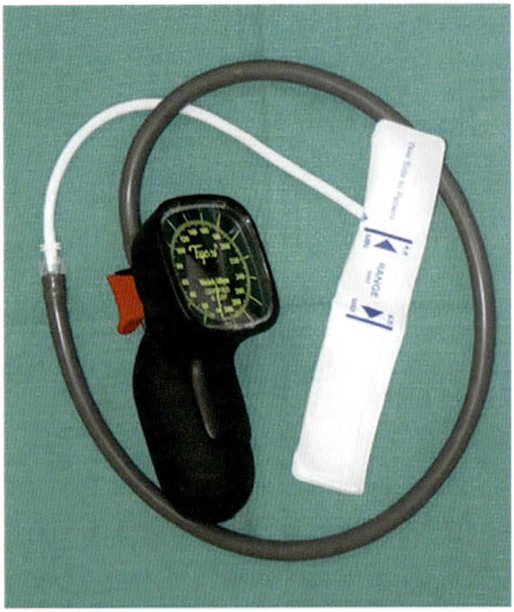

Fig. 8.5. Sphygmomanometer and small cuff.

described previously and the cuff is placed proximal to it, either around the humerus (Fig. 8.6) or tibiotarsus. The cuff is then inflated to a suprasystemic pressure (until the Doppler signal stops). The cuff is then slowly deflated until the signal returns. This is the systolic pressure.

Realize that the size of the cuff and the location can dramatically affect the readings. In addition, indirect measurements do not correlate well with direct measurements, so it is important to monitor the *trends* and not focus on the actual values as much. A decreasing BP trend (Table 8.2) can indicate hypovolemia, hypothermia, and/or blood loss, so the appropriate measures (i.e. fluid therapy, heat, etc.) should be taken.

Maintenance of Anesthesia

The oxygen flow should be at least *1 liter/min/kg*. The isoflurane percentage should be adjusted constantly, as needed, always seeking the lowest

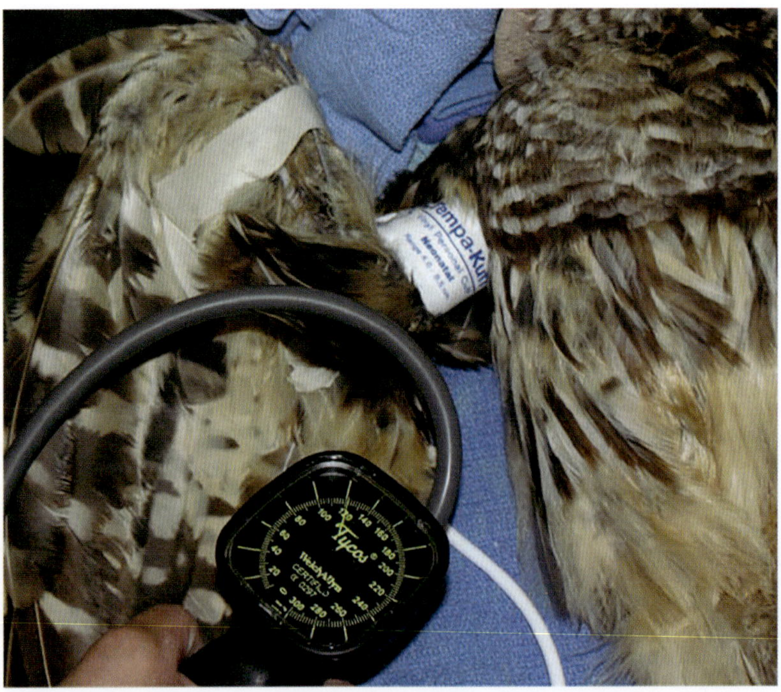

Fig. 8.6. A BP cuff placed around the humerus of a barred owl.

Table 8.2. BP values. Note that these are only general guidelines. The *trends* observed during anesthesia are much more important.

Species	Systolic pressure (mmHg)
Normal awake	120–180
Anesthetized	90–150
Hypotension	<90
Hypertension	>200

possible concentration. Premedication with butorphanol helps to lower your gas requirements. Typical procedures can be completed with a setting between 2 and 3% but each case is unique and should be treated as such.

Raptor Tip

Oxygen flow rate should be 1 liter/min/kg.

It is difficult to clearly state "normal" heart and respiratory rates since they vary so much with the species, the individual, and stress level. In general, larger birds have a lower heart rate than smaller birds (Table 8.3). In addition to the heart rate, one must always listen for the "quality" of the heart beat as well as for arrhythmias.

The respiration rate should be deep and should be around 15–20 breaths per min.

All patients should be given a few deep breaths manually each minute, by compressing the bag attached to the anesthetic circuit.

A ventilator is very handy to have as apnea is not uncommon in birds. Pressure-based machines such as the Vetronics VT-9093 Small Animal Ventilator (BASi-Vetronics, West Lafayette, IN, USA) are useful and allow the depth of inhalation to be controlled. A snug ET tube is needed for proper operation since an airtight seal is required between the tube and the glottis. These types of ventilators can also help keep smaller-diameter ET tubes from clogging. A potential problem with pressure-based ventilators is that a partially obstructed or kinked ET tube may not be noticed since the machine will continue to deliver gas at a preset pressure but at a reduced volume. Monitoring $ETCO_2$ as described above will allow this problem to be discovered quickly.

A word of caution: be very careful to slowly wean your patient off the ventilator as hypoventilation and death can occur if the bird is not able to breathe independently.

Warmed crystalloids are very beneficial in maintaining BP when given at a rate of *10 ml/kg/h* through an IV or IO catheter. A fast bolus of about 5–10 ml/kg at the beginning of the procedure is helpful as are *boluses of 5–10 ml/kg during periods of hypotension*. For stable patients and short, elective procedures, SQ fluids can be given at 30–40 ml/kg prior to induction.

It is a good practice to maintain your patient on oxygen after the procedure is over. This should continue until visible signs of recovery are evident.

Table 8.3. Target heart rate.

Species	Heart rate (bpm)
Eastern screech owl	200
Red-shouldered hawk/barred owl	180
Red-tailed hawk/great-horned owl	170–180
Black vulture/turkey vulture	120–150
Bald eagle	140–150

Emergency Drug Dosages

Epinephrine: 1:1000 = 1 mg/ml
Dosage: 0.5 mg/kg = 0.5 ml/kg IV
Atropine: 0.54 mg/ml
Dosage: 0.1 mg/kg = 0.2 ml/kg IV
Doxapram: 20 mg/ml
Dosage: 10 mg/kg = 0.5 ml/kg IV, IM
For epinephrine and atropine, triple the dosage for the IM route.

Theory and Practice

In theory, it should be possible to hook up every instrument and monitor a whole host of

Page 1 of __

Anesthesia Record

Patient Id Cody | Date 12/2/15

Species HAHA | Weight 718 g

Procedure Toe Amputation | ET tube size 3

Premeds Fluids LRS 35 SQ | Flow rate 1 L\min O_2

Analgesia Torb 0.15 Im | IO Catheter ______

Antibiotics on enrofloxacin | Vent - Max pressure ______

Post Op enro ½ cc SQ, meloxi 0.07 Im | Exp length ______

Time Intubation: 1:53 pm Start: 2:02 pm SX Stop: 2:13 Extubation: 2:22 pm

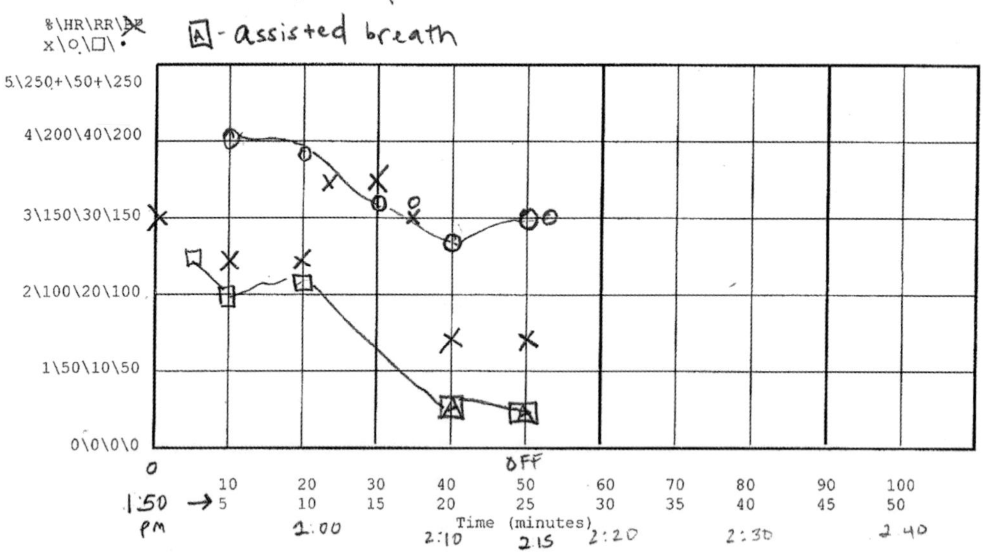

Emergency drug dosages	
Epinephrine (1:1000): 0.5 ml\kg IV =	1.05 IM
Atropine: 0.05 ml\kg IV =	0.42 IM 2:11 pm
Dopram: 0.5 ml\kg IV, (IM) SQ =	0.35 2:18 pm

2:11 atropine

2:15 isoflurane off

2:20 awake

2:18 Dopram

Fig. 8.7. Sample anesthetic record.

parameters. In practice this is not always possible and in fact, in some situations, it is inadvisable. It can often take quite a bit of tweaking and adjusting to get everything working properly and it does not make sense to spend more time setting up your monitors than it takes to complete the entire procedure. Additionally, it is very easy to get distracted by countless alarms and inaccurate or fluctuating measurements. It is safer and more efficient to stick to the basics:

- Heart rate monitoring with esophageal stethoscope ± Doppler flow.
- Respiratory rate and depth monitoring—watch the bag inflate and the chest rise and fall. Manually bag the patient once or twice each minute.
- Provide supplemental heat.
- Have IV/IO access ready for fluids and emergency drugs.
- Record your measurements on an anesthetic log (Fig. 8.7) so trends are obvious.

In addition, the following are helpful:

- Monitor $ETCO_2$.
- Intermittent BP measurements.

Bibliography

Ceulemans, S.M., Guzman, D.S., Olsen, G.H., Beaufrère, H. and Paul-Murphy, J.R. (2014) Evaluation of thermal antinociceptive effects after intramuscular administration of buprenorphine hydrochloride to American kestrels (*Falco sparverius*). *American Journal of Veterinary Research* 75(8), 705–710.

Mans, C.I., Guzman, D.S., Lahner, L.L., Paul-Murphy, J. and Sladky, K.K. (2012) Sedation and physiologic response to manual restraint after intranasal administration of midazolam in Hispaniolan Amazon parrots (*Amazona ventralis*). *Journal of Avian Medicine and Surgery* 26(3), 130–139.

Ritchie, B.W., Harrison, G.J. and Harrison, L.R. (1994) *Avian Medicine: Principles and Application*. Wingers Publishing, Inc., Lake Worth, FL, USA.

Rupiper, D.J., Mashima, T.Y., James, W. and Carpenter, G. (2001) *Exotic Animal Formulary*, 2nd edn. W.B. Saunders Company, Philadelphia, PA, USA.

9 Soft Tissue Surgery

Learning Objectives

1. Creating a sterile field.
2. Instruments and suture material required.
3. Dealing with barbed-wire injuries.
4. Abdominal approaches and procedures.
5. Toe amputation.

Preparing the Surgical Field

The feathers are of vital importance. Therefore, always pluck as few feathers as possible to create a sterile field. It is always preferable to pluck feathers, rather than to clip them, since this encourages feather regrowth and minimizes the time required before eventual release. However, some feather clipping instead of plucking may be necessary in cases where the skin is badly traumatized and torn.

A sterile field can be created using masking tape in a border around the surgical field (Fig. 9.1). Masking tape forms a nice margin, does not leave a sticky residue on the feathers, and can be surgically prepared prior to the placement of traditional drapes.

The surgical field should be prepared with scrubs of iodine or chlorhexidine-based antiseptics alternated with either alcohol or saline. Be careful when using alcohol around existing wounds. In addition, alcohol has a significant cooling effect and can cause hypothermia in small birds, or even in large birds, if used on the body wall or abdomen.

Suture and Instruments

Braided, absorbable suture such as polyglactin 910 (Vicryl®, Ethicon, Somerville, NJ, USA) is ideal for working with thin bird skin. It is very flexible, has excellent knot security, and the absorption time (approximately 21 days) is usually long enough for most avian applications. Reports in the literature regarding excessive tissue reaction have not been noticed by this author. A swedged-on, taper needle is preferred over a cutting needle since a cutting needle is not necessary for avian skin/tissue and can lead to undesirable tears when under tension. The most useful suture size is 4-O, but 3-O and 5-O should also be available as needed. Monofilament, absorbable suture such as polydioxanone (PDS®, Ethicon, Somerville, NJ, USA) has very little drag but it is very stiff and has poor knot security. In addition, its absorption period (180 days) is often much longer than is required.

Following general surgical guidelines, a monofilament suture should be used when dealing with an organ with a lumen such as the GI tract, in order to prevent wicking and leakage of fluid.

Avian surgery does not necessarily require different surgical instruments, but smaller, more delicate instruments than typically found in small animal packs are very helpful. Every surgery pack should have the following:

- Two high-quality Brown-Adson forceps. Use them with a very gentle touch to minimize tissue damage.
- Small, high-quality, curved iris scissors and at least one small, curved hemostat.

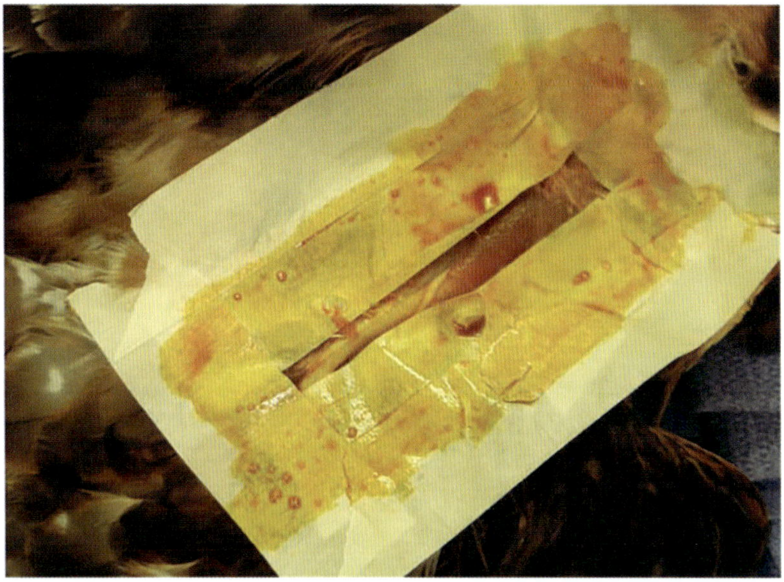

Fig. 9.1. Establishing a clear surgical field with masking tape.

- One 4½″ (11.4 cm) needle driver. Olsen-Hegars are best because they have integrated cutting edges.
- Sterile, cotton-tipped applicators.

General Wound Care

Birds have very little subcutaneous tissue. Scabs that may appear superficial may actually penetrate deeply to the underlying structures (i.e. bone, tendon, etc.). Therefore, "no good scab should go unpicked" and repeated surgical debridements under general anesthesia should be performed as needed.

Standard wound care principles should be followed which include wet-to-dry debriding dressings, followed by non-adherent dressings such as Telfa™ pads (Covidien, Dublin, Republic of Ireland). Once necrotic tissue has been removed, granulation tissue will develop quickly, and staged, partial closure of wounds can be attempted. Hydrocolloid dressings such as Duoderm® (Convatec, Greensboro, NC, USA) work very well to prevent desiccation when applied to wounds with exposed bone and other delicate tissue such as tendons. Oil emulsion dressings such as Adaptic® (Johnson & Johnson, New Brunswick, NJ, USA) or Curity™ (Convatec, Greensboro, NC, USA) are excellent for covering granulated wounds and Tegaderm™ (3M, St Paul, MN, USA) is great for all types of wounds and for securing the other dressings in place (Fig. 9.2). SSD cream (Ascend Laboratories, Parsippany, NJ, USA) works very well as a topical treatment for all sorts of wounds.

> **Raptor Tip**
>
> For wounds that are not healing well, try mixing 1 ounce (30 ml) of SSD cream with 100 units of regular insulin.

Barbed-wire Injuries

Barbed-wire injuries are often extremely serious. They can result in devastating loss or destruction of tissue, typically on the ventral side of the humerus, elbow, and ulna/radius. Owls are most commonly affected, due to their preference for hunting at night often in areas where barbed wire is commonly used (Fig. 9.3).

The barbs are often tightly wrapped into the patagium and the ligamentum propatagialis may be devitalized or transected. Treatment is as follows:

- Supportive care including fluids, analgesics, antibiotics, and anti-inflammatories should be given.
- The wire barbs must be removed and the tissue untwisted as soon as possible in order to restore the blood supply. Needle-nosed wire cutters are useful to cut the barbs out from both sides of the wing.
- The tissue should be cleaned and flushed.
- Any exposed tendon or bone should be covered immediately. Close any available skin wounds or use hydrogel dressings to prevent desiccation if tendon is exposed.
- Place wing in a figure-8 wrap for support.

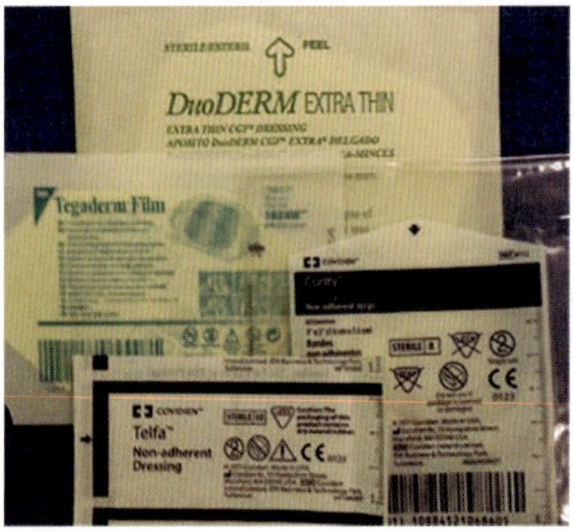

Fig. 9.2. Dressings that are very useful for treating avian wounds.

Raptor Tip

Give barbed-wire injuries some time to heal before attempting to repair.

It may take several days or a week for the full extent of the damage and necrosis to become evident. Surgical repair of major defects in the patagium web or patagial tendon should not be rushed because attempts to repair too early may result in dehiscence.

Extensive scar tissue formation can result during the healing process, so repeated PT should be carried out to ensure full ROM is maintained.

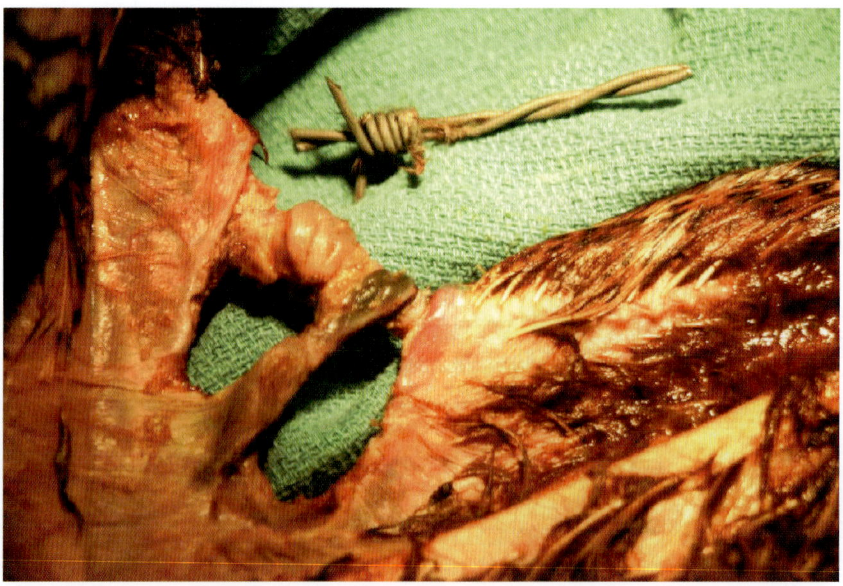

Fig. 9.3. A typical barbed-wire injury in a great-horned owl. This wound involves the propatagium and the ligamentum propatagialis.

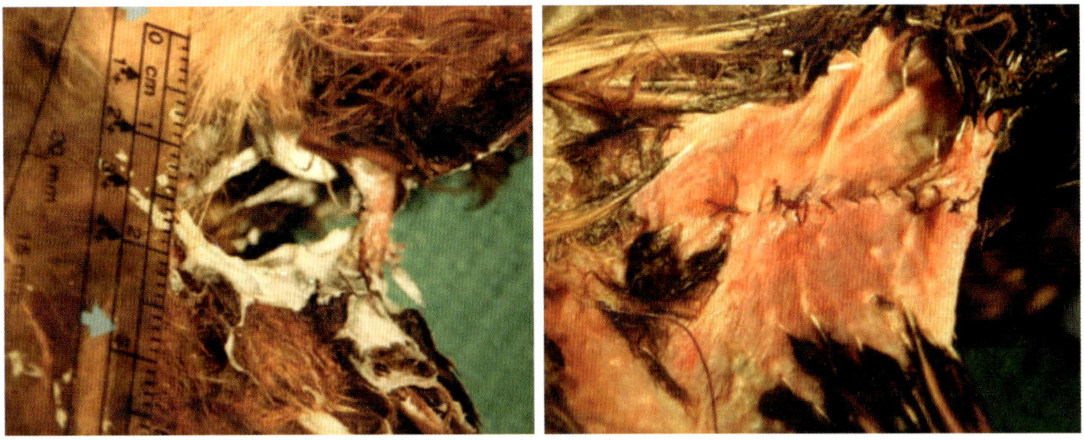

Fig. 9.4. Before (left) and after pictures (right) of a barbed-wire injury. The patagial tendon was intact in this case.

The blood supply to the patagium is not extensive so be sure to create fresh, bleeding edges before suturing. Defects should be sutured on the ventral and dorsal aspects of the web (Fig. 9.4).

If the damage is not extensive, the ends of the ligamentum propatagialis can be freshened and reconnected. Be sure to get healthy tissue edges before reconnecting the tendon. It is better to lose a few more millimeters of tendon than to attempt to reconnect non-viable tissue. Use 6-O, absorbable, monofilament suture (e.g. PDS®) and a tension-relieving pattern such as the Bunnell pattern (Fig. 9.5). The wing must be immobilized for several weeks. With careful post-op PT, losses of a few centimeters of tendon can be accommodated and full extension may be regained (see Chapter 10 regarding PT).

Some of these wounds cannot be repaired and the patagium and tendon must be resected. It has been stated that an intact patagium and ligamentum propatagialis are required for flight and successful release. However, some birds with radical resections (Fig. 9.6) can actually fly very well. Therefore, resection and flight cage testing should be tried, whenever possible (Scott, 2011). The potential for scarring and contracture is great, so repeated assessment of ROM and PT will be required and should be continued long after the wound has superficially healed. Note: the loss of extensive patagial surface area will probably be of more significance to soaring birds such as vultures, so this may not be a useful option in those species. In addition, the sound level will more than likely be affected, so be sure to carefully evaluate all owls before release.

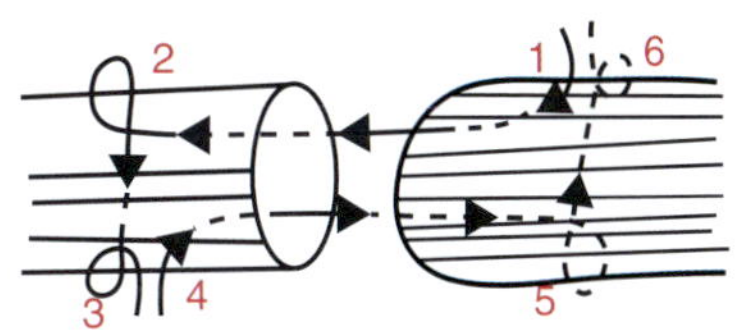

Fig. 9.5. Bunnell pattern for tendon repair. The loose ends at 1 and 6 are tied as are the ends at 3 and 4.

Many patagium wounds will include full-thickness defects, or "portholes" (Fig. 9.7). The defects are often impossible to close, especially when the wing is undergoing PT. Luckily, these portholes will contract over time and they rarely pose a problem. Therefore, attempting to close these defects is not necessary. As stated above for the radical resection, the ROM of the elbow and wrist should be periodically assessed. PT may be required, and performed frequently, since scar tissue formation and contracture are likely. The prognosis for these injuries is very good.

Celiotomy

There are several different approaches to gain access to the abdominal space and the choice depends on the target organ. Any approach will necessarily penetrate the air sacs and this will lead to leakage of anesthetic gas and potential difficulty in maintaining anesthesia by inhalation anesthetics. The surgical site should be packed with saline-soaked gauze to prevent as much gas escape as possible. In addition, the head should be elevated to prevent fluids used for flushing from draining into the respiratory tract.

The patient should be fasted for 12 h, if possible, and should be allowed to produce a pellet before surgery as this will reduce the size of the ventriculus and greatly enhance exposure to the abdomen.

In all cases, the incision should be made by tenting the skin off the body wall musculature, making a small stab incision in the skin, and then extending the incision with scissors. This is then repeated with the body wall, with the muscular layer tented above the underlying organs. A sweeping incision with a scalpel blade is dangerous and can lead to lacerations of the viscera. The body wall and skin should always be closed separately in two layers.

Raptor Tip

Be very careful to not lacerate the viscera when entering the abdominal cavity.

Ventral approach

This approach is useful for access to the cloaca, ventriculus, and small intestine. This is also a good approach for liver biopsies and in treating cases of egg binding.

- A ventral midline or trans-abdominal (either cranial, mid-abdominal, or caudal) incision can be made. In addition, the two incisions can be combined to form a flap for increased access (Fig. 9.8).
- A typical ventral midline incision extends from the caudal border of the sternum to the cranial extent of the cloaca. A cranial trans-abdominal incision should be made at least 5 mm from the caudal border of the sternum to allow enough muscle wall to close the incision. The caudal trans-abdominal incision is made 1–2 cm cranial to the vent.

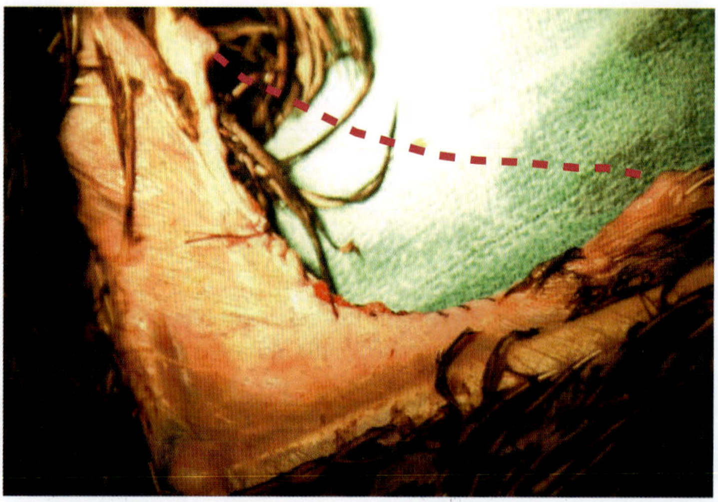

Fig. 9.6. Same bird as in Fig 9.3 after resection of necrotic tissue. The dotted line indicates the extent of the wing web before the injury. This bird healed and flew very well.

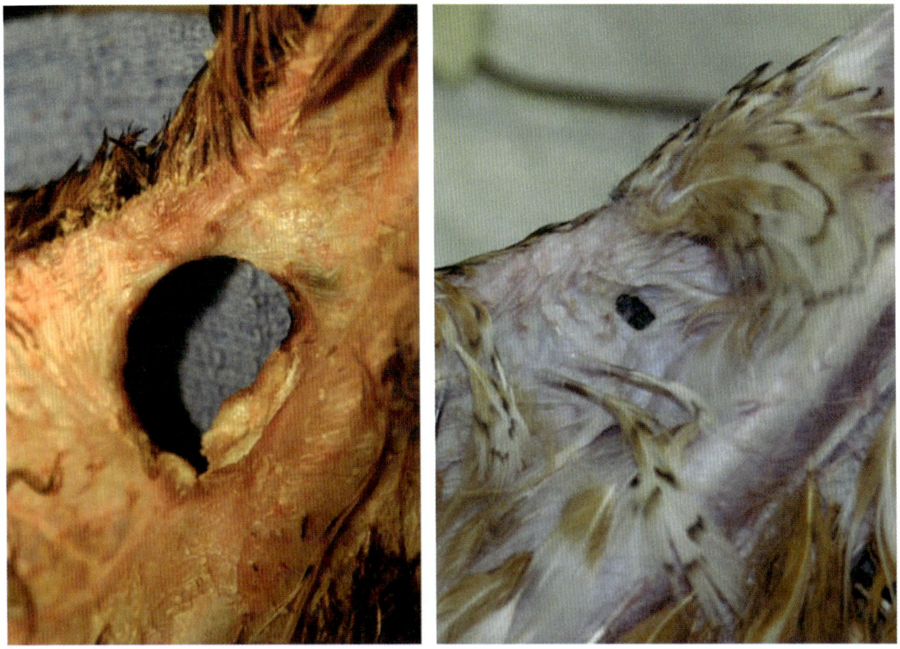

Fig. 9.7. Porthole contraction in great-horned owl with a barbed-wire injury.

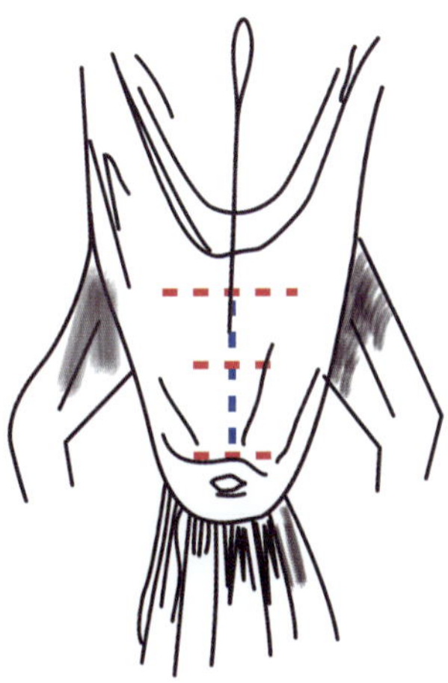

Fig. 9.8. Ventral abdominal approaches. The ventral midline (blue) incision can be combined with a trans-abdominal incision (red).

Left lateral approach

This approach is useful for access to the female reproductive tract, left kidney, proventriculus, and spleen. Note that the actual exposure afforded by this entry is quite limited and this approach can be challenging. Make this approach as follows:

- Place the bird in right lateral recumbency.
- Pull the left leg caudally and dorsally as far as it will go.
- Locate the cranial extent of your incision which is over the second-to-last (7th) rib approximately ¼ to ⅓ of the distance from dorsal to ventral.
- Locate the caudal extent of your incision which is at a 45° angle caudal ventrally and is as far caudally as you can go before running into the thigh muscles. This path should describe a diagonal line through the paralumbar fossa (Fig. 9.9).
- Make a skin incision as described previously by tenting the skin and using scissors. In raptors, the thigh does not pull very far caudally, so the incision may be quite short. It can be extended caudally by incising the skin of the leg web underneath the knee.
- Locate and ligate the superficial femoral artery and vein as they course dorsally to ventrally from the hip joint. Note that a ligation

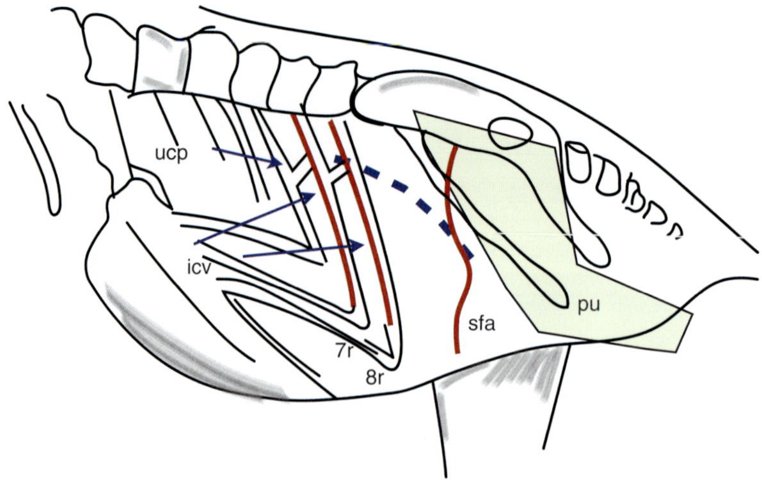

Fig. 9.9. Left lateral celiotomy: pubis (pu), superficial femoral artery and vein (sfa), 7th and 8th ribs (7r, 8r), uncinate process (ucp), intercostal vessels (icv). The incision is indicated by the dashed line. The green shaded region shows how far the leg can be pulled back.

should be made dorsally and ventrally to the intended incision to minimize blood loss.

- Make an incision in the body wall following the same path described above.
- Transection of the 8th and possibly the 7th rib may be necessary for adequate exposure. Ligate the intercostal vessels that run on the cranial edge of the ribs, then transect the rib with scissors. Note that the ribs are simply transected and pushed aside; they are not removed. In raptors, rib transection seems to be necessary more often than not, since the exposure afforded through the paralumbar fossa is quite limited.
- Use a retractor to improve exposure and complete the procedure while paying close attention to the potential for escaping anesthetic gas.
- Transected ribs are generally not reattached. They are placed back into a normal position and are left to heal naturally.
- Close the body wall and skin separately.

Cloacal ventplasty

A ventplasty procedure is used to reduce the diameter of the vent and may be helpful in cases of recurrent cloacal prolapse due to atony of the vent sphincter. This procedure is generally not appropriate for wild raptors in a rehabilitation setting but may be needed to treat a captive permanent resident.

To perform this procedure:

- One or two wedges of skin and subcutaneous tissue are removed. The size of the wedge depends on the severity of the prolapse.
- The tissue is dissected away from the cloaca itself and the cloaca is not penetrated.
- The incisions are closed with simple interrupted sutures.
- A single midline wedge can be removed, or alternatively, two smaller wedges at the 1 o'clock and 11 o'clock positions can be removed.

Cloacopexy

A cloacopexy procedure is used to fix the body of the cloaca in position and is required in cases of recurrent prolapse. This procedure is not appropriate for wild raptors in a rehabilitation setting but may be needed to treat a captive permanent resident. Several methods have been described but the procedure described here seems to work well and is the least technically challenging:

- The cloaca is pushed cranially with a red-rubber feeding tube, sterile swab, or other blunt probe, and it should be positioned so that the vent is slightly inverted. This technique allows the cranial extent of the cloaca to be identified before the skin incision is made.

- A ventral incision is made near the cranial extent of the cloaca. The incision can be either on the midline or transverse.
- Any fat is bluntly dissected away from the body wall and surface of the cloaca.
- The body wall is closed and the wall of the cloaca is incorporated into the closure. Monofilament, absorbable suture is used and it is passed full-thickness into the lumen of the cloaca.
- Optionally, the cloaca serosa can be incised so that the cloacal submucosa heals directly to the body wall. This often yields the best results.
- The skin is closed separately (Fig. 9.10).

Liver biopsy

Liver biopsies are indicated in cases of suspected liver disease (e.g. radiographic hepatomegaly or significant elevations of BA). With the patient in dorsal recumbency, a 5–10 mm incision is made parallel to and 5 mm caudal to the caudal margin of the sternum. The incision is extended through the body wall. A normal liver does not extend beyond the border of the sternum. In cases of hepatomegaly, the liver will bulge past the sternum and be easily accessible via this approach (Fig. 9.11).

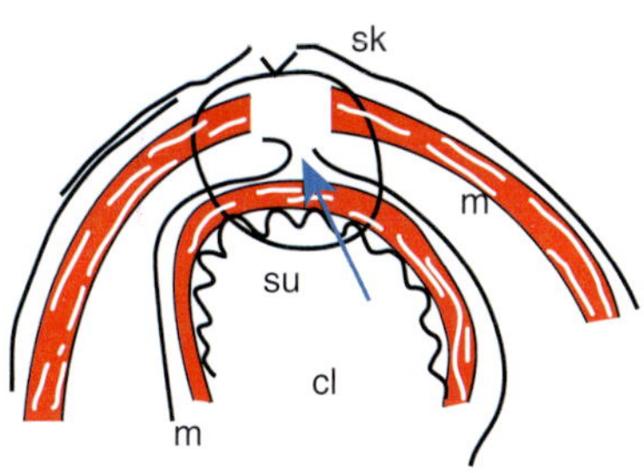

Fig. 9.10. Incisional cloacopexy: skin (sk), muscular layers of cloaca and body wall (m), cloacal lumen (cl), suture closing the body wall with the subserosal layer of the cloaca (su), incision in cloacal serosa (arrowhead).

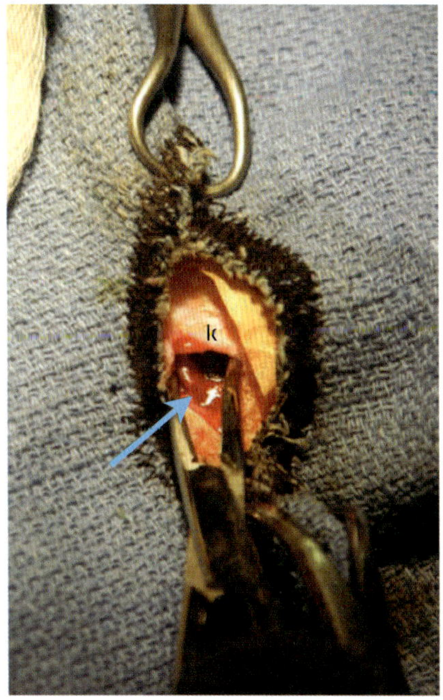

Fig. 9.11. Liver biopsy. The edge of a liver lobe is about to be grasped with hemostats. Edge of keel (k), liver (arrowhead).

To collect a biopsy sample:

- A curved hemostat is used to gently grasp the liver and to isolate a section along the edge of the lobe.
- The sample is sharply separated with a scalpel blade. The cut edge is monitored for a minute or so to check for bleeding.
- Hemorrhage is rare, so the liver edges do not typically need to be sutured.
- The body wall is closed routinely in two layers.

Ocular Evisceration

This procedure is described in Chapter 5.

Proventriculotomy/ Ventriculotomy

A proventriculotomy is indicated primarily to remove foreign bodies from the proventriculus or to gain access to the ventriculus. This procedure is not without risk, therefore endoscopic retrieval should be attempted first.

- A left lateral approach is required for this procedure. Refer to the Celiotomy section, above.
- Stay sutures are placed at the proximal and distal end (near the isthmus) of the proventriculus (Fig. 9.12).
- The proventriculus is gently elevated up into the opening of the incision and saline-soaked gauze is packed around and underneath to prevent accidental leakage into the abdomen. Blunt dissection of the suspensory ligaments may be required to mobilize the proventriculus.
- The incision is made across the body of the proventriculus, starting at the isthmus and continuing cranially. Avoid any major vessels if possible.
- Use a retractor to open the incision. The proventriculus can be delicate so extra care is needed to prevent unnecessary trauma.
- Remove the foreign body and carefully check that the lumen is clear.
- Close in two layers with 4-O or 5-O monofilament absorbable (PDS®) suture. Use a continuous pattern followed by an inverting layer.

Fasting after surgery is not recommended, although smaller, more frequent meals may help prevent over-distention.

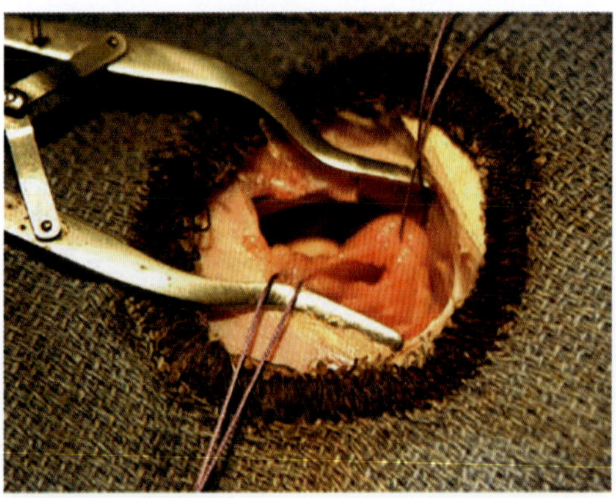

Fig. 9.12. Proventriculotomy via a left lateral approach.

Direct entry into the ventriculus can also be attempted since, in raptors, the muscle wall is thin and holds suture well. A cranial trans-abdominal or ventral midline approach can be used.

Ruptured Crop

A ruptured crop is common in hawks suffering blunt trauma (e.g. hit-by-car) after ingesting a large meal. Immediate surgical repair is best and healing is usually rapid. If repair is delayed, then repeated tube-feeding will be required. This is stressful and, in general, unnecessary.

- Remove all contents of the crop. The contents can be grasped with long forceps orally but it is usually easier to access the crop through the wound. Flush the crop with warm saline until clear.
- Surgically prepare the area and gently pluck the feathers around the wound to create a good margin.
- Using blunt dissection around the wound, separate the crop from the surrounding skin.
- Debride the edges of the crop wound and ensure there is a fresh edge around the entire perimeter of the wound.
- Close the crop in two layers. Absorbable, monofilament suture in a simple interrupted or simple continuous pattern works well. The mucosa tends to evert so be careful to get good apposition. Use an infolding mattress pattern to close the second layer.
- Debride the skin edges and close with a continuous pattern.

There is no need to withhold food, but all food should be boneless or be cut up into small pieces for 1 week. Avoid force-feeding or tube-feeding if possible.

Toe Amputation

Severely damaged digits are not an unusual finding on intake exams. Ruptured tendons can present in two different ways. If the flexor tendon is damaged, then the digit will be hyper-extended and somewhat flaccid. If the extensor tendon is damaged, then the digit will be curled under and may have an abrasion or wound on the dorsal surface. In addition, swollen joints and osteoarthritis are also common findings. In many cases, amputation of the affected digit is the best option. In general, digits 1 and 2 are the most important (Fig. 2.5) and amputation of these digits, especially the hallux (digit 1), will generally rule out release. This must be considered before proceeding. Possible exceptions to this rule are vultures since they do not use the hallux to make a kill or to carry food.

Raptor feet are very dirty, so be especially careful when preparing the site for surgery. A tourniquet is very helpful in controlling bleeding. An assistant applying pressure to the vessels running along the medial tarsometatarsus is often enough. A radiosurgical unit (Ellman International, Hicksville, NY, USA) is also helpful in limiting blood loss, especially when making the skin incision and dissecting through the deeper structures.

Raptor Tip

A tourniquet can be made easily from a Penrose drain. Loop it around the limb, tighten, and secure with a hemostat.

- Make the skin incision so that skin from the plantar surface can be pulled around dorsally over the tip of the digit. This results in a much more resilient stump and keeps the incision out of direct contact with the ground (Fig. 9.13).
- Always preserve as much of the digit as possible by amputating as distally as the wound or lesion will allow. This will provide for optimal weight bearing on the foot and leads to the best long-term prognosis. Amputations are typically performed by disarticulating the digit at the most distal joint that is proximal to the lesion.

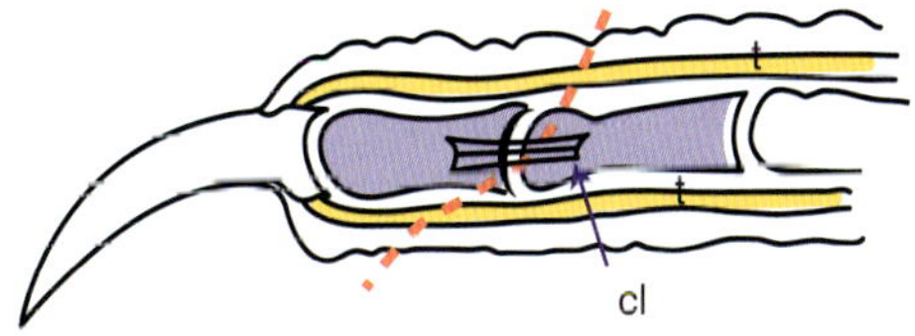

Fig. 9.13. Disarticulation amputation: flexor and extensor tendons (t), lateral collateral ligaments (cl), skin incision is indicated by the dotted line.

- Extend the skin incision dorsally and centered over the joint.
- Bluntly dissect the subcutaneous tissue to reveal the lateral collateral ligaments. Cutting them should mobilize the distal phalange.
- The flexor and extensor tendons are pulled distally and then cut. The intact proximal portions of the tendons will retract back proximally into the sheath. Alternatively, the cut ends of the tendons can be pulled around the end of the bony stump and sutured to each other. This can help create a tough tissue pad at the end of the digit and may result in better functionality for the remaining digit.
- The remaining attachments are bluntly dissected and any vessels should be clamped or ligated if possible. In reality, the vessels are quite small and can rarely be identified, but bleeding can be significant.
- The distal digit is discarded and all soft tissue tags are removed. Every effort should be made to remove any remnants of the joint capsule, which may have the potential to secrete joint fluid.
- The articular cartilaginous surface of the distal condyle should be removed with rongeurs until a bleeding bed of bone is revealed.
- Remove any resulting bone spurs and flush the wound.
- A few drops of lidocaine placed on the stump before closing the skin may provide some post-op analgesia.
- Close with an interrupted pattern by pulling the skin up from the plantar surface. There should be little to no tension on the suture line if enough skin was left when the initial incision was made.

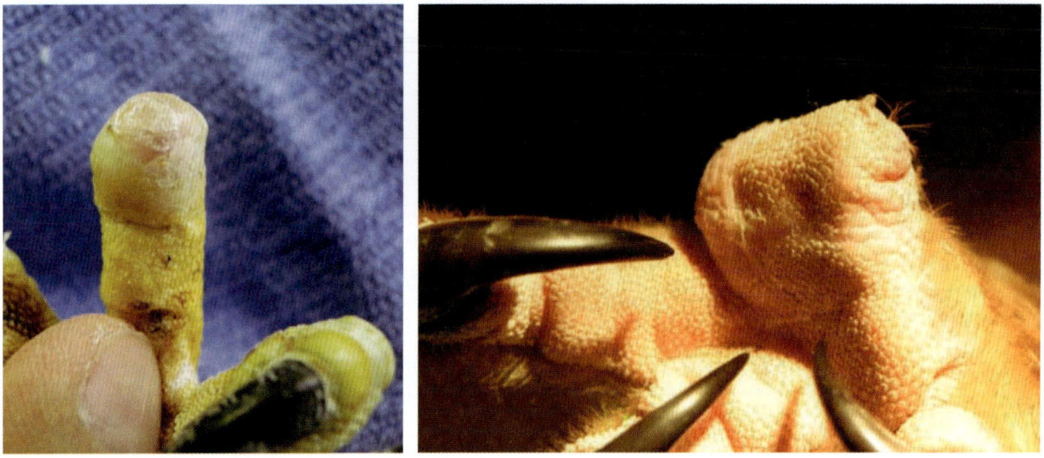

Fig. 9.14. Healed amputations. The stump on the left is still very fragile because the original wound would not allow for the tough plantar skin to be pulled up over the tip. Compare to the stump on the right.

- Place a padded bandage on the stump and secure it by looping elastic bandage material around the ankle. Change the bandage every 3–4 days for 10 days until healed (Fig. 9.14).

Note: if amputation of the hallux (digit 1) is necessary (in a resident bird or a vulture, perhaps), it may be necessary to remove the proximal phalange as well as the distal end of metatarsal 1, since these bones, if left intact, can form a pressure point and may lead to chronic bumblefoot.

Tracheotomy

This procedure is used to access the syrinx or tracheal lumen in cases of obstruction due to a foreign body or a mass such as a fungal granuloma. It is necessary in cases where endoscopic access is not possible or practical, especially in very small patients.

In general, anesthesia should be provided via air sac cannulation since the trachea will be obstructed during the procedure.

- The bird should be placed on a diagonally elevated board to aid in viewing down into the trachea.
- A feeding tube can be passed down the esophagus to aid in identifying and avoiding that structure.
- A skin incision is made over the lesion, or in the thoracic inlet if the target is the syrinx.
- In species with a crop, the crop may need to be elevated and retracted away to improve exposure to the trachea.
- Stay sutures may be used to help elevate the trachea. In addition, a blunt hooked instrument can be used to gently pull the syrinx cranially for better visualization.
- A transverse incision is made between two tracheal rings. The incision should not extend beyond 50% of the tracheal circumference.
- The tracheal incision is closed with two or three simple interrupted sutures of absorbable monofilament material (PDS®). The sutures should incorporate one or two rings on each side of the incision and the knots should be tied outside the tracheal lumen.

Bibliography

Altman, R.B., Clubb, S.L., Dorrestein, G.M. and Quesenberry, K. (1997) *Avian Medicine and Surgery*. W.B. Saunders Company, Philadelphia, PA, USA.

Chitty, L. (2008) *BSAVA Manual of Raptors, Pigeons and Passerine Birds*. BSAVA, Gloucester, UK.

Ford, S., Chitty, J. and Jones, M. (2010) Surgical aspects of raptor feet. Handout. *31st Conference of the Association of Avian Veterinarians, August 2010, San Diego, CA, USA*. Association of Avian Veterinarians, Teaneck, NJ, USA.

Redig, P. and Ponder, J. (2010) Raptors: Practical information every avian practitioner can use. *Proceedings of the 31st Conference of the Association of Avian Veterinarians*. Association of Avian Veterinarians, Teaneck, NJ, USA, pp. 171–180.

Scott, D. (2011) Return to flight after radical resection of the patagium. *Proceedings of the 11th Conference of the European Association of Avian Veterinarians, Madrid, Spain*. European Association of Avian Veterinarians, pp. 120–121. Available at: www.eaavonline.org (accessed February 2016).

10 Orthopedics

Learning Objectives

1. Proper triage: what can be repaired and what cannot?
2. Placing IM pins with and without an ESF tie-in.
3. The importance of post-op care.
4. Repair of humerus fractures.
5. Repair of ulna/radius fractures.
6. Repair of tibiotarsus fractures.

When treating avian fractures, we are often dealing with relatively acute cases in otherwise healthy birds that have simply had an unfortunate accident. Because of this, the prognosis can be quite good and recovery can be dramatic.

Unfortunately, fresh injuries are not always present on admission and sometimes you have to deal with a very thin or emaciated bird with an old, poorly healed fracture. This is particularly true with vultures that seem quite able to survive for weeks or months with a fracture or other injury.

Triage and Stabilization

Always provide analgesia and sedation prior to your examination and workup. An initial examination, including palpation of all long bones, examination of the head and eyes, as well as a VD radiograph, should take less than 10 min if you are properly prepared:

- Provide analgesia (butorphanol 2 mg/kg IM).
- Palpate all long bones. Use alcohol to dampen the feathers in order to check for bruises but be careful to avoid any open wounds.
- Identify any open wounds or bone exposure.
- Examine eyes, oral cavity, and ears for evidence of head trauma. It is easy to focus on the obvious fracture and miss serious trauma elsewhere. There is no use in repairing a fracture in a blind bird.
- Anesthetize and take a VD radiograph.
- Stabilize with fluids (SQ or IO, if necessary) and meloxicam.
- If there is bone exposure and/or contamination, a combination of enrofloxacin and clindamycin is very effective and should be started immediately.
- Flush all wounds with warm saline. Remember the humerus and femur are connected to the air sacs so do not flush directly into the proximal ends of fractures affecting these bones.
- To prevent desiccation of the bone fragments, the bone ends should be thoroughly cleaned, flushed, and tucked under the skin if possible. Temporary sutures can be used to close the wound. SSD and a hydrogel dressing (e.g. Duoderm®, Convatec, Greensboro, NC, USA) work well when all exposed structures cannot be completely covered by skin.

Raptor Tip

Remember to examine the eyes and do a complete physical exam to make sure your patient is a good surgical candidate.

> **Raptor Tip**
>
> The goal of triage is to prevent desiccation of the bones and to immobilize the fracture.

Apply the appropriate bandage based on the location of the fracture:

- Humerus: figure-8 + body wrap.
- Ulna/radius/metacarpal bone: figure-8 wrap only.
- Clavicle/coracoid/scapula: body wrap. Note that the body wrap may be incorporated into and continued from a figure-8 wrap.
- Femur: very difficult to splint. Make a deep "donut" nest with towels to keep the bird as comfortable and as quiet as possible. Surgical repair as soon as possible is very important.
- Tibiotarsus: make a splint with roll cotton and elastic bandage material. You can stiffen the splint with a metal coat-hanger sidebar or tongue depressor. Sidebars on the medial side can cause inadvertent rubbing and wound formation on the body wall so only apply them on the lateral/cranial side. Since the leg web comes almost to the knee joint in most birds, it can be very difficult for the splint to extend much above the knee and therefore stabilization with this type of splint is not always very effective. This is especially true of proximal tibiotarsus fractures. If required, repair as soon as possible.
- Tarsometatarsus: make a splint similar to the tibiotarsus. Extend it proximally above the hock joint. The splint can be continued distally and combined with a foam shoe to stabilize the ankle joint.
- Digit: a foam shoe/wrap that extends up above the ankle works well.

Surgical correction of fractures should be attempted within 24 h if patient status allows.

Radiographic Views

In many cases, two orthogonal radiographic views should be obtained in order to properly manage a fracture. It is very common for a poorly aligned fracture to look well aligned on one view (Fig. 10.1). In these cases, you may erroneously opt for conservative treatment when surgical intervention is required. This is especially true of tibiotarsus and ulna fractures.

Prognostic Factors

Bone exposure

Open, contaminated fractures are not uncommon in birds. Remarkably, osteomyelitis is rare, but it does happen. Careful attention to detail when cleaning the wound initially and when debriding it during the repair is critical to success. The use of clindamycin is very helpful in preventing or treating osteomyelitis.

Healthy bone has a pinkish satin appearance. Devitalized or dead bone can either look dark or appear bleached white. In either case, it must be removed. If the devitalized area is only a few millimeters at the tip of a long oblique fragment, then it can simply be removed. If the affected area is larger or encompasses the entire circumference of bone, then the fracture may not be repairable.

Proximity to a joint

Fractures involving the elbow or carpus typically do not do well. The ROM of these joints needs to be essentially perfect for flight and this is rarely possible with these types of fractures. Proximal humerus fractures, especially those involving the pectoral crest, are tolerated well in owls but not at all in diurnal birds such as red-tailed hawks. Fractures involving the leg joints are similar as far as prognosis is concerned but there is more leeway regarding diminished ROM. However, with fractures of the leg, it is important to guarantee equal or similar weight bearing to ensure that bumblefoot will not develop in the future.

Chronicity

An old, poorly healed fracture in an emaciated bird does not generally lend itself to repair (Fig. 10.2). Resetting a poorly healed fracture by breaking

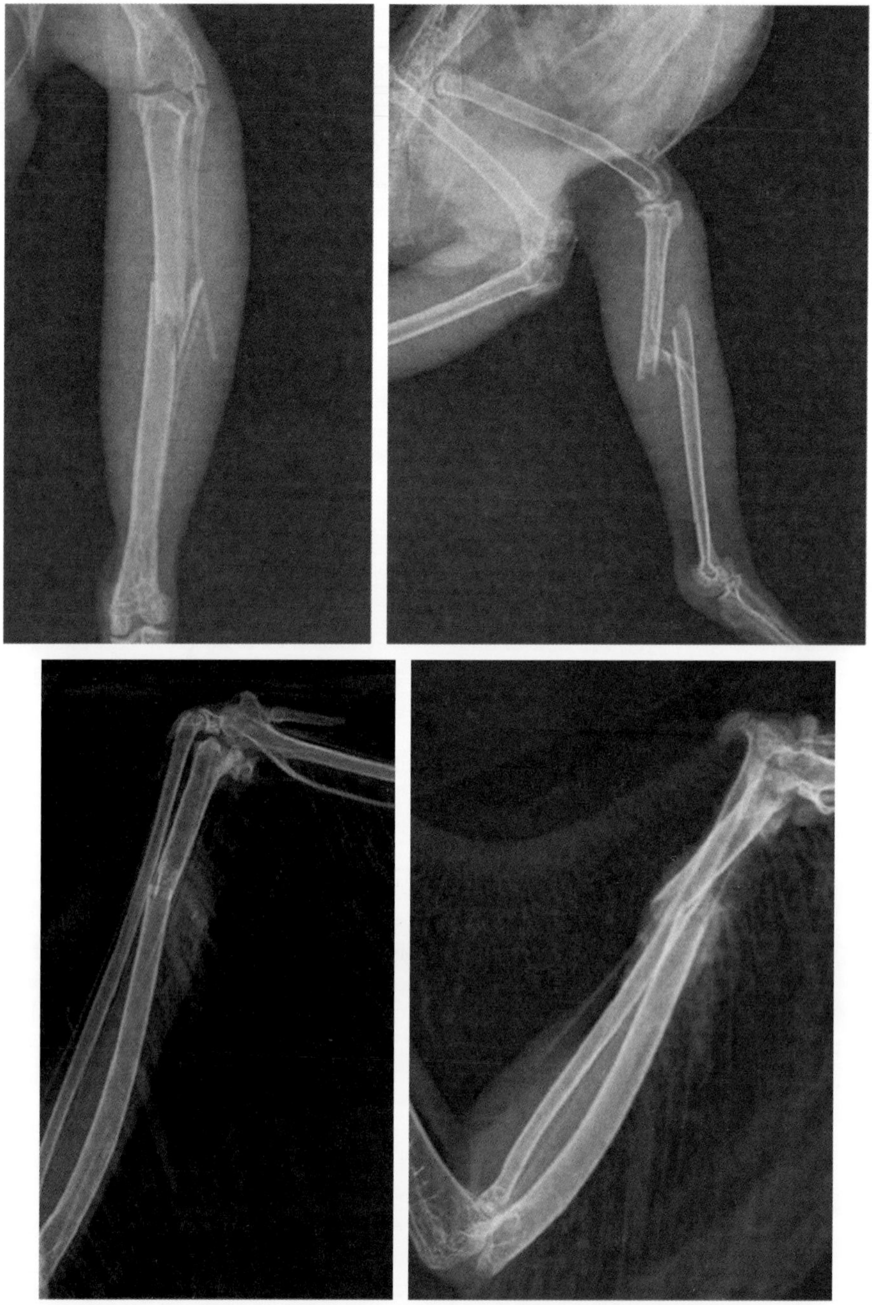

Fig. 10.1. Two radiographic views are often needed. This tibiotarsal fracture looked well aligned on the VD view (top left) and may have been simply splinted if a lateral view (top right) was not obtained. Similarly, this ulna fracture (bottom left) may have been treated with just a figure-8 wrap if the orthogonal view (bottom right) had not been obtained.

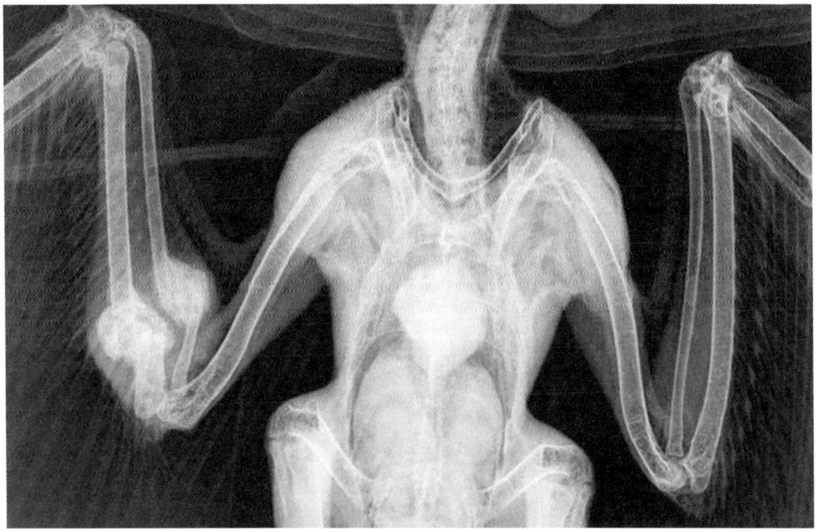

Fig. 10.2. Some birds defy all the odds. This black vulture was admitted with a keel score of 1.5/5 and old, poorly aligned, healed fractures of the ulna and radius. The extension of the wing, however, was quite good. After 2 months of good food and exercise, this bird flew beautifully, and was eventually released.

down a callus and re-aligning the bone ends is sometimes possible but is much more difficult than it looks on a radiograph. In addition, the existing scar tissue and poor extension which usually accompany these cases do not generally allow for a successful outcome or release. Chronic leg fractures are much easier to deal with than any fracture involving the wing.

Typical Timeline and Protocol

An orthopedic case is a large commitment in time and resources. The actual surgery, if indicated, is only the first step in a long process. This process is outlined in Table 10.1.

Post-op care

Maintenance of pins

Maintenance of pin tracts is very important and it is not uncommon for them to be a little bloody and drain for a day or two. However, they should be clean and dry by the end of the first week. Take the time to clean the pins with betadine, flush with saline, and apply triple-antibiotic ointment whenever the bird is handled for PT. This procedure should continue until the pins are clean and dry. Continued drainage may indicate a problem with either a loose implant or osteomyelitis. Immediate evaluation and radiographs are indicated in these cases.

A loose fixation is usually worse than none at all. It should be removed immediately and replaced if possible.

Begin treatment for osteomyelitis immediately if it is suspected. Antibiotic choice should always be based on culture and sensitivity, if possible, but clindamycin can be a very effective choice when a culture is not possible.

> **Raptor Tip**
>
> The goal should always be to get surgery done as soon as possible. However, in cases of head trauma, it is often much safer to wait a few days before any prolonged anesthesia.

PT

The importance of PT for wing fractures (whether the fracture was surgically repaired or not) cannot be overstated. Realize that surgery is just the first step in a long process to get a bird to release.

PT is always done under general anesthesia and each session should only take 10–15 min including induction and recovery (Fig. 10.3).

The elbow is stabilized with the thumb and forefinger on one hand. The wrist is grasped with the other hand with the forefinger pressing on the area around the radial carpal bone.

The elbow and carpus are extended and flexed together repeatedly and also held in extension for short periods.

A goniometer is helpful to accurately and objectively measure the extension of the joints (Fig. 10.4). It is critical that the swivel point of the goniometer be held exactly over the elbow or wrist joint, otherwise inaccurate measurements will be obtained.

The elbow joint angle is formed by the center axis of the humerus and the ulna and ideally measures at least 140–150°. Some species such as the osprey can extend beyond that angle. If ever in doubt, measure the extension of the opposite wing.

Raptor Tip

Elbow extension: 140–150°+.
Wrist extension: 180°.

The carpus joint angle is formed by the ulna and the major metacarpal bone. The joint should extend to 180° so that the ulna and metacarpal bones form a straight line.

PT does not seem to be as necessary for leg fractures. Normal daily use and weight bearing is adequate to maintain good ROM.

PT is started on day 3 post-surgery, continues three times weekly for a week or two, and is continued or tapered as needed. Note that it is much easier to lose degrees of ROM than it is to get them back, so err on the side of too much or too frequent. Also, doing PT is really more of an art than a science. It takes some practice to know how far or how hard you can push any given bird. It is also very important to have consistency in the staff performing the therapy for any given bird, since it is easy to go too far or not far enough if the person is not accustomed to working with the individual patient.

It is critical to record the starting *and* ending angles of the elbow and carpus (Fig. 10.5). The

Table 10.1. Typical timeline for a humerus fracture.

Day/week	Activity or milestone
0	Admission and triage
0–2	Butorphanol IM BID then switch to tramadol
0–10	Meloxicam PO BID
0–14	Start on antibiotics as appropriate. Enrofloxacin plus clindamycin works well
1	Surgery
2	Clean pins and apply triple antibiotic. Repeat q3d for the first 7–10 days as needed
3	Start PT under general anesthesia. Remove wing bandage if an IM–ESF tie fixation was used
3–14	Continue PT three times weekly for 2 weeks
10	Radiograph every 10–14 days
2–4 weeks	Decrease PT as needed
5 weeks	Remove fixation and move to small cage to allow limited exercise
8–10 weeks	Move to flight cage and begin forced exercise
12–16 weeks	Release!!

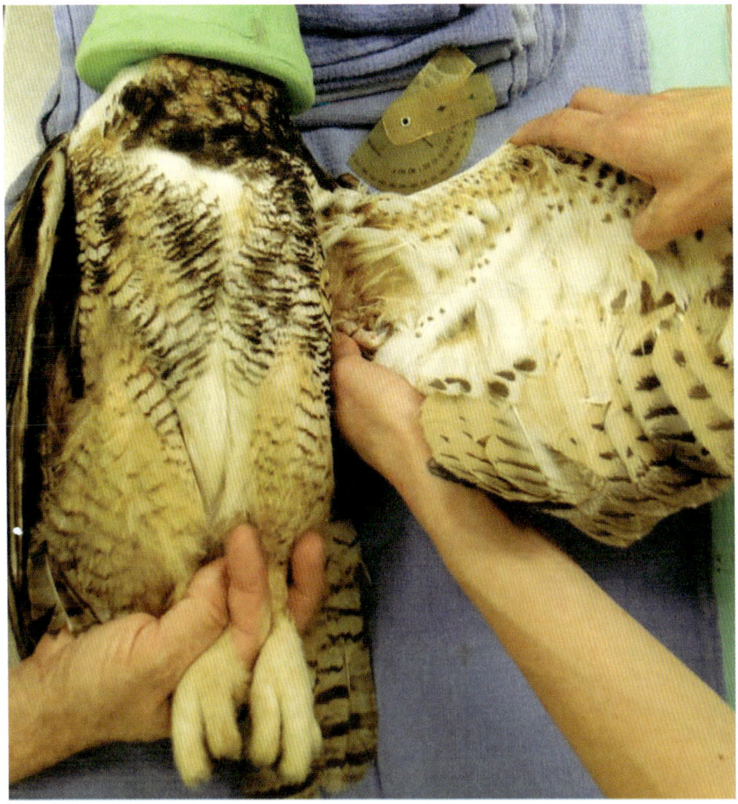

Fig. 10.3. Doing PT. Note that the bird's feet are properly restrained even when under general anesthesia.

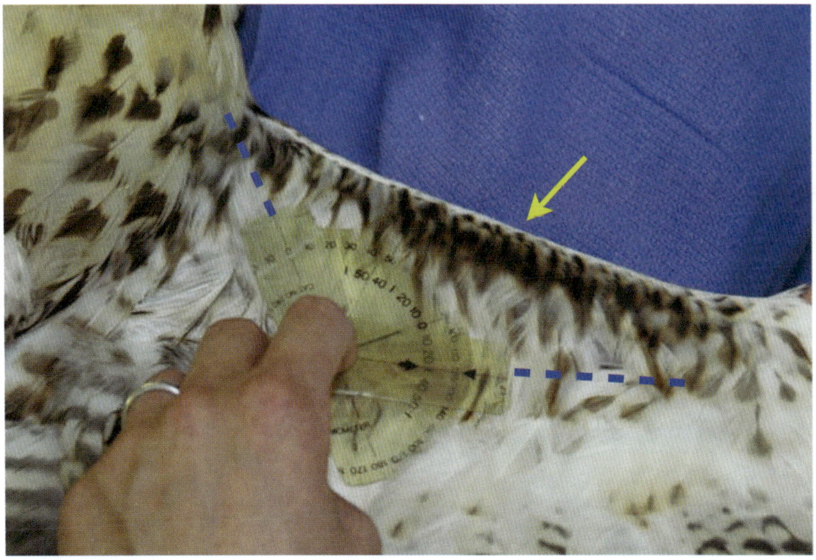

Fig. 10.4. Using a goniometer to measure ROM of the elbow. The arrow is pointing to the patagium and the dotted lines are over the humerus and ulna. The goniometer is centered on the elbow joint.

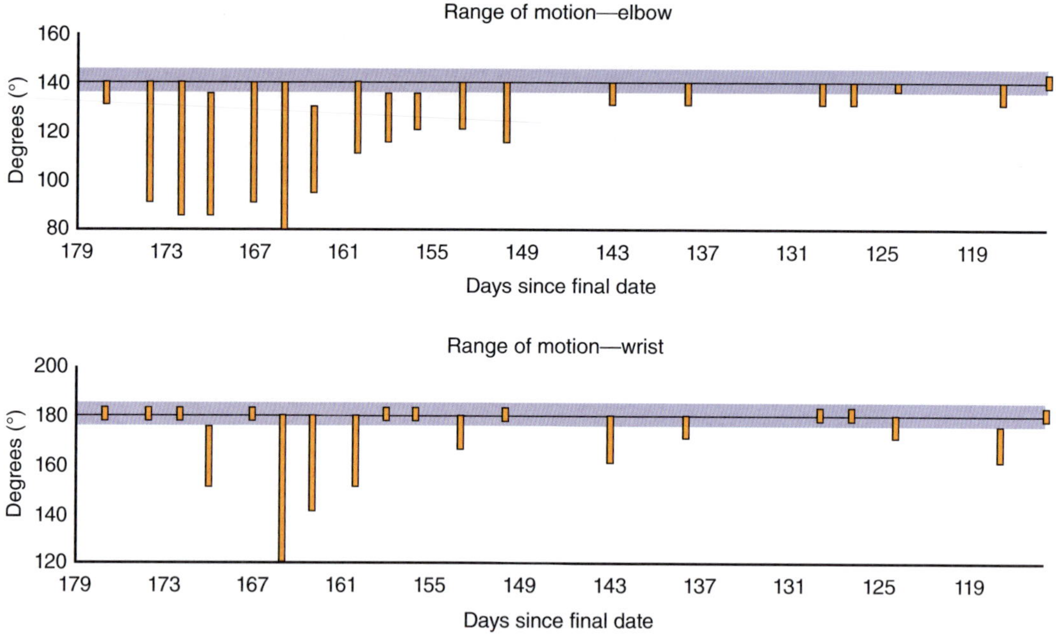

Fig. 10.5. Graphs of PT measurements displayed by the RaptorMed™ medical records software. The orange bars indicate the starting (bottom) and ending (top) angles for the elbow and wrist. The violet horizontal bands represent the desired/target measurements. When the orange bars are completely and consistently within the violet band, you have finished with PT.

beginning angle is important since it indicates how well the bird can extend its joints on its own without external pressure. The ending angle is also important because it demonstrates how far the joint is able to extend. When the starting angle and ending angles are at or near the desired angle, PT can be discontinued.

Removal of implants

Implants are removed when the fracture is stable on palpation *and* there is good radiographic evidence of bone healing. There is no set schedule for this but here are some guidelines:

- Most implants can be removed after 4–6 weeks.
- Young birds (less than 4 weeks old) heal rapidly and implants in neonates can usually be removed after 10–14 days.
- Fractures of the leg can take longer to heal so implants may sometimes be left in a bit longer.
- Cerclage wires cannot usually be removed and shuttle pins are never removed.
- IM pin–ESF tie-in constructs can be removed in stages but this is generally not necessary.
- Induce general anesthesia to remove all implants.

Raptor Tip

Primary bone healing does not typically occur in birds; therefore a large callus should be palpable and visible on a radiograph when a fracture is healing properly.

Aseptically clean/prepare all implants before removal. This is especially true of external fixator cross pins which will need to be pulled through the bone in order to remove.

The resulting pin holes usually seal over quickly and do not need to be covered.

Exercise

Once the fracture is healed and PT has been completed, it is time for exercise and flight training. Birds with fractures or other injuries will lose condition quickly and will develop muscle atrophy in the 3–4 months that they have been in rehab. It takes an appropriate-sized flight cage (see Chapter 15 for details) or a creance line and a progressively more strenuous exercise regimen to return them to fitness. While some studies seem to indicate that creance line training is a more effective method of exercise, it is also very resource-, time-, and staff-intensive, and is not without significant risk of injury. Because of this, exercise in a flight cage is often more practical and can still be very effective. The exception to this rule is for peregrine falcons, which should be free flown by an experienced falconer.

A typical protocol may start at 2–3 cage lengths daily and gradually work up to 14–15 lengths once or twice daily over a 2-week period. This program is continued for an additional 2 weeks with the bird's flight constantly monitored and evaluated. Some things to look for:

- Ability to glide: a red-tailed hawk or vulture should be able to glide for the final 30–40% of the cage length as it approaches a perch landing.
- There should be no noticeable labored or open-mouthed breathing. Keep in mind that stress and warm temperatures can easily make a bird breathe hard, so it is important to differentiate these causes from exercise intolerance.
- There should be no noticeable asymmetry when viewed from the front, side, or behind. See Chapter 17 for possible exceptions.
- It should only take a few wing beats to get into a smooth flight pattern and level flight should be maintained.
- There should not be an excessive amount of feather noise in hawks and owls should be essentially silent after the first couple of wing beats.

Supplies and Instruments

It does not take a large kit of expensive instruments to repair most fractures in birds. The cortices of avian bone do not hold screws well, so plating procedures are generally not appropriate. However, most fractures can be repaired nicely with IM pins, external fixators, or a combination of the two. In addition to the standard soft tissue instruments required for any surgery, an orthopedic pack (Fig. 10.6) should include:

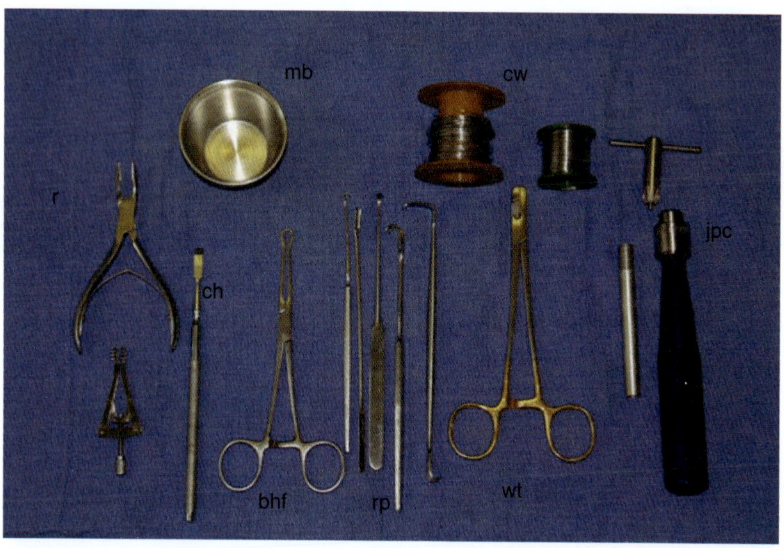

Fig. 10.6. Orthopedic instruments: Jacob's pin chuck (jpc), cerclage wire (cw), wire twister (wt), mixing bowl (mb), ronguer (r), chisel (ch), bone-holding forceps (bhf), various retractors and pry bars (rp).

- A small Jacob's pin chuck.
- Bone-holding forceps. Brown-Adson forceps work well for many smaller bones. Human phalange forceps are perfect for larger bones.
- Stainless-steel cerclage wire (26-gauge) and a wire twister/cutter.
- Small 4″ (10 cm) ronguers. Dental extraction forceps make an effective and inexpensive alternative.
- Various retractors and pry bars.
- A bone chisel.
- A small, metal mixing bowl.
- A pin cutter with sufficient strength to cut through pins as large as ⅛″ (3 mm) in diameter.

Steinmann pins and K-wires

Steinmann pins and K-wires are used extensively for both intramedullary placement and for cross pins in external fixators (Fig. 10.7). In general, 9″ (23 cm) smooth pins with a trocar tip on both ends are the most useful. Frequently used sizes (in inches) include: 0.035, 0.045, 0.062 (1/16), 5/64, 3/32, 7/64, and ⅛ (0.9–3 mm). Note that the unused ends of these pins can be recycled and used as cross pins in external fixators. IMEX (IMEX Veterinary Inc., Longview, TX, USA; www.imexvet.com (accessed May 2020)) has a great selection of pins, K-wires, and orthopedic instruments.

IMEX also has very small "stick pins" which have a positive-profile thread on one end, come in diameters from 0.03 to 0.062″ (0.9–1.6 mm), and are ideal for the cross pins used in an IM–ESF fixation.

Sidebar material

Some sort of material will be needed to create external fixator sidebars. Options include various two-part epoxies and acrylics that are mixed and formed. Veterinary thermoplastic (VTP) is also a

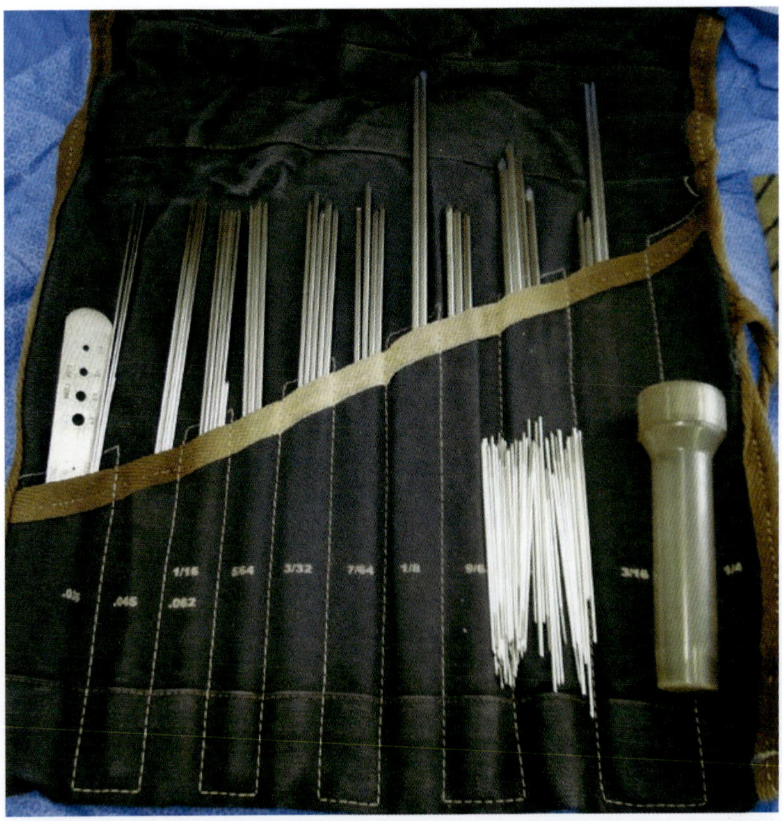

Fig. 10.7. A typical pin pack.

great option (Fig. 10.8). It comes in many forms including rolls (X-Lite®, Allard International, Helsingborg, Sweden; www.allardint.com (accessed June 2020)) and fiberglass-reinforced sheets. It is softened in hot water and molded into place to incorporate the stainless-steel pin. It sets up quickly but still allows enough time to mold it. Its other big advantages are that it is transparent on radiographs, it is not messy or exothermic, and it can be cut and added to later, if needed.

Techniques

IM pins

Intramedullary pins are great for achieving proper alignment of long bone fractures and are excellent at resisting bending forces. However, they provide no rotational stability and are often combined with an external fixator in a tie-in procedure for this reason.

When selecting a pin for placement, the pin should fill approximately ½ to ⅔ of the medullary space.

Always blunt the trocar tip when driving an IM pin toward a joint to prevent inadvertent penetration. By blunting the tip, it is much harder to penetrate the metaphysis into the joint space. This is particularly important when driving toward the stifle in a femur, toward the carpus in an ulna, and toward the elbow in a radius.

ESFs

External fixators provide very good bending and rotational support but it is difficult to get good end-to-end alignment of the bone fragments. A bilateral fixator can only be used for fractures of the tibiotarsus and tarsometatarsus. In the case of the tibiotarsus, an IM pin is usually combined with an ESF. A unilateral ESF combined with an IM pin is generally used for most other fractures (see below). When using an ESF alone, the general rule is that at least two cross pins will need to be placed above and two pins placed below the fracture. When an IM pin is combined with an ESF, usually only one cross pin is required above and below the fracture.

The pins should be placed as close to the fracture as possible but far enough away to avoid any fissures and to ensure that the pin penetrates solid bone. It is better to be further from the fracture in order to ensure a solid placement than to be too close and have an unstable pin.

The sidebars should be as close to the skin surface as possible but also must allow room for swelling. This is particularly true of tibiotarsus fractures, which often swell significantly after surgery. In these cases, leave at least 1 cm of space between the skin and sidebar.

Positive-profile (PP) threaded pins have a much tighter junction with the bone than smooth pins. They also have superior pull-out resistance; however, they can be difficult and dangerous to

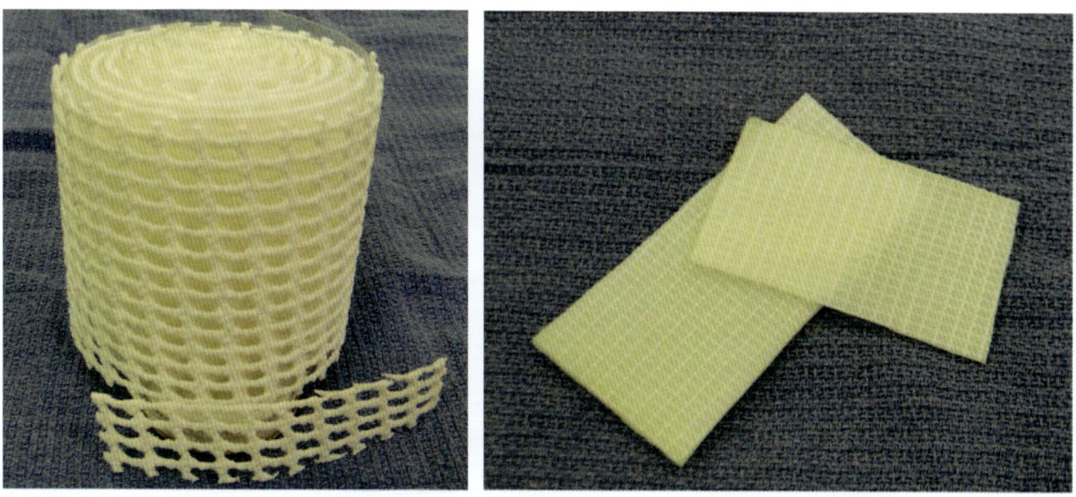

Fig. 10.8. VTP in rolls (X-Lite®) and sheets.

place since the threads can entrap adjacent soft tissue and cause serious damage. Therefore, when using threaded pins, the threads must be carefully isolated from the surrounding soft tissue. This can be achieved with a tissue-protecting sleeve or simply by having an assistant pull the surrounding soft tissue aside with hemostats.

Another option is to use all smooth pins instead. In the author's experience, this works well and they are much easier to place and to remove. One technique to "lock" the pins into place and achieve a stable fixation is to vary the angles at which the pins penetrate the bone (Fig. 10.40). If all the pins are parallel to each other, then the entire fixator can slide back and forth. However, if the pin angles are varied, the fixator is rigidly held in place.

When placing a cross pin with a pin chuck, minimize wobble to ensure a tight contact between the pin and the bone. To do this:

- The chuck should be rotated back and forth, not in a full circle. This only applies to smooth pins since threaded pins clearly must be placed with full rotations.
- The chuck should be rotated with your fingertips, not with your wrist, since this allows for finer control.

IM pin with ESF tie-in

This combination provides excellent fixation, resists bending, compression and rotational forces, and allows for very good alignment of bone fragments. It is the procedure of choice for most humeral and femur fractures and is also useful for many tibiotarsus and ulna fractures. This construct consists of an IM pin with an external fixator made from two cross pins that are bent and joined together with a sidebar (Fig. 10.14). When this construct is used, a wing wrap is unnecessary. This author, however, generally uses a wrap for 3 days post-op to provide some comfort and support, and to avoid damage to the feathers if there is a wing droop.

Shuttle pins

A shuttle pin is a form of internal fixation that works well on transverse or short oblique fractures of the ulna and tibiotarsus. The advantages of using a shuttle pin are:

- The procedure is relatively quick and easy.
- Excellent end-to-end alignment can be achieved.
- There are no penetrating pins to be managed, which can be a potential source of infection.
- There is no risk of further damage that can result from the placement of the traditional IM pin.

The disadvantages are:

- The shuttle pin becomes a permanent implant which cannot be removed.
- The pin does not resist rotational forces as well as other methods and requires placement of a wing wrap for several weeks.

Shuttle pins are made from polypropylene rods (Fig. 10.9). This plastic is biologically inert,

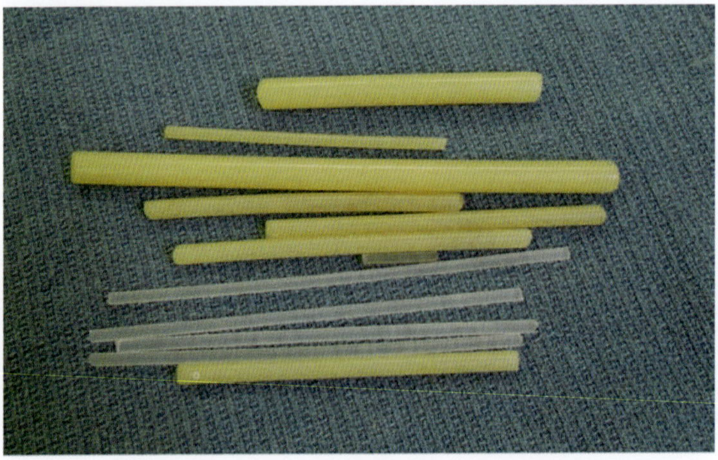

Fig. 10.9. Raw polypropylene rod stock.

flexible, easy to work with, and is completely transparent on radiographs. The pins can be autoclaved and included in your pin pack. Typical diameters of common use are from ⅛″ to ½″ (3–13 mm). These pins are most useful in transverse, non-comminuted fractures of the ulna and tibiotarsus. In the tibiotarsus, they may be used alone but are typically combined with an external fixator. They can also be useful in midshaft ulna fractures in young, developing birds. In these cases, placing an IM pin can cause damage to the developing proximal ulna. Using a shuttle pin instead can avoid these potential problems.

Shuttle pins are typically short and need only span the fracture by approximately 1 or 2 cm on either side. However, a longer shuttle pin will result in a more rigid fixation due to increased friction with the endosteal surface of the bone. Regardless of the length, the entire length of the shuttle pin must be able to slide *completely* into one of the bone fragments (Fig. 10.10c).

When placing the shuttle pin, there must be enough cross-sectional space in the medullary cavity for the shuttle pin and *two* lengths of suture (Fig. 10.10c) to fit comfortably. The pin must slide easily inside the medullary cavity, as a tight fit may lead to endosteal bone necrosis and a delayed or non-union. The suture needs to be large (such as 2-O or larger) to reduce the chance of breaking. This is important since the shuttle pin may become trapped inside one bone fragment if the suture breaks while the pin is being slid across the fracture (Fig. 10.10e). The risk of the suture breaking is increased if the fracture is oblique with sharp edges, so repair of these fractures should not be attempted with a shuttle pin. Thin stainless-steel suture can be used to decrease the chance of the suture breaking in these cases.

Cerclage wires

Cerclage wires are useful when dealing with a long oblique fracture, especially in the humerus. They are rarely used alone and are usually combined with an IM pin. Various textbooks state that cerclage wires should always be placed in pairs. This is not always possible and this author has found a single wire to be very helpful as part of an overall fixation in many situations. Cerclage wires are useful because they allow for the application of compression across the fracture. This is not possible with IM–ESF fixations alone.

Placement of a cerclage wire can be technically challenging. You must ensure no tissue (especially vessels, nerves, or tendons) is entrapped between the wire and the bone.

Always bend the wire tip over into a loop before passing it around the bone. This keeps it from getting snagged on the surrounding soft tissue and makes passing it around the bone *much* easier.

When twisting the wire, always apply traction to the wire ends since this ensures equal tension on each side of the loop. Do not attempt this with needle holders. Get a good pair of wire twisters (they are worth the cost).

The twist must be bent over and wire ends cut off short, since there is usually very little soft tissue

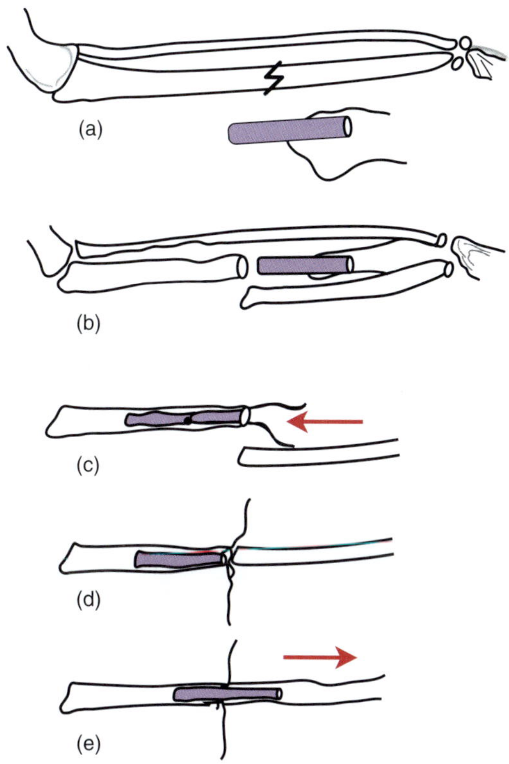

Fig. 10.10. Shuttle pin placement in an ulna fracture. A shuttle pin is cut to size, a hole is drilled through the center with a K-wire, and suture is passed through the hole (a), the bone ends are distracted (b), the shuttle pin is slid completely into one fragment (c), the bone ends are re-aligned (d), and the shuttle pin is slid back across the fracture line by applying traction on the suture (e). The suture is then removed.

to cover the wire ends. Penetration of the wire ends through this skin is the biggest complication seen with cerclage wire placement. To minimize this risk, use the thinnest gauge wire possible (22-gauge is often too large, but 26-gauge wire works well). Absorbable, monofilament suture can also be used as a cerclage. This suture does not allow you to achieve any compression, but it can be useful to help hold loose fragments in place.

Fractures of the Wing

Humerus

Humeral fractures are very common and there are many possible presentations including proximal, midshaft, and distal (up to and including the elbow joint). These fractures are often long oblique, highly comminuted, open fractures accompanied by massive soft tissue trauma. In more chronic cases, there can be significant scar tissue formation and contracture. Bone exposure is very common.

In addition, massive soft tissue swelling distal to the elbow can result from a torsion at the fracture site. The prognosis is very poor in these cases.

Humeral fractures are approached dorsally (Fig. 10.11). There is very little soft tissue (just skin) covering much of the distal half of the humerus. The radial nerve is a very large nerve which runs diagonally over the dorsal–lateral aspect of the humerus. This nerve should be identified before your incision is made and then protected from trauma and desiccation during the repair. Note that this nerve may be difficult to locate due to the swelling and inflammation that can accompany a humeral fracture.

In some cases, there may be a large wound with bone penetration on the ventral surface.

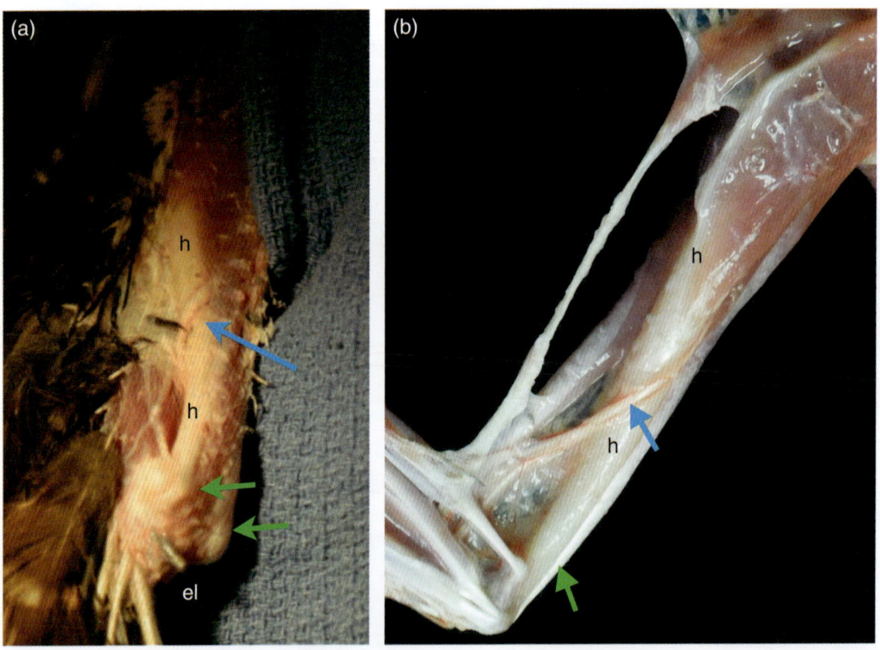

Fig. 10.11. The dorsal approach to the humerus. The distal humerus (h) is only covered by skin in much of this area. The radial nerve (blue arrow) runs over the surface of the bone about ⅔ of the distance to the elbow (el). The paired triceps tendons (green arrows) are also quite visible and must be avoided when placing an IM pin. In (a), no dissection was done prior to this photo. The skin is just wet with alcohol and radial nerve is clearly visible through the skin. In (b), only the skin was removed.

These wounds should be cleaned, debrided, and closed before attempting to repair the fracture from the dorsal side.

Midshaft humerus fracture

A typical midshaft fracture of the humerus is repaired as follows:

- The bird is placed in ventral recumbency.
- The dorsal humerus from the shoulder to just past the elbow is plucked and aseptically prepared.
- The radial nerve is identified and an incision is made over the fracture site.
- The wound, if present, is debrided and flushed.
- The bone ends are identified and brought up into the incision. The bone ends are debrided and freshened as necessary.
- An appropriately sized smooth IM pin is selected and placed. The pin diameter should fill ½ to ⅔ of the medullary canal.

There are two options for placement:

- Drive from the elbow toward and across the fracture (Fig. 10.13). The *paired* triceps extensor tendons (Fig. 10.12) are pushed aside and the trocar tip of the pin is placed *between* them at a 90° angle against the bone. The pin is driven until it just barely penetrates the bone and then is slowly angled into the medullary cavity while continuously driving and rotating the pin through the cortex. The initial entry point of the pin is critical and should be situated just distal to the normal curvature of the distal humerus. This position allows the IM pin to be guided into the medullary canal. Placement in this way is also important since it will not interfere with the ROM of the elbow and it avoids traumatizing the articular surface of the joint (Fig. 10.14). If the pin is placed any further distally, then it will impinge upon the olecranon when the elbow is extended.
- The pin can also be driven proximally from the fracture site to exit at the proximal humerus near the shoulder (Fig. 10.15). This necessarily penetrates the large muscle mass over the shoulder but appears to cause very few problems. The trocar tip at the distal end of the pin is blunted, the bone ends are aligned, and the pin is driven across the fracture into the distal

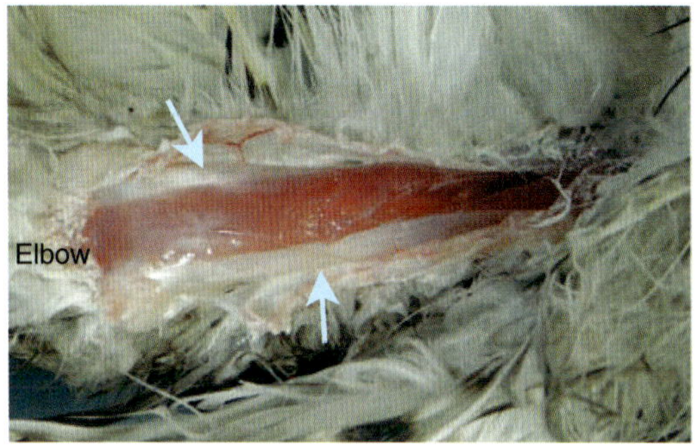

Fig. 10.12. The caudal view of a humerus in a red-tailed hawk showing the paired triceps tendons (arrows).

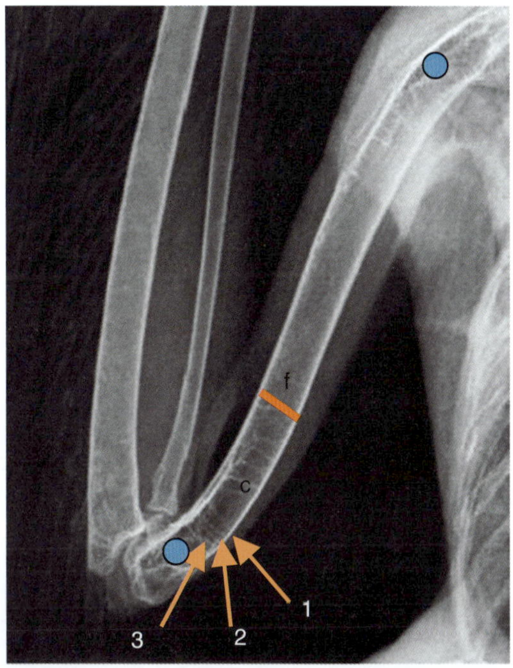

Fig. 10.13. Driving an IM pin from the elbow to repair a midshaft fracture (f). The pin is started perpendicular to the bone (1). Once the pin has a slight "bite", it is slowly re-directed (2, 3) as the trocar tip penetrates the cortex. The pin is placed distal to the natural curve (c) present in the humerus. The blue dots indicate the placements for the cross pins.

> **Raptor Tip**
>
> Do not flush up into the proximal humerus fragment since it is connected to the air sacs.

fragment. This option is simple and eliminates any chance of damage to the elbow joint or the triceps tendons. *This is definitely the preferred method.*

The wound is flushed, any loose fragments are arranged and packed back into the fracture site, and the incision is closed and covered with a sterile dressing.

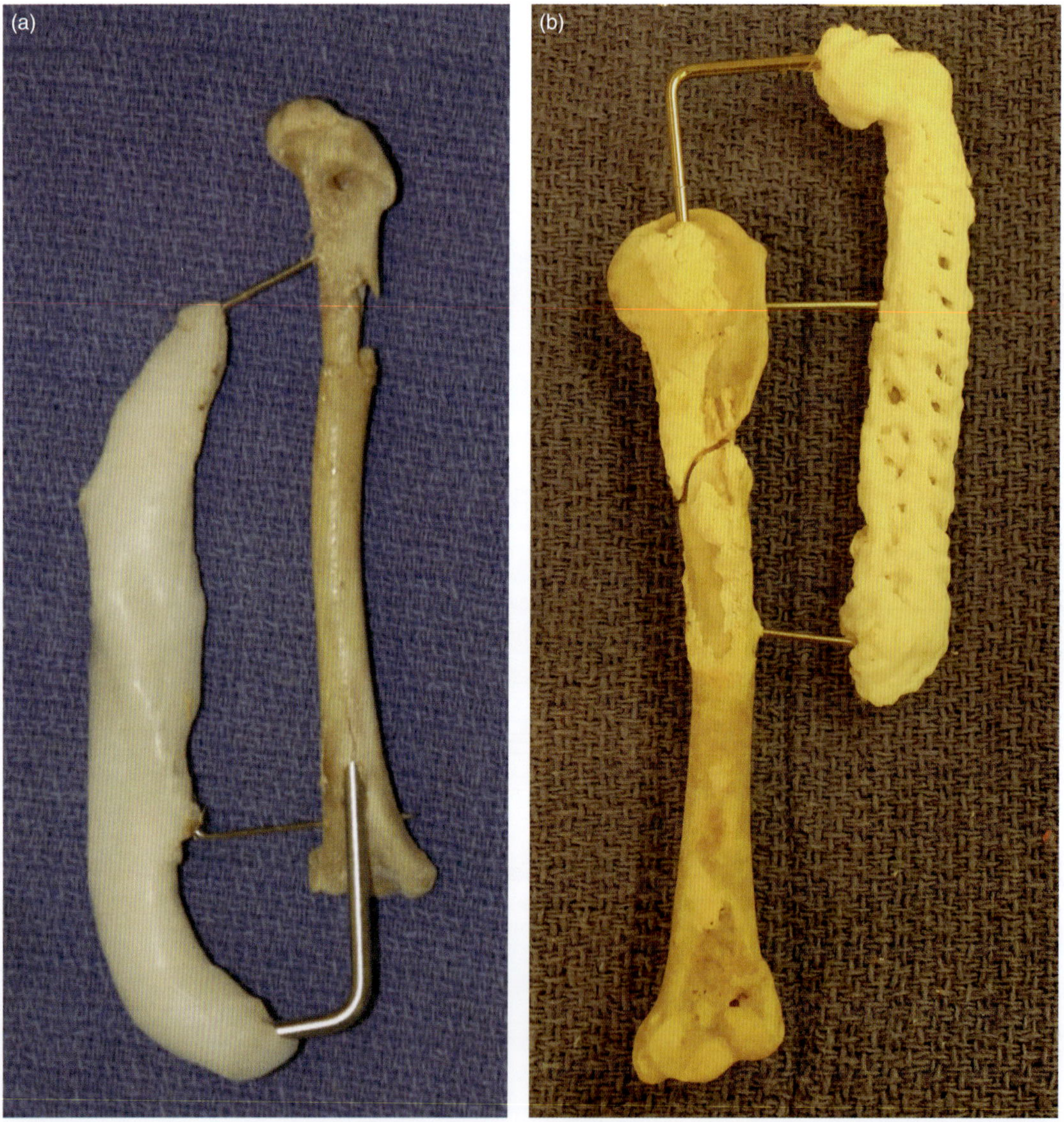

Fig. 10.14. An IM–ESF tie-in construct with the IM pin exiting distally near the elbow in (a) and proximally near the shoulder in (b). The sidebars are made from two different types of VTP.

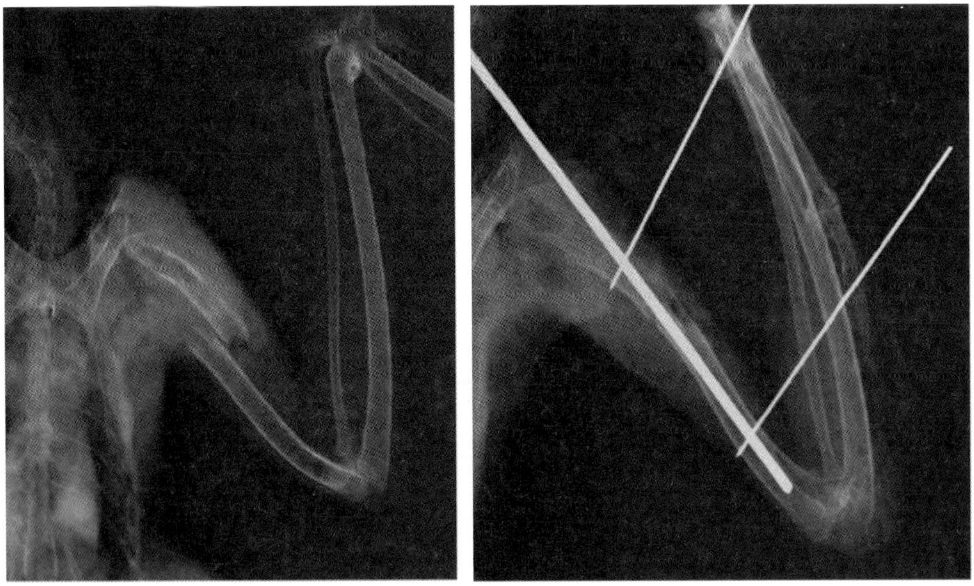

Fig. 10.15. A typical midshaft humeral fracture repaired with an IM–ESF tie-in. The IM pin exits at the shoulder.

Two cross pins are placed from the *dorsal* side perpendicular to the humerus. The pins are aligned dorsally and are placed proximal and distal to the fracture (approximate locations are indicated in Fig. 10.13). The cross pins do not fully penetrate the cortex on the ventral side. Instead, they are driven until the trocar point is just barely palpable coming through the cortex. They should not penetrate the skin. If the proximal cross pin is placed very close to the shoulder, it may not be possible to palpate the tip as it penetrates the ventral cortex. In this case, it is simply driven until it is firmly in place. Take care to not drive the proximal pin too far since it can cause serious trauma to the soft tissues in the axilla.

An intra-operative radiograph should be taken to verify pin placements. Of particular importance is the IM pin, which may need to be advanced or withdrawn.

While the bird is in *ventral* recumbency, the rotational alignment of the fracture is checked by comparing the orientation of both elbows and both pectoral crests (Fig. 2.2).

Once the proper rotation is confirmed, the cross pins and the IM pin are bent so that they overlap, and a sidebar is constructed to complete the fixation (Fig. 10.14). It is critical that the pins are carefully stabilized with large pliers or vise grips while the pins are bent.

The pin sites are covered with triple-antibiotic ointment and the wing is immobilized with a figure-8 and body wrap.

Begin PT on day 2 or 3 and remove the wrap at that time.

Long oblique humerus fracture

Long oblique fractures are usually open fractures with large amounts of exposed bone. These fractures are repaired in the same way as transverse fractures; however, these fractures can benefit from the use of cerclage wires (Fig. 10.16). While most references state that a minimum of two wires are required for any effect, this is not always possible in such small patients. Oftentimes even a single wire, when used in conjunction with an IM pin, can dramatically improve the rigidity of the repair.

Distal humerus fracture

Distal humeral fractures pose a unique challenge since the distal fragment can be quite short. In these cases, a single IM pin cannot be used as it

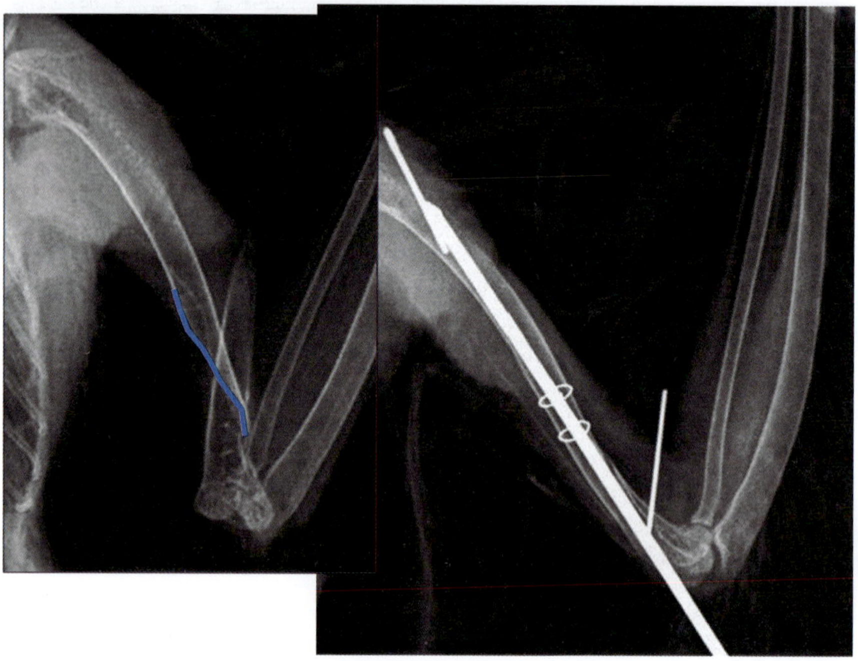

Fig. 10.16. A long oblique fracture repaired with cerclage wires. The wires locked the fracture ends together and almost perfect alignment was achieved. An ESF was also used. The blue line outlines the edge of the proximal fragment.

would have to exit very close to or in the elbow joint. Conversely, if the IM pin exits at the shoulder and is simply driven into the distal fragment, there may not be enough contact/friction with the distal fragment to provide much stability. To repair these fractures:

- A pair of thin, flexible K-wires are driven from the fracture into the distal fragment (Fig. 10.17). They are driven such that they exit on opposite sides of the humerus through the condyles (Fig. 10.18).
- The trocar tips on the proximal ends of the pins are blunted.
- The bone ends are aligned and each pin is driven, a little at a time, in an alternating fashion into the proximal fragment. Since the pins are thin, flexible, and blunt, they should arch off the endosteal surface of the proximal fragment.
- A single cross pin is placed in the proximal humeral fragment, as described previously. A distal cross pin is not required, since the two IM pins function well together to prevent any rotational and bending forces.
- The two IM pins and the cross pin are bent and a sidebar is constructed dorsally as described above.

Highly comminuted fracture

Some severely comminuted fractures (Fig. 10.19) can be repaired using a combination of techniques. Some helpful hints:

- Clean, flush, and debride the wound extensively. All loose but viable bone fragments should be collected and saved in a saline-soaked gauze. Non-viable (i.e. off-color) fragments should be discarded.
- When the IM pin is placed, these fractures tend to collapse and the overall length of the limb is reduced. To correct this problem and restore the length, pull the distal and proximal fragments apart along the IM pin. It is difficult to know exactly how far to separate

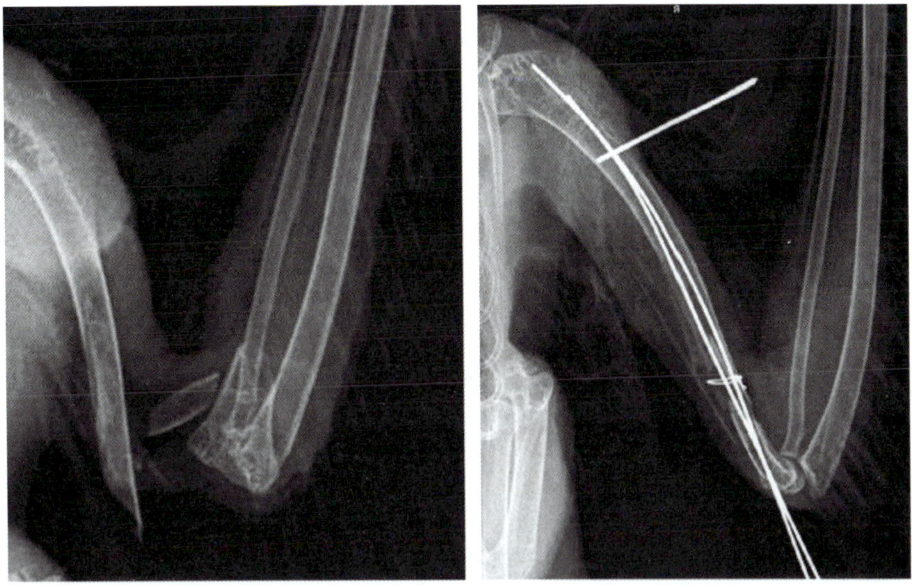

Fig. 10.17. Distal humerus fracture repaired with two flexible IM pins and an ESF tie-in. The fracture was only about 18 mm from the elbow. Notice how the thin IM pins are curved up into the proximal fragment.

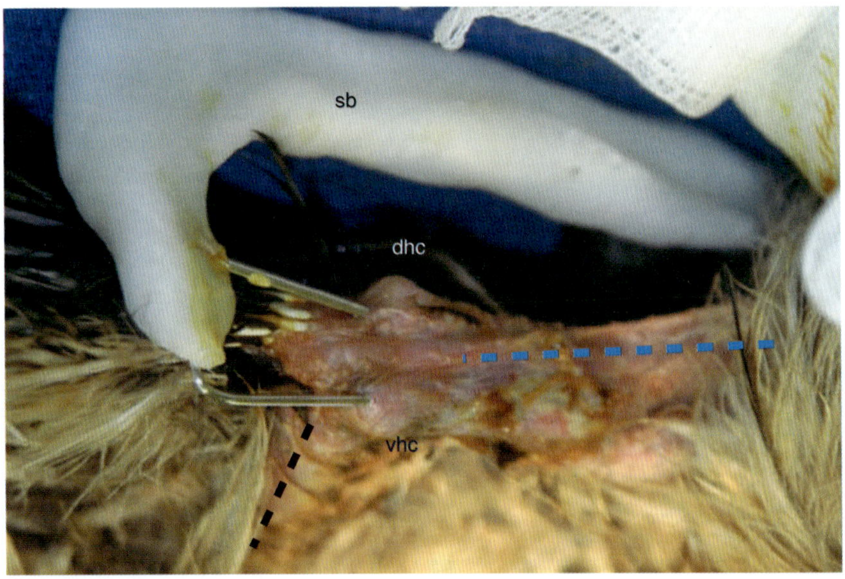

Fig. 10.18. Repair of distal humeral fracture (same bird as in Fig. 10.17). The flexible IM pins can be seen exiting the dorsal and ventral humeral condyles (dhc, vhc). The blue dotted line outlines the humerus and the black dotted line outlines the ulna. The sidebar (sb) is on the dorsal side and incorporates both IM pins and the proximal cross pin (not shown).

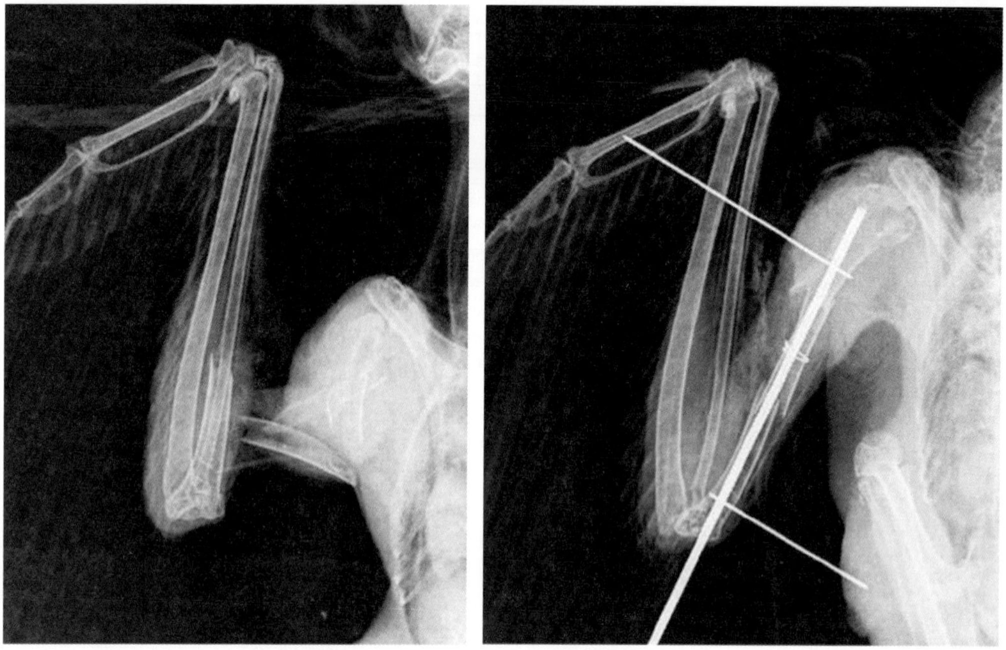

Fig. 10.19. This highly comminuted fracture was repaired with an intramedullary IM–ESF tie-in, a cerclage wire, and IMEX TR Matrix bone implant material. This bird healed well and was released. Note that the pins have not been bent yet to form the sidebar.

them, but taking an intra-operative radiograph can be helpful in making this determination.

- Pack all loose fragments around the IM pin to fill any gaps and attempt to reconstruct the bone column. For fragments that are still partially attached by soft tissue, try to handle them as little as possible and do not separate the fragments from any soft tissue connections that may still be present. Be sure to place the fragments so the curvature of each piece is wrapped around the pin in a more anatomic arrangement. Realize that it is usually not possible to get the fragments to fit back together like "puzzle pieces". Cerclage wires can be very helpful in these cases.
- Do not be afraid to experiment. Try new techniques or combine several together.

Humerus fractures in small birds

While the IM pin–ESF tie-in is the ideal fixation for most humeral fractures, placement of cross pins can be technically challenging in small birds such as kestrels and screech owls. In these cases, a simple IM pin may suffice, and a return to full flight is still possible. While some references state that a return to flight and release is not possible with an IM pin-only fixation, this is simply not true (Fig. 10.20) and should be attempted if no other option exists.

> **Raptor Tip**
>
> The tip of the pin exiting near the elbow must be covered at all times. It is hard to believe, but some birds, especially owls, can get the IM pin stuck between their mandibles!

With just an IM pin for stabilization, there is nothing counteracting rotational forces (i.e. the external fixator). Therefore, you must be especially careful when doing PT to not induce any rotation. In addition, the figure-8 and body wrap

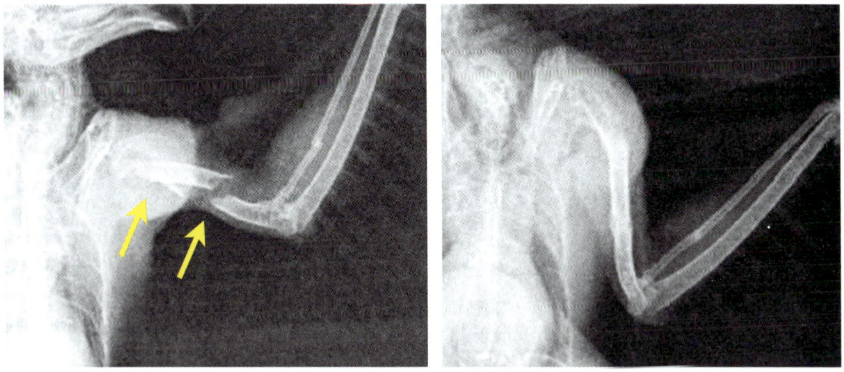

Fig. 10.20. This double humerus fracture (arrows) in an American kestrel was repaired with just a single IM pin. The pin was removed in exactly 30 days and this bird flew very well.

should remain in place for at least 3 weeks (and possibly longer) instead of the usual 2–3 days.

Proximal humerus fracture

Proximal humeral fractures can be difficult to repair surgically. The large muscle mass in the area can make it challenging to expose the bone ends. In addition, the proximal bone fragment may be too short to accept an IM pin and it is no longer a tubular structure so it can be hard to align when attempting to place the pin. Luckily, these fractures are not very common. Some options include:

- A single IM pin exiting at the shoulder.
- A tension band wire placed over two K-wires placed in a crossed configuration. This is an advanced procedure that requires extensive elevation of muscle tissue to get adequate exposure (see Samour, 2008 for details).
- A simple figure-8 and body wrap with PT and cage rest may suffice in some cases.

Prognosis for releasability varies depending on the fracture and the species but can only be determined after evaluation in a flight cage. Owls can do surprisingly well (Fig. 10.21) but diurnal birds such as large hawks rarely heal properly.

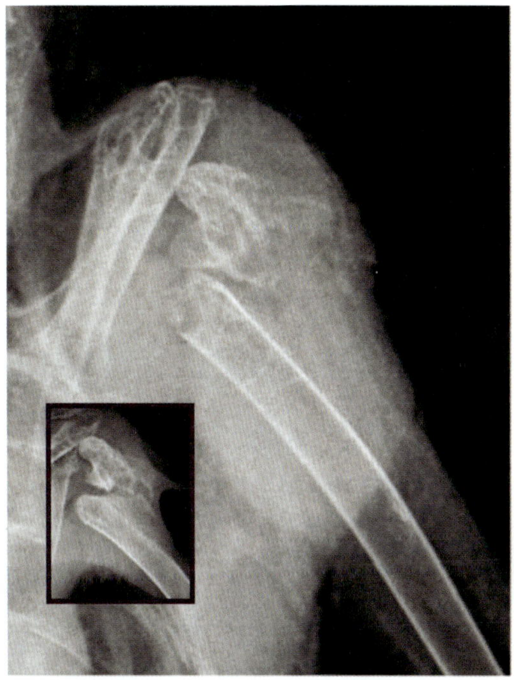

Fig. 10.21. Proximal, very poorly aligned humerus fracture in a barred owl. It was treated with a body wrap, cage rest, and PT. A bridging callus formed after 3 weeks (inset) and this bird eventually regained near-perfect flight and was released.

Ulna and radius

The most commonly seen fractures involve the ulna. They are either solitary or present with a radius fracture. Solitary radius fractures are relatively uncommon. When either bone is intact, the intact bone functions as an internal splint and maintains the overall length of the limb. The wing should be stabilized with a figure-8 wrap prior to surgery.

There are several options for treatment, depending on the severity and location of the fracture(s):

- In general, surgical correction of fractures should be performed as soon as possible. However, there are cases where surgery is not the best option. For example, in simple ulna fractures where the bone ends overlap by at least 50%, a figure-8 wrap can be quite effective. In other cases in which the alignment is not ideal, waiting a few days can improve the situation substantially. This is especially true in highly comminuted midshaft ulna fractures. In these cases, the natural forces exerted by the tendons and other soft tissues against an intact radius can pull many of the bone fragments back into correct alignment (Fig. 10.22).
- In this author's experience, most solitary ulna fractures generally do quite well without surgery. A figure-8 wrap and careful PT are all that many of these cases need (Fig. 10.23).

Ulna fracture repair with an IM pin ± ESF tie-in

The most common repair technique for ulna fractures is to place an IM pin:

- A dorsal approach is recommended. The advantage of the dorsal approach is that the ulna is directly accessible underneath the skin and this approach facilitates the placement of an ESF tie-in. However, the secondary feather follicles overlie the area and must be avoided when the incision is made.
- An incision is made over the fracture site and the fracture ends are identified. These fractures are usually accompanied by large blood clots which need to be removed and the area flushed clear.
- Place the IM pin. The pin is typically introduced at the proximal ulna just distal to the olecranon and it is driven toward the fracture. The pin must be placed so it does not interfere with the elbow joint. Fortunately, the ulna in most raptor species has a gentle curve just distal to the elbow which allows the pin to be placed and driven into the medullary canal without affecting the elbow joint (see arrow in Fig. 10.24). The pin is placed in a manner similar to that described for the humerus fracture (Fig. 10.13) where the pin is initially driven perpendicular to the bone surface then the angle is gradually changed to direct the pin up into the medullary canal.

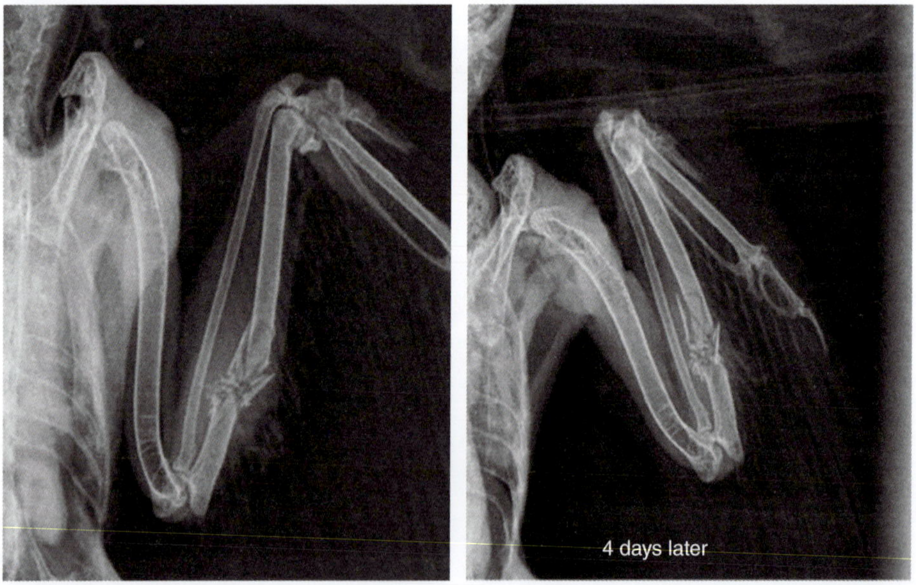

Fig. 10.22. This misaligned ulna fracture looked much better 4 days later. Surgery was not required and figure-8 bandage worked well.

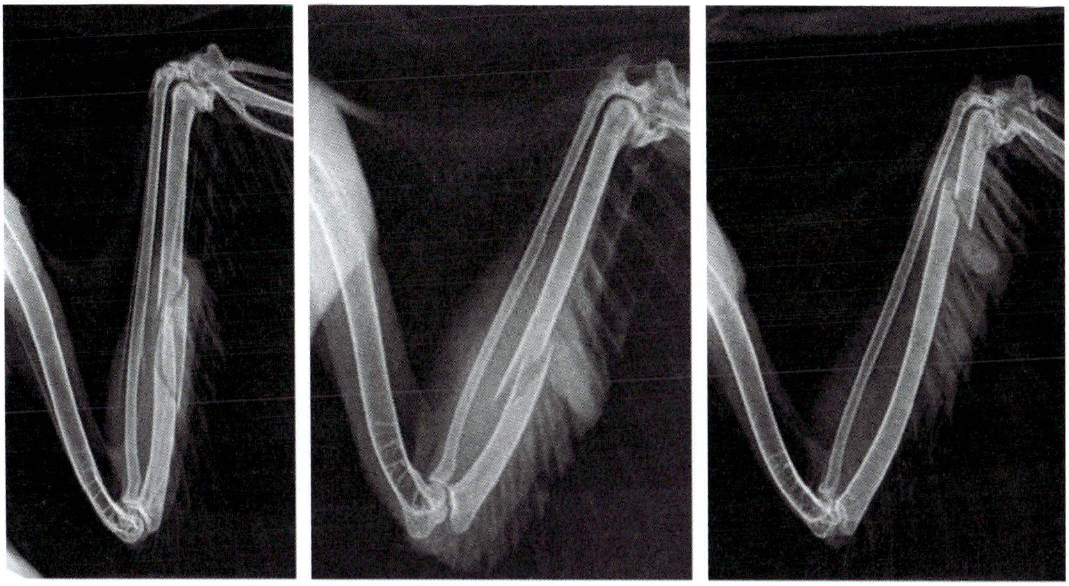

Fig. 10.23. All these ulna fractures were treated conservatively with a figure-8 wrap and PT. All birds were eventually released.

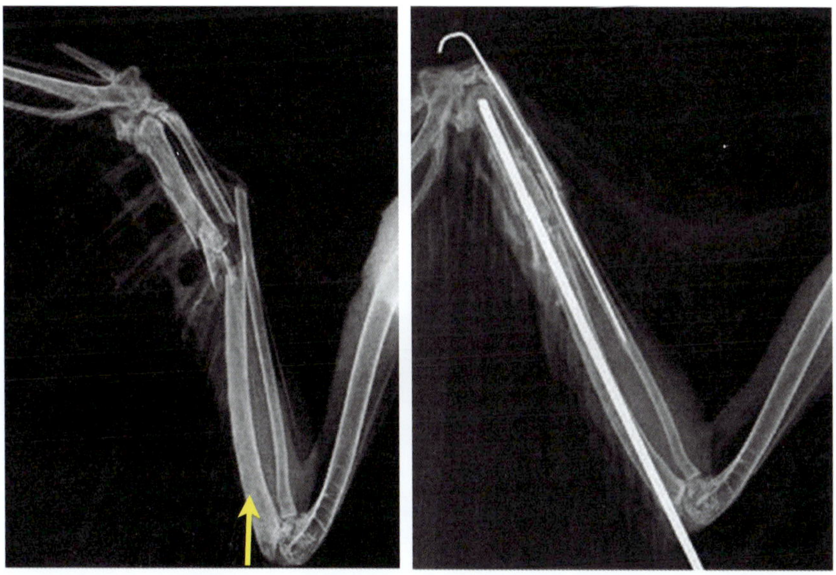

Fig. 10.24. Badly comminuted, open combination radius/ulna fracture. Both fractures were repaired with IM pins. The yellow arrow indicates where the IM pin should be driven into the ulna. As can be seen on the right, the ulna pin may be a little too close to the elbow joint.

This technique only works well for midshaft and distal fractures.

- The pin is driven until the tip is visible at the fracture. The trocar tip is blunted and the bone ends are aligned.
- The pin is driven across the fracture into the distal fragment.
- The wound is flushed and closed (usually in two layers).
- A radiograph is taken to verify pin placement and the pin is adjusted as needed.
- The pin is cut off at the elbow, leaving enough exposed so it can be grasped when it is time to be removed.
- The wing is placed in a figure-8 wrap and the wrap is maintained for 3 weeks while PT is performed. Be careful as the IM pin can loosen and migrate out from the entry point.
- The addition of an ESF in a tie-in procedure is also possible. A single cross pin is placed proximal and distal to the ulna fracture from the dorsal side. The addition of the ESF neutralizes all rotational forces and also prevents the IM pin from migrating. Therefore, a wing wrap is not required. Because the wing is not confined to a wrap, much less PT is required and you can expect a quicker overall healing time (Fig. 10.25). Because of this, *this is the preferred method of fixation*. However, this procedure is technically challenging in smaller birds and there is a chance of inadvertent damage or fracture when the cross pins are placed.

Radius fracture repair with an IM pin

The only repair technique for radius fractures is to place an IM pin (Figs 10.24, 10.26, and 10.27). These are probably the easiest fractures to repair because the bone is readily palpable and visible directly under the skin along much of its entire length. Unlike ulna fractures, all fractures involving the midshaft or distal radius should be repaired. This bone is highly mobile and a non-union is likely if these fractures are not stabilized appropriately.

- A dorsal or ventral approach can be used.
- An incision is made over the fracture and the bone ends are identified.
- Place the IM pin. With the carpus fully flexed, the pin is introduced at the fracture site and is driven distally to exit at the wrist. Flexion of the carpus allows the radial carpal bone to be avoided when the pin exits. Be sure to surgically prepare the area.
- The trocar tip is blunted and the bone ends are aligned.
- The pin is driven across the fracture into the proximal fragment.
- The wound is flushed and closed (usually in one layer).

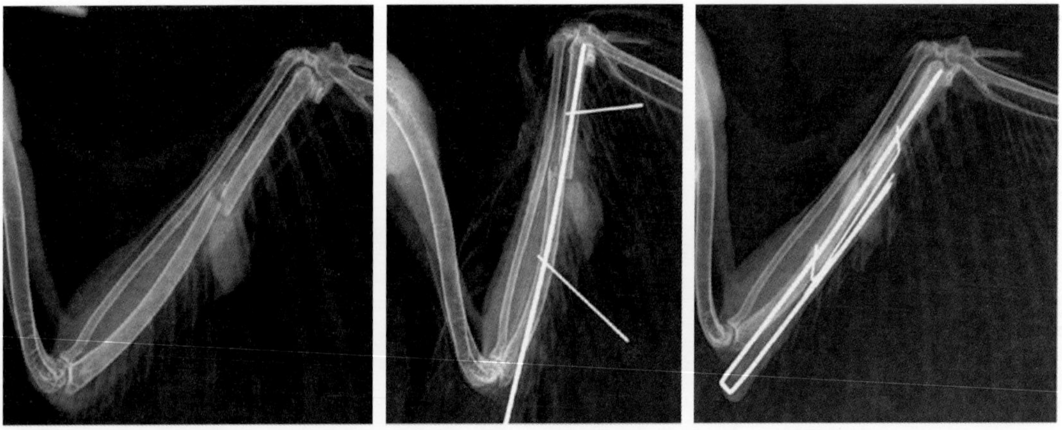

Fig. 10.25. Displaced ulna fracture repaired with an IM–ESF tie-in.

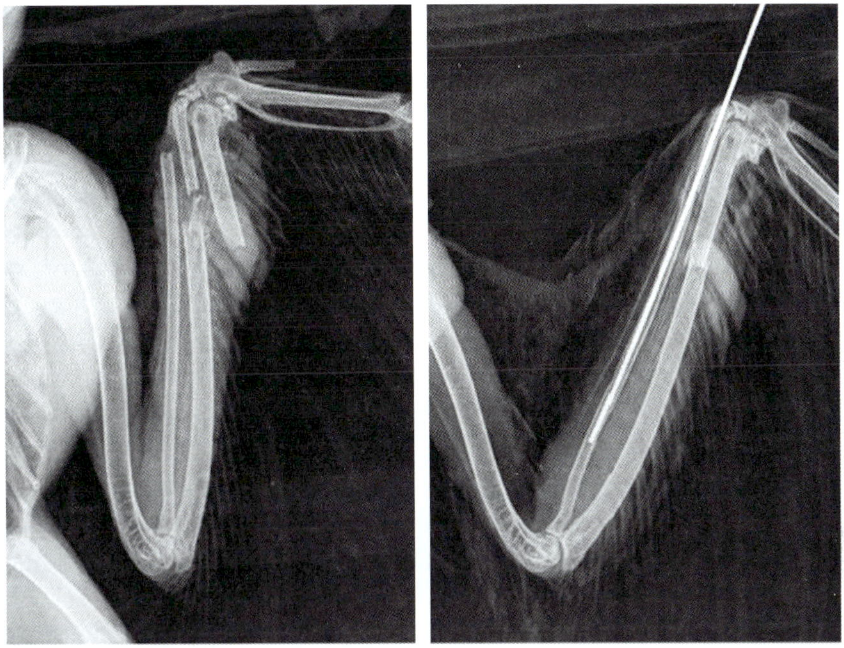

Fig. 10.26. Combination ulna/radius fracture. The radius was repaired with a standard IM pin and a translucent polypropylene shuttle pin was used in the ulna. Shuttle pins work very well in transverse fractures such as these, and the stability of this type of repair can be excellent.

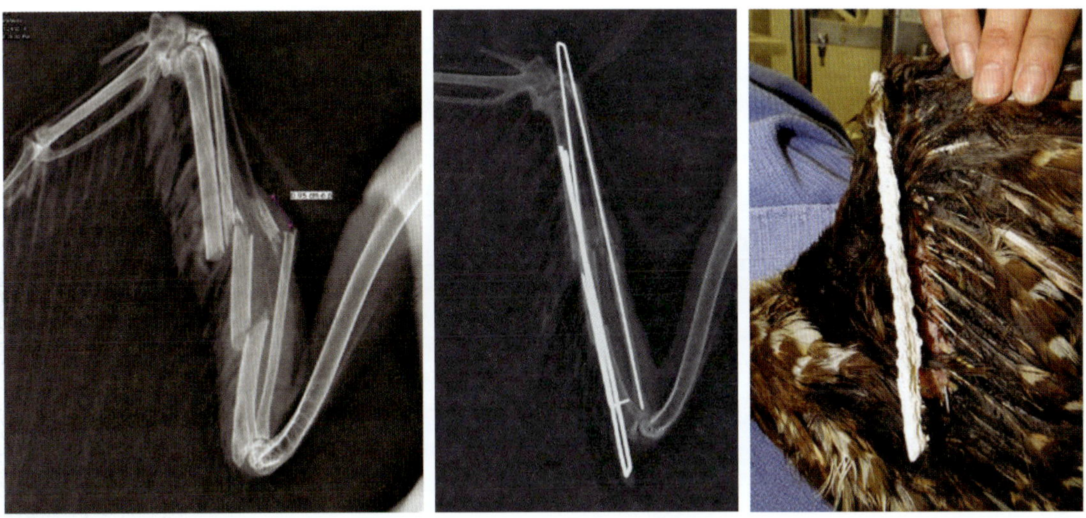

Fig. 10.27. Combination ulna/radius fracture repaired with an IM–ESF tie-in. Note that the radius IM pin is bent back and incorporated into the sidebar, and that the ulna IM pin could probably have been driven in a little further. The color photograph shows the sidebar as viewed from the dorsal side of the wing.

- A radiograph is taken to verify pin placement and the pin is adjusted as needed.
- The pin is cut off at the wrist, leaving enough exposed so that it can be grasped when it is time to remove it.
- The wing is placed in a figure-8 wrap and the wrap is maintained for 2 to 3 weeks while PT is performed. The pin end protruding at the wrist must be covered at all times since it can easily cause severe eye trauma if left uncovered.

Notes

The IM pin in the radius may not allow complete ROM in the carpal joint so remove this pin early (at approximately 2–3 weeks).

This procedure necessarily penetrates the joint space, so extra care and attention must be taken to ensure the pin exit is kept clean.

For smaller birds such as the screech owl or sharp-shinned hawk, 20–22-gauge spinal needles 2–3″ (5–7.6 cm) in length make excellent IM pins.

Ulna fracture repair with a shuttle pin

For midshaft, transverse fractures of the ulna, a shuttle pin can be an excellent choice (Fig. 10.26). They are particularly helpful in young, developing birds, as mentioned previously.

Combination ulna and radius fracture

With these fractures, all structural integrity of the wing is gone, the limb is entirely unstable, and there can be massive amounts of soft tissue damage and swelling of the distal limb (Fig. 10.26). A figure-8 wrap is necessary pending surgery, but the wrap cannot stabilize these fractures effectively. Surgery should be performed almost immediately after the patient is stabilized. In these cases, both bones will require surgical stabilization (Fig. 10.27). The recommended procedure is to use an IM–ESF on the ulna and an IM pin in the radius. The radius IM pin is bent back dorsally and incorporated into the ulna fixation sidebar.

Highly comminuted ulna fractures

Some highly comminuted fractures are better treated without surgical intervention (Fig. 10.28). Attempting to place an IM pin or other internal fixation may damage the already tenuous blood supply and make matters worse. In these cases, attending to the soft tissue wounds, immobilization with a figure-8 wrap, and PT may be all that is needed.

Metacarpal fractures

Metacarpal fractures can be difficult to treat. Usually both the major and minor metacarpal bones are fractured (Fig. 10.29). There is very little soft tissue covering the bones, so exposure and desiccation of vital structures is a serious risk. In addition, these fractures may take a longer time to heal when compared to other fractures and this may be due to limited soft tissue coverage in the area. Options for treatment are shown below.

Figure-8 wrap over a padded splint

This method can actually be very effective and is oftentimes the best choice, but PT of the carpal joint can be difficult to perform without placing stress across the fracture gap. This is especially true if the fracture is close to the wrist joint. There is an increased likelihood of a non-union resulting in fractures treated in this manner, but sometimes there are few other good options. A figure-8 wrap can be augmented with a splint made from various materials:

- SAM splint material (Fig. 10.30) is very helpful for these applications since it can be molded and is padded with foam.
- VTP is also useful and can be molded to create a very secure splint (Fig. 10.31).

IM pin

An IM pin (Fig. 10.29) provides a more stable fixation and resists bending so PT can be carried out more easily. However, injury to the carpal joint can occur since the pin must pass through it. In addition, the ROM of the carpus may be decreased

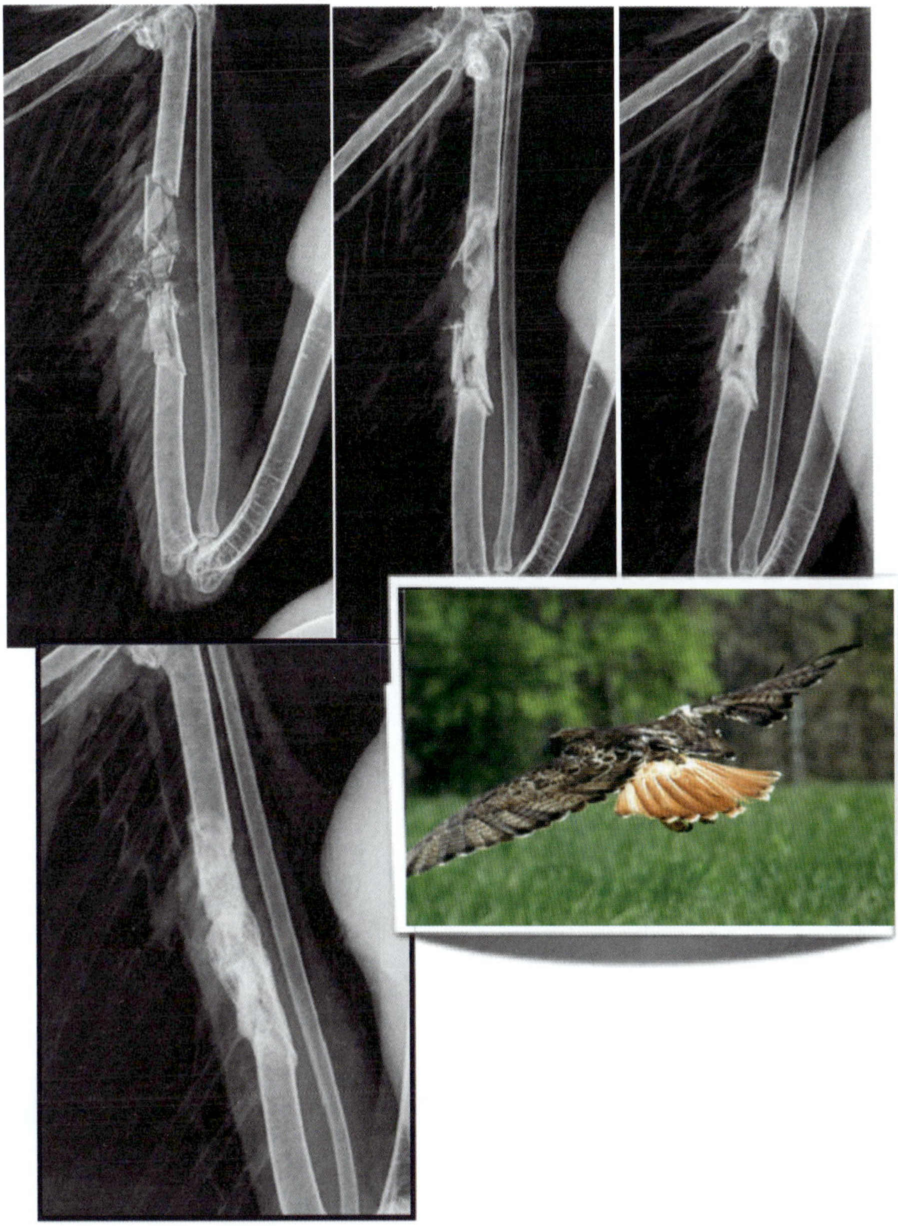

Fig. 10.28. A highly comminuted ulna fracture in a red-tailed hawk was treated conservatively and healed nicely over a period of 16 weeks. She had a gap from two missing secondary feathers but otherwise flew well and was released.

so these pins should be removed as soon as possible (i.e. 2–3 weeks).

To place the IM pin in the major metacarpal bone:

- A ventral or dorsal approach can be used and this can depend on whether there is an existing open wound or not.
- Identify and isolate both bone ends.

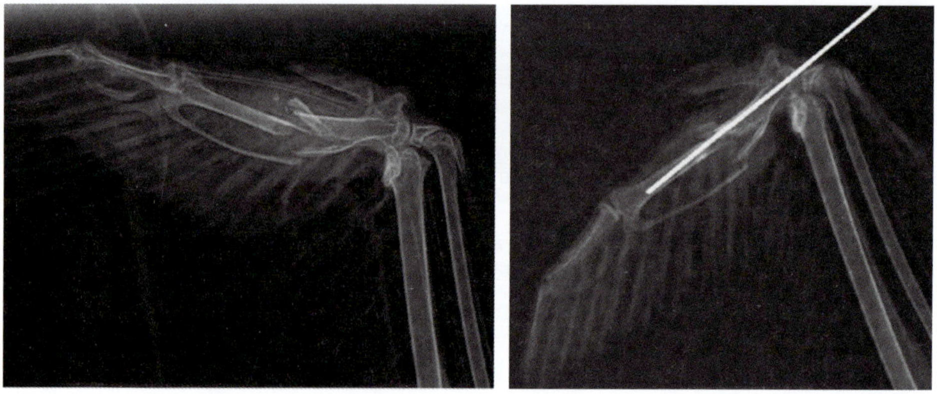

Fig. 10.29. A typical metacarpal injury with fracture of both the major and minor bones. This was very unstable with an open wound. The fracture was repaired with an IM pin.

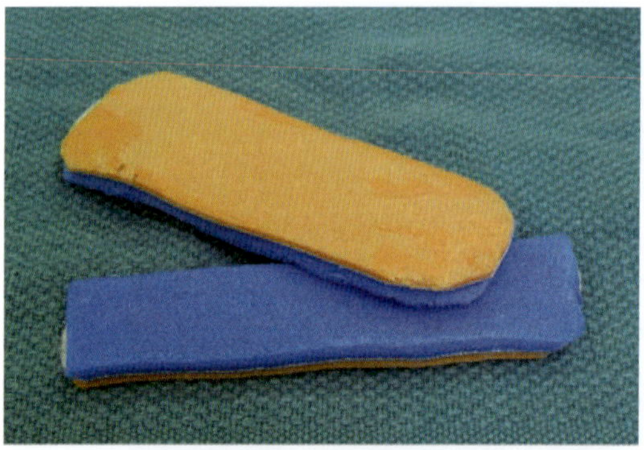

Fig. 10.30. SAM splint material is a thin layer of bendable aluminum sandwiched between foam. It is very useful for metacarpal fractures.

- Fully flex the wrist joint and drive the pin from the fracture proximally to exit at the wrist.
- Blunt the trocar tip facing the fracture and drive it across the fracture into the distal fragment.
- Close the wound and place a figure-8 wrap.
- Do frequent PT and remove the pin after 2–3 weeks.

Fractures of the Leg

With any leg fracture, close attention should be paid to the development of bumblefoot on the opposite foot. In order to reduce the chances of bumblefoot developing, leg fractures should be repaired as soon as possible and, with appropriate analgesia, weight bearing is often seen within 48 h after surgical repair.

Handling of these birds is complicated because the fractured leg should never be grabbed directly. Plan your treatments to minimize the need to handle the bird and utilize a "body grab" when handling is required.

Femur

Femur fractures are generally closed due to the large amount of muscle mass covering the bone. Midshaft fractures (Fig. 10.32, for example) can be repaired with an IM pin–ESF tie-in as follows:

- A lateral approach is used.
- The large muscle masses are separated along fascial planes.
- The bone ends are identified and blood clots are removed.
- An IM pin is introduced at the fracture and driven proximally to exit through the greater trochanter on the lateral aspect of the hip joint (Fig. 10.33).
- The trocar tip facing the fracture is blunted and the pin is driven distally across the fracture. Be very careful to not drive the pin too far (i.e. into the stifle joint). The blunted trocar tip helps as you will feel resistance once the tip enters the metaphysis.

- The wound is flushed and the incision is closed in two layers.
- A cross pin is placed from the lateral to medial side of the distal femur just proximal to the femoral condyles. The femur is supported with two fingers from the medial side and the pin is driven until it can just be felt penetrating the cortex on the medial side. This pin can be placed distal to the most distal extent of the IM pin. In this case, this pin can be larger as it does not have to share medullary cavity space with the IM pin.
- Another cross pin is placed from lateral to medial proximal to the fracture. Be careful not to place it into or near the femoral neck and acetabulum. It is sometimes difficult to palpate the pin on the medial side, so it is often driven "by feel" until the trocar tip firmly engages the medial cortex. Since this pin must share medullary space with the IM pin, it is typically smaller than the distal cross pin and must be placed very carefully to avoid creating additional fractures.
- The cross pins and the IM pin are bent laterally and incorporated into a sidebar (Fig. 10.33).

Raptor Tip

Do not flush into the proximal femur fragment since it is connected to the air sacs.

Note

Many references indicate that a proximal cross pin placed near the acetabulum is always necessary. The intent of this pin and the need for a full external fixator is to prevent rotation and to maintain the overall length of the femur. In this author's experience, there is more than sufficient muscle mass to prevent most rotation, and many femur fractures tend to be transverse, so the risk of the fracture collapsing down on itself is minimal. In addition, the placement of this proximal cross pin can be technically challenging, especially in small birds, and can result in significant damage if improperly placed (i.e. iatrogenic fractures, penetration of acetabulum, etc.). For these reasons, a modified construct

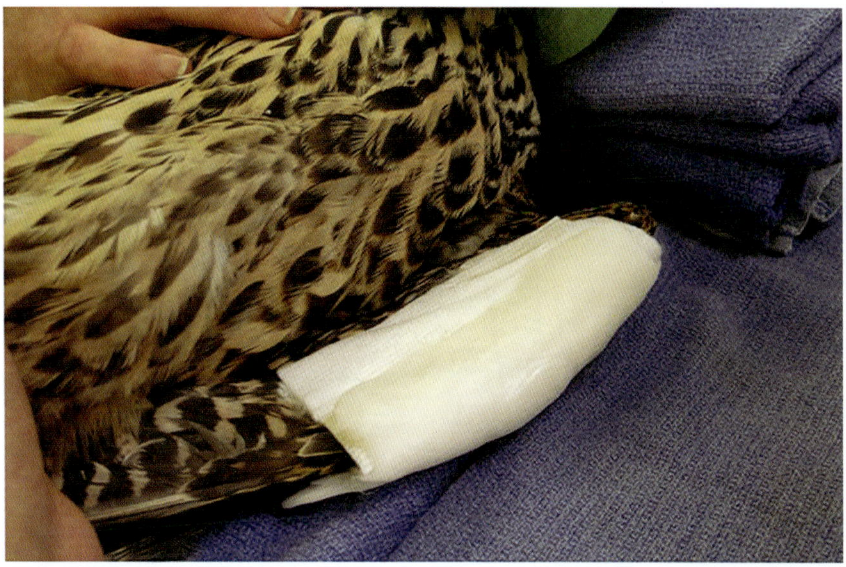

Fig. 10.31. A metacarpal splint created with VTP can be molded around the ventral and dorsal sides to create a very stable environment for bone healing.

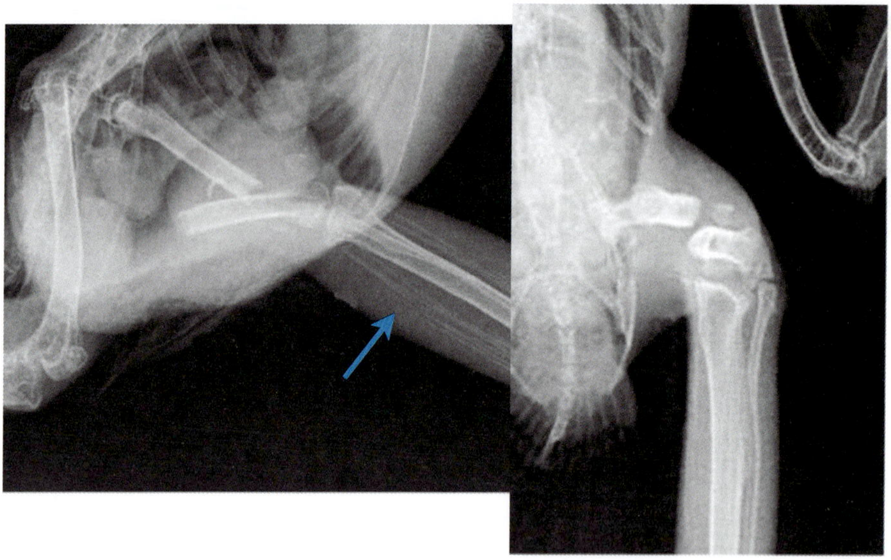

Fig. 10.32. A typical transverse, midshaft femur fracture. A lateral view is very helpful when planning your repair. Note that many tendons in owls are calcified (arrowhead).

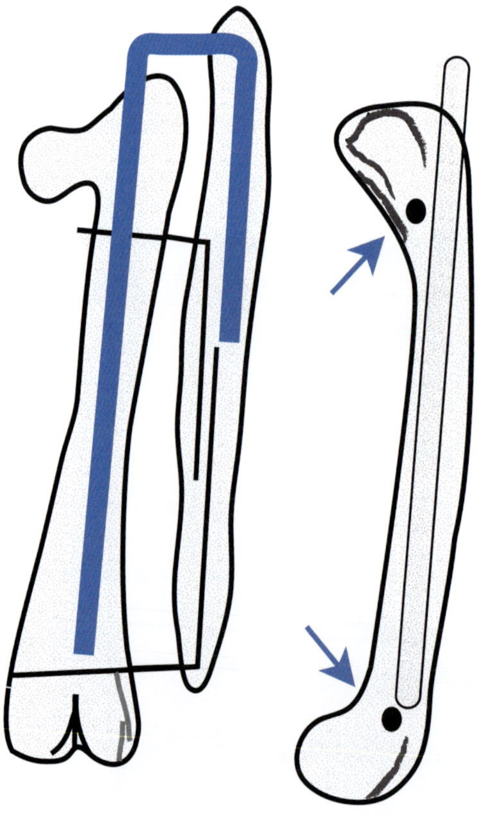

Fig. 10.33. Placement of an IM–ESF fixation for a femur fracture. The arrows are pointing to the cross pins on the lateral view.

(Figs 10.34 and 10.35) that skips the proximal cross pin can often be used in smaller birds or in simple, transverse fractures in birds of all sizes. In these cases, the single distal cross pin is placed simply to prevent the IM pin from migrating out at the hip. This fixation is easy to place and has been very effective in many fractures and in many species.

Femoral head fractures

These fractures are usually managed with cage rest and may heal with the formation of a false/fibrous joint. However, formation of bumblefoot in the opposite foot may occur. In addition, some cases can result in degenerative joint disease and may ultimately require a femoral head osteotomy (FHO). In fact, performing an FHO early may lead to a quicker return to function and a better overall outcome (Burgdorf-Moisuk *et al.*, 2011).

Tibiotarsus

Tibiotarsal fractures are very common. Luckily, many tend to be located in the midshaft region and are therefore more likely to be surgically repairable.

There is a large amount of soft tissue surrounding much of the tibiotarsus bone. This prevents

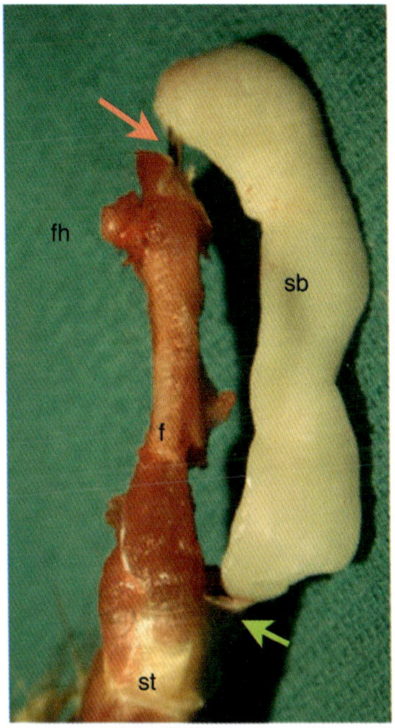

Fig. 10.34. External fixator on femur from a cadaver. Femoral head (fh), midshaft fracture (f), sidebar on lateral aspect (sb), stifle joint (st), IM pin (orange arrow), distal cross pin (green arrow).

bone exposure, but it can also result in massive swelling after the initial injury and post-operatively. The swelling can make placement of cross pins challenging, as palpation of the bone becomes more difficult. In addition, the cross section of the tibiotarsus presents a thin, almost knife-like edge laterally, so it can be difficult to place cross pins when utilizing an external fixator (Fig. 10.36).

There are many options when managing tibiotarsus fractures (Fig. 10.37) and they depend on the location and complexity of the fracture as well as the age and size of the patient. Some options include:

- A simple padded splint. These are appropriate for well-aligned, transverse fractures, and in very young birds. Splints do not work well for proximal fractures.
- An IM pin exiting at the tibial crest. These are appropriate and work well in young birds with mostly transverse fractures. If the fracture is oblique, this fixation may allow the bone ends to collapse into one another resulting in a loss of overall length.
- An ESF works in some cases but, when used alone, it can be difficult to get good end-to-end

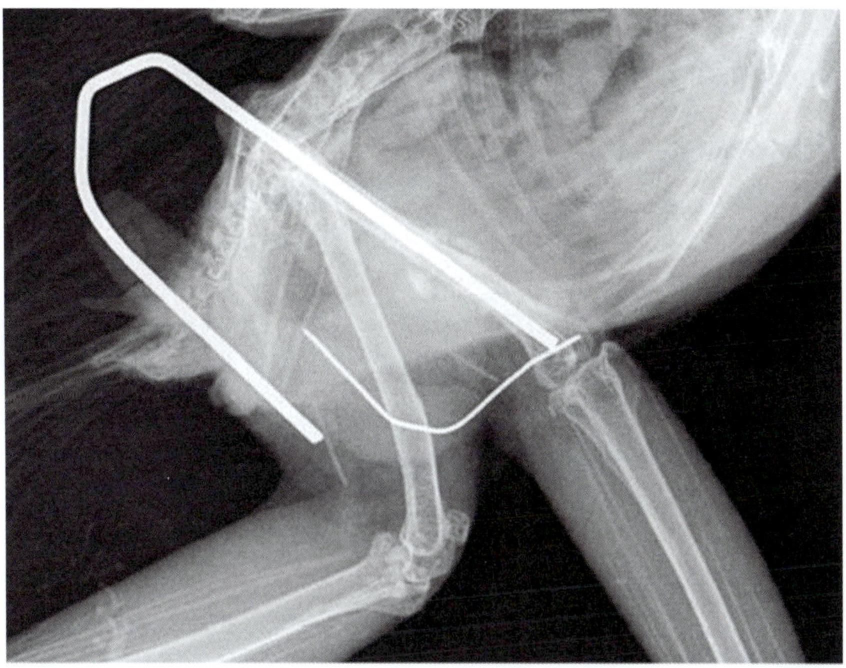

Fig. 10.35. Transverse femur fracture repaired with an IM pin and an ESF tie-in. Note that only a distal cross pin was used. Both pins are bent to connect into a sidebar on the lateral side.

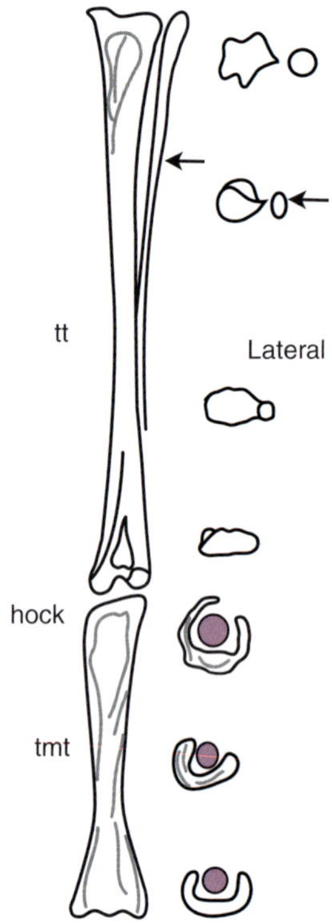

Fig. 10.36. Cross section of the lower leg in a barred owl. The lateral aspect of the tibiotarsus (tt) is quite sharp, partly due to the fibula (arrowheads). The caudal tarsometatarsus (tmt) forms a concave channel that contains the flexor tendons and vessels (purple circle).

alignment of the bone fragments. This is *not* recommended.

- ESF + IM pin tie-in (Fig. 10.38) allows for very excellent rigidity and alignment but the stifle joint must be penetrated. Although this sounds like it would lead to complications, this works quite well and it is the suggested method of repair in most cases. It is often possible (and recommended) that the IM pin be removed early (after 3 weeks).
- ESF + shuttle pin (Fig. 10.39) also allows for excellent rigidity and alignment and it does not require involvement of the stifle joint.

IM pin placement

To place an IM pin:

- A closed procedure can be attempted by placing the IM from the tibial plateau in much the same way that one would place an IO catheter (Fig. 4.8). This can be difficult as swelling, and the large amount of soft tissue, can make getting good end-to-end alignment of the bones very difficult. This is much easier for proximal fractures. An open procedure is usually a better choice and does not result in any noticeable post-operative problems.
- For an open procedure, a medial approach usually provides the easiest access to the fracture as it avoids the fibula and the tibial nerve on the lateral side and it is relatively easy to

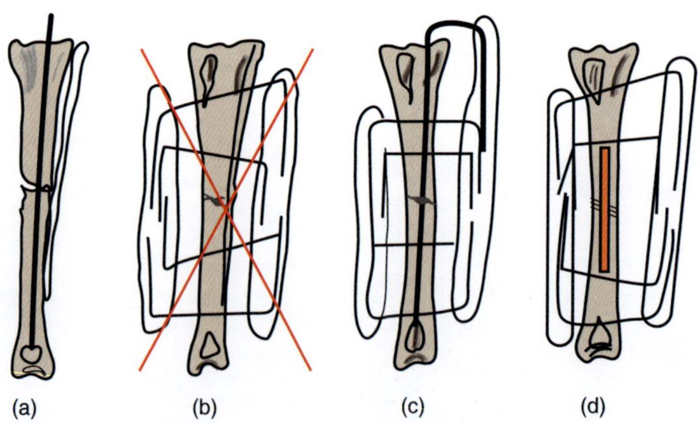

Fig. 10.37. Fixation options for tibiotarsal fractures. An IM pin alone (a), a standard bilateral ESF (this option is *not* recommended) (b), an IM pin + ESF tie-in (c), and an ESF plus a shuttle pin (d).

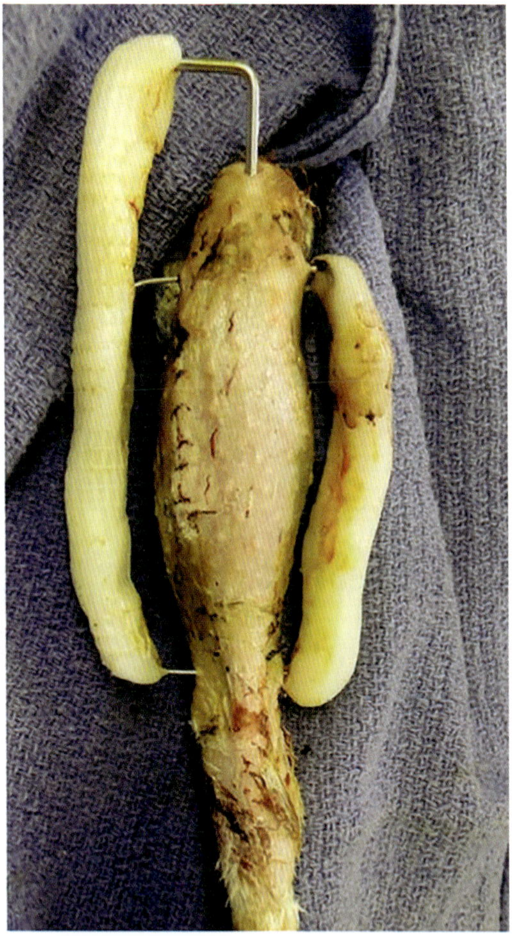

Fig. 10.38. ESF–IM tie-in repair of tibiotarsal fracture.

atraumatically dissect between the large muscle bellies of the gastrocnemius and the cranial tibial muscles. However, the approach can and should be made wherever the bone ends are most easily palpable under the skin.

- An incision is made over the fracture and the muscle bellies are divided along fascial planes, if possible.
- The fracture bone ends are identified.
- The knee joint is *maximally* flexed and a pin is driven from the fracture proximally, exiting at the tibial plateau.
- The distal trocar tip is blunted and the pin is driven into the distal fragment.
- The wound is flushed and closed in two layers.
- The pin is cut off at the stifle so that enough pin is left exposed to allow it to be grasped with a pin chuck when it is time to be removed. If an ESF is to be incorporated, the IM pin is left long and is not cut off.
- A padded splint (Chapter 4) is applied to cover the pin and for additional support and protection (if needed). Note: the exposed pin end should never be left uncovered.

IM–ESF tie-in

As stated above, an ESF alone is not a good option as it is very difficult to achieve good end-to-end alignment at the fracture site. Because of this an IM–ESF tie-in (Fig. 10.38) is usually the best choice. The IM pin is placed before the ESF as described above. To place an ESF:

- The entire leg from the stifle to just past the hock must be plucked and aseptically prepared. The foot should be covered in a sterile wrap to reduce the chance of contamination.
- For the IM–ESF tie-in procedure, usually only a single pin is needed above and below the fracture. In larger birds (e.g. vulture or eagle) or in cases where the ESF is used alone, a total of four cross pins are required.
- The cross pins are usually placed from lateral to medial.
- The proximal pins are generally more difficult to place since there is more soft tissue covering the bone. Also, the lateral edge is very thin and has a knife-edge profile that must be penetrated with the trocar tip (Fig. 10.36). It is sometimes helpful to approach the bone from the cranial–dorsal aspect so that the pin does not have to directly penetrate the sharp, lateral edge. The proximal-most pin should angle distal-medially. This angle keeps the proximal end of the medial sidebar away from the body wall when the bird is in a normal perch position.
- The distal pins are easier to place since the bone is more rounded and much easier to palpate. The distal-most pin should be placed proximal to the condyles to avoid damage to the collateral ligaments.
- The IM pin is now bent around on the *lateral* side.

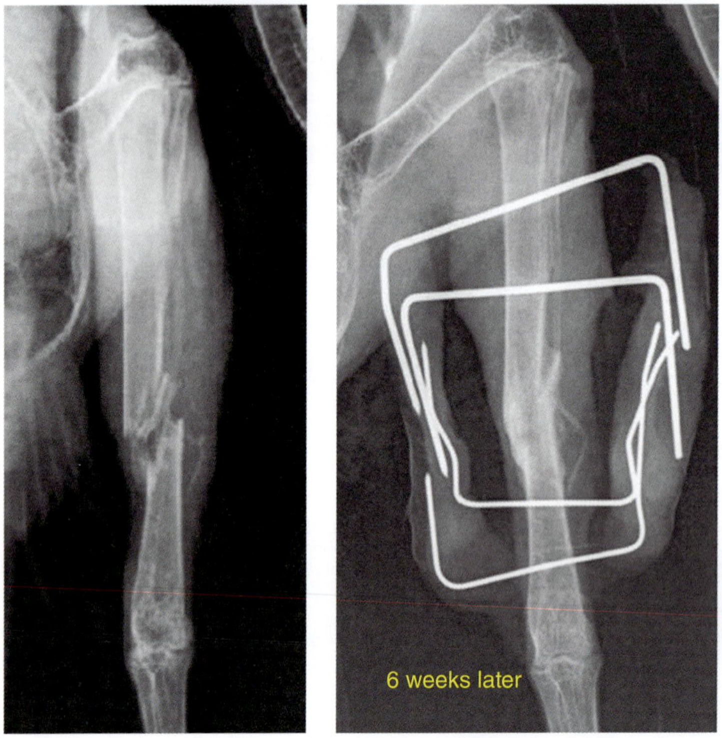

Fig. 10.39. Tibiotarsal fracture in a turkey vulture. An ESF + shuttle pin achieved good alignment and the fixator was removed after 6 weeks.

- The stifle and hock joints are aligned, the cross pins are bent, and the sidebars are created. It is very important that enough space (at least 8–10 mm) is left between the skin and the sidebars since substantial post-op swelling is common.
- The fixation is kept covered with elastic bandage material for 10 days to keep it clean, and the pin tracts should be cleaned periodically and coated with triple-antibiotic ointment for the first week.

Tarsometatarsus

Tarsometatarsal fractures are relatively uncommon. When they do occur, there may be significant swelling of the foot and digits. This is due to the almost complete lack of soft tissue covering in the area and resultant compromise to the vasculature. There are few options for repairing these fractures:

- A splint may be effective in very young or small birds.
- External fixation (Fig. 10.40). This is the one case where a bilateral external fixator without an IM tie-in is the treatment of choice.

The unusual cross section of this bone (Fig. 10.36) with a large concave channel rules out the possibility of using a shuttle pin or IM pin. When placing the cross pins for the ESF, it is critically important that the pins are placed through the cranial aspect to avoid traumatizing the tendons and vessels that are located within the channel. Note that the concavity is not as pronounced in hawks as in the barred owl pictured in Fig. 10.36, but the aforementioned cautions still apply. Also, take care to avoid the medial metatarsal vein when placing the cross pins.

Coracoid, Clavicle, and Scapula

Coracoid fractures are very common after blunt force trauma such as a hit-by-car or window-strikes.

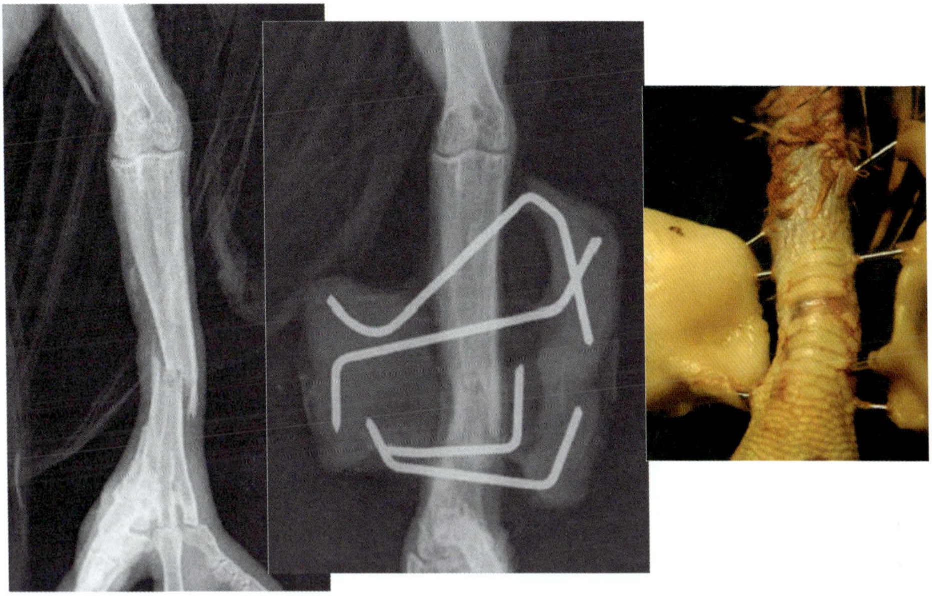

Fig. 10.40. Tarsometatarsus fracture in a red-tailed hawk. It was repaired with a standard ESF using VTP for sidebars. Note the intentionally diverging angles of the cross pins.

Cooper's hawks commonly strike windows when chasing prey and will present with a coracoid fracture (Figs 10.41 and 10.42). Oftentimes, the only clinical signs evident are the inability to fly and a wing droop. If the injury is fresh, there may be bruising over the chest and coracoid area. Some of these fractures can be palpated with a finger placed in the furcular hollow, but this can be difficult in small birds.

These fractures are usually visible on a VD radiograph and typically are of one of two types:

- Midshaft fracture with medial displacement of the distal fragments.
- Luxation of the synovial joint where the coracoid attaches to the sternum.

In severe cases, the fracture may be comminuted and the head of the humerus dropped. Remember it is very important that you have good positioning when taking VD radiographs. The keel and spine must be overlaid very well in order to properly evaluate the coracoid bones.

In the past, treatment consisted of the placement of IM pins. This surgery is no longer recommended since it is a potentially dangerous procedure and surgery is usually unnecessary. Recent studies (Redig, 2009) have shown the odds of return to flight and release are very high (>98%) with conservative therapy alone.

A typical coracoid fracture protocol is:

- Oral meloxicam and tramadol for 10 days.
- Weeks 1–2: immobilization of wing with a body wrap. Perform PT under anesthesia 1–2 times weekly to prevent stiffening of the elbow and carpus.
- Weeks 3–4: remove wrap and move to small cage allowing limited exercise.
- Weeks 5–6: move to flight cage and slowly begin forced exercise.
- Release evaluation after 6–8 weeks. The prognosis is good even with badly displaced or comminuted fractures.

Scheelings (2014) has shown that simple cage rest for 3 weeks (without a body wrap or PT) can also be very effective.

Clavicle and scapula fractures are much less common than coracoid fractures. In any case, they are managed in the same manner as coracoid fractures and both have a very good prognosis.

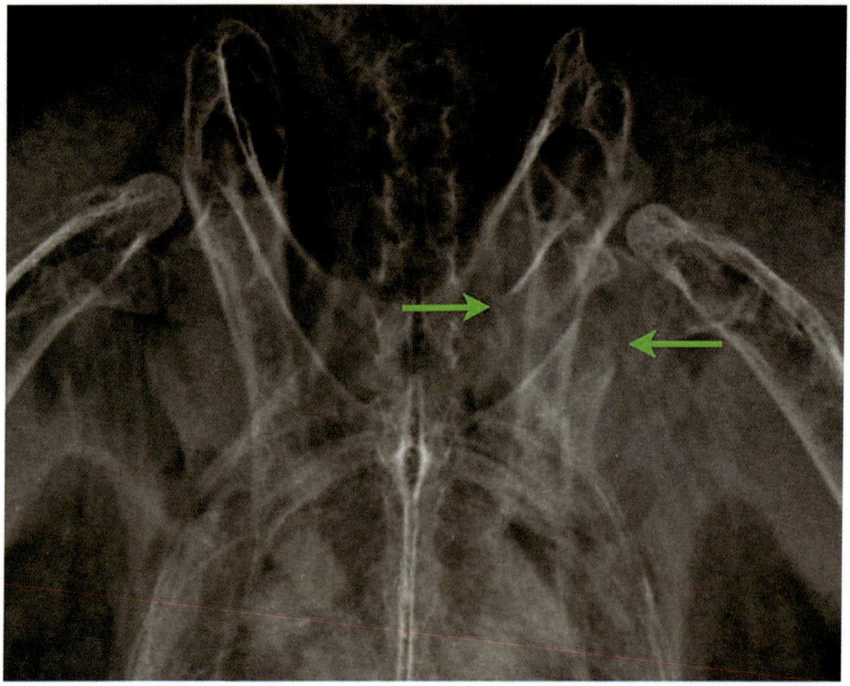

Fig. 10.41. A left coracoid fracture. The distal end is displaced medially as is typically the case. The arrows are pointing to each side of the fracture.

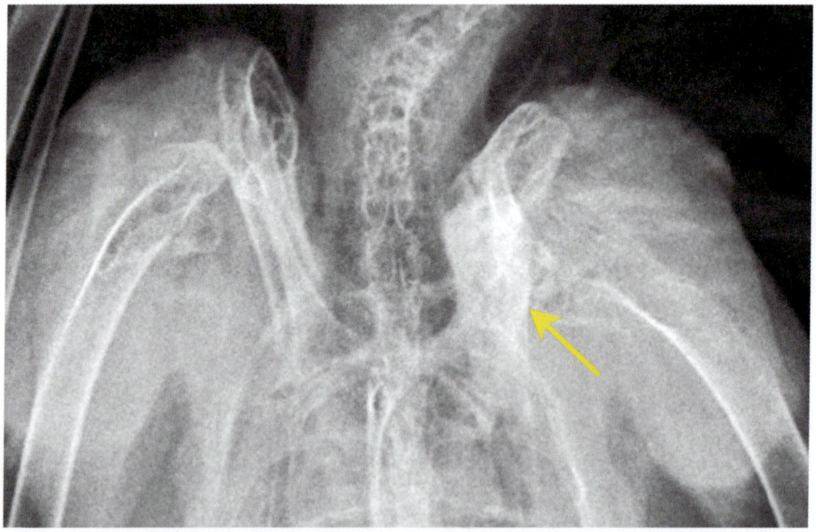

Fig. 10.42. A left coracoid fracture. This one has evidence of chronicity. It is very bright and sclerotic due to the callus and bony proliferation (arrow).

Pelvic Fractures

Pelvic fractures are generally well tolerated and can occur in the pubis, ileum, or ischium (Fig. 10.43). The weight-bearing path from the leg is through the femur to the acetabulum, to the ileum, and then to the synsacrum and spine. Therefore, fractures *not* involving this pathway should have minimal impact on weight bearing, although the associated pain may definitely produce lameness.

Since the acetabulum is formed by the fusion of the caudal aspect of the ileum with the cranial edge of the ischium, a fracture in either of these bones may lead to a damaged joint.

Treatment is non-surgical and usually consists of appropriate analgesia/anti-inflammatories and cage rest as in the case of femoral head fractures. Besides bumblefoot, a complication to be aware of in female birds is the potential for future egg binding and dystocia, especially in the case of displaced pubis fractures.

Fractures of the Beak

The beak in a raptor is composed of a thin layer of keratin overlaying the maxilla and mandible bones. Any impact sufficient to cause a fracture

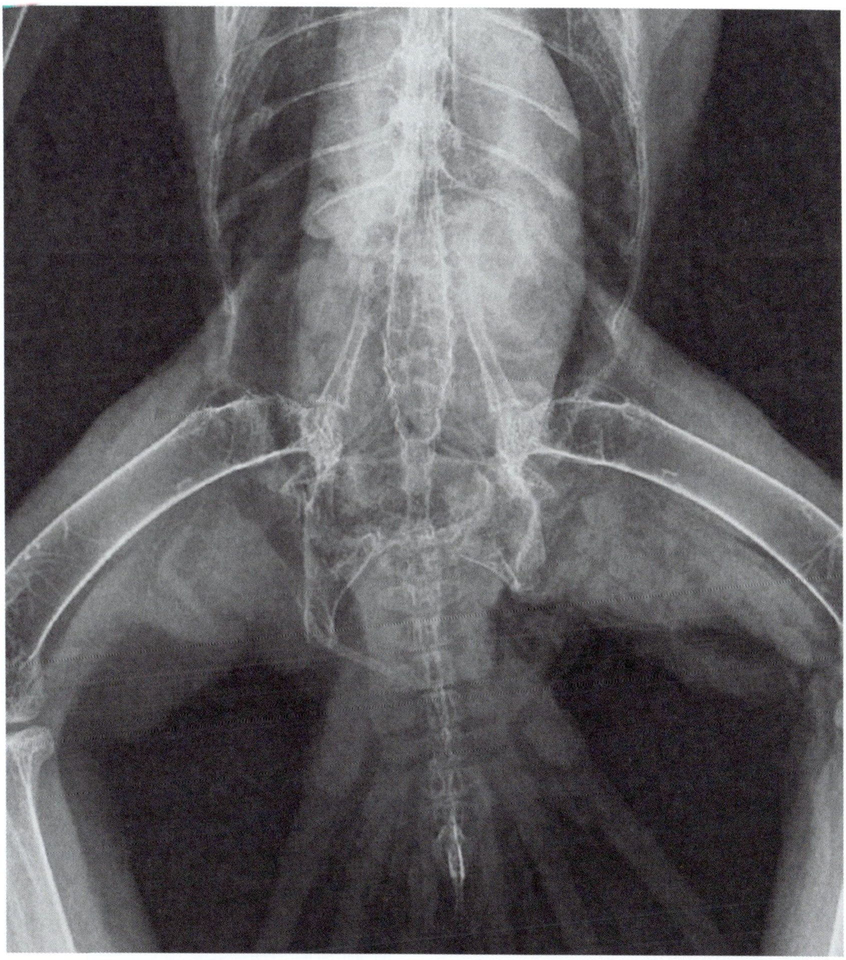

Fig. 10.43. A left pelvic fracture. The ischium and pubis are both fractured with significant displacement. The acetabulum appears intact.

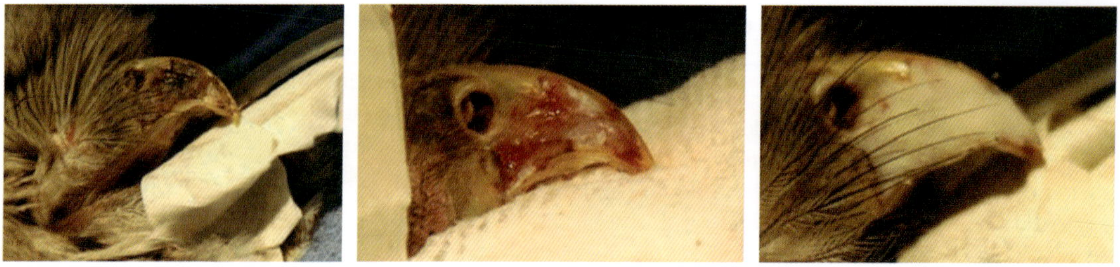

Fig. 10.44. A slab fracture of the beak in a barred owl. The fracture is debrided down to a healthy soft tissue bed. Ellman Temp-Plus™ is used to fill the defect.

or crack in the beak keratin will most certainly affect the underlying bones.

Beak trauma usually involves the tip but can also affect the main body (Fig. 10.45) of the maxillary beak and cause large slab fractures (Fig. 10.44). It is hard to predict how these fractures will heal but, in general, if the beak's germinal root tissue (near the base of the beak and cere) is not affected, then the beak fracture can heal and the keratin can regrow. Patience is required as beak regrowth can take several months. In addition, frequent coping may be required in order to keep proper occlusion when the mouth is closed. If a bird does not have a beak that closes properly, it cannot be released, as the beak will not wear properly and will ultimately overgrow, leading to the inability to eat.

Beak fractures are treated as follows:

- Clean and debride any loose or devitalized tissue. This must be done with the bird anesthetized through an ET tube so that you can have proper access to the beak.
- Any defects are repaired with a filler/epoxy. The filler is also used to stabilize any loose fragments, particularly at the tip. If successful, the bird should be able to eat normally while the fracture heals and the keratin regrows. One good product to try is Temp-Plus™ dental acrylic (Ellman International, Oceanside, NY, USA). It is a two-part acrylic (powder + liquid) that can be mixed to various consistencies for different applications. The filler will slough as the keratin grows and may need to be replaced.

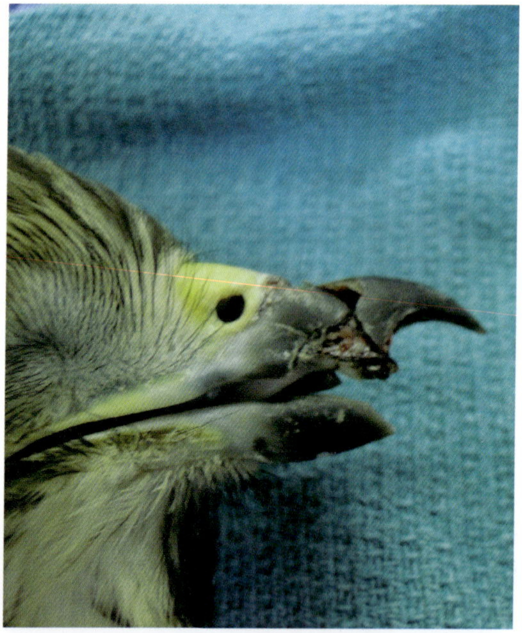

Fig. 10.45. A fracture of the distal 50% of the entire maxillary beak in a hawk. The underlying bone is undoubtedly affected. This is a non-releasable injury and this bird was euthanized.

Luxation of the Elbow

Elbow luxations present with a wing droop, a very swollen joint, and a poor ROM. The most common dislocation occurs when the radius is displaced dorsally from its articulation with the dorsal humeral condyle. The head of the radius can be palpated projecting from the dorsal surface of the elbow. Luxations of the ulna can also occur but are less common (Fig. 10.46).

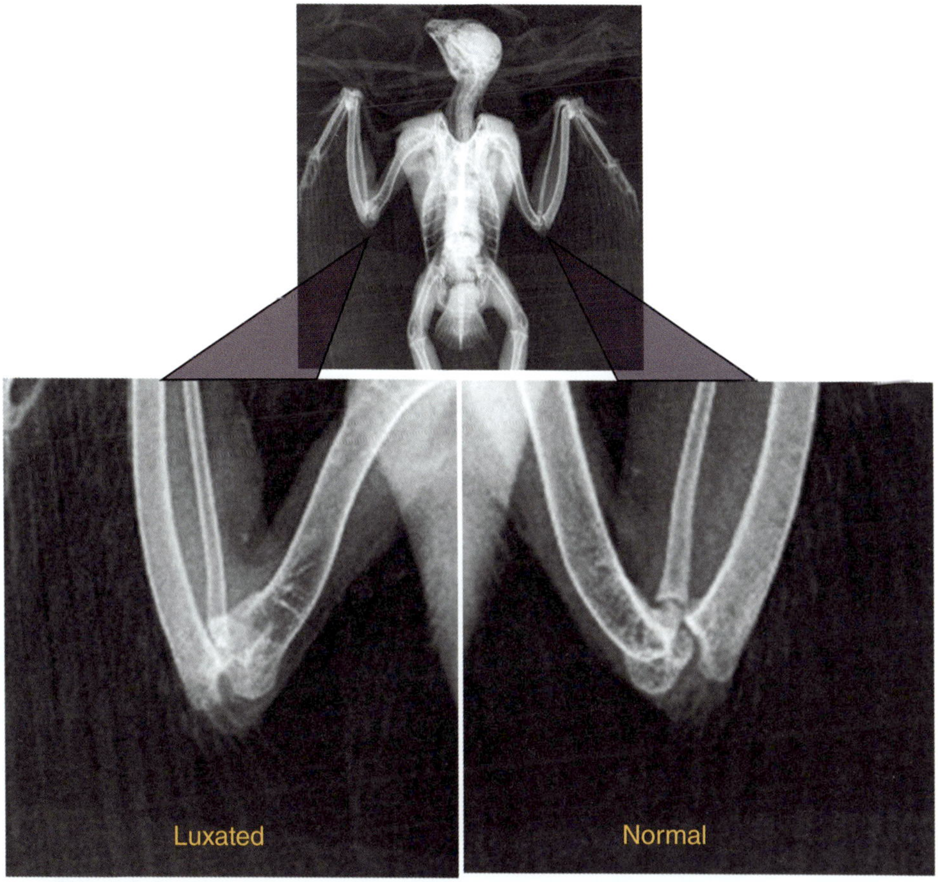

Fig. 10.46. Dorsal luxation of the radius. The proximal radius is overlapped by the dorsal humeral condyle rather than articulating smoothly with it.

It is very important that these injuries be treated immediately. Even a few days of scar tissue formation can prevent correction. To reduce simple radius luxations:

- Induce general anesthesia.
- Flex and extend the elbow while applying pressure to the dorsal aspect of the radius to force it back into articulation with the humerus.
- If repositioned properly, the joint should regain full ROM. This should be confirmed radiographically.
- The wing should be immobilized with a figure-8 wrap for 2 weeks. PT can be done once weekly but use extreme caution to avoid re-luxating the radius. In many cases, it is safer to simply skip the PT during this period.
- The bird should be confined to a small enclosure/kennel for another 2 weeks before slowly starting to exercise in a flight cage.

Prognosis is fair to good if treatment is initiated promptly (within days of the initial injury).

In cases with severe ligament disruption, the joint may be very loose and luxation can recur easily. In these cases, an imbrication procedure and/or the creation of a pseudo-collateral ligament on the dorsal aspect of the elbow may be required. In addition, trans-articular fixation with an ESF may be necessary. The prognosis for return to normal function and full ROM is poor for these cases. These advanced techniques have been described (Ackermann and Redig, 1997).

Fractures in Young Birds

The joints in young birds are just a cartilaginous model for what will become a mature joint when fully developed (Fig. 10.47). Although it varies greatly with species, the maturation process is generally complete at approximately 6–8 weeks of age. This has clinical significance since it affects how fractures can be repaired in these young patients. Specifically, it is important to avoid disruption of the developing areas in the metaphyseal regions, so we sometimes need to get creative when dealing with these fractures.

Fortunately, due to the amazing growth rate and metabolism of young birds, a good outcome can be achieved with a less than ideal fixation. In addition, the implants can often be removed in as early as 7–10 days. Some tips when repairing these fractures:

- For humerus fractures, the IM pin should exit at the shoulder to avoid interfering with the elbow joint's development. An ESF tie-in is usually not necessary and is not recommended since placement of the cross pins can result in inadvertent damage to the soft, growing metaphyseal regions.
- Exiting an IM pin at the distal radius in a developing bird does not seem to cause a problem and can be done if necessary.

> **Raptor Tip**
>
> To avoid feather damage, figure-8 wing wraps should be used very sparingly, or never, in growing birds.

Be especially careful when placing ulna IM pins from the elbow, as damage to the growth plate near the olecranon is possible. These fractures may do fine without surgery if the radius is intact. Using a shuttle pin is also a good option for midshaft ulna fractures in young birds.

- Tibiotarsus fractures do very well with just an IM pin exiting at the stifle joint.

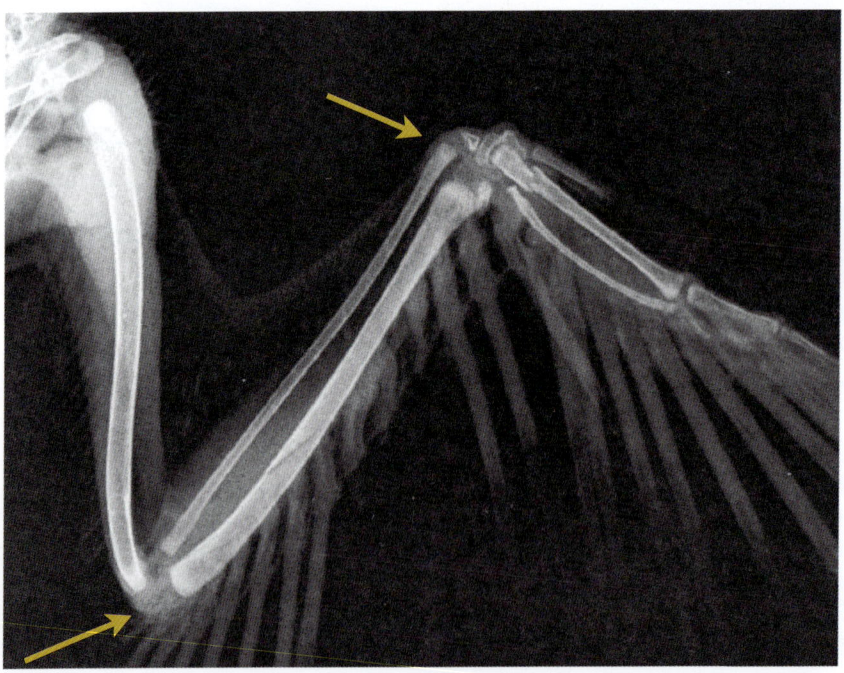

Fig. 10.47. Normal elbow and carpal joints in a 2–3-week-old bird. Note the large radiolucent gaps at the ends of the long bones where the joints are still forming (arrows). Also note that all flight feathers are in blood.

- Due to the massive number of developing blood feathers, a figure-8 wrap is not recommended and can seriously damage growing feathers. These wraps should be avoided and a simple splint made from a loop of masking tape around the wing is usually sufficient.
- The medullary cavities in the long bones of young birds may not always be hollow and are mostly filled with soft bone at this age. Therefore, the cavity may need to be pre-tapped before placing an IM pin.
- Habituation and imprinting are serious concerns when treating these young patients. Take all precautions to minimize contact while treating these fractures (see Chapter 12).

Raptor Tip

Habituation and imprinting are serious concerns in young patients. Take all precautions to minimize contact when treating these fractures.

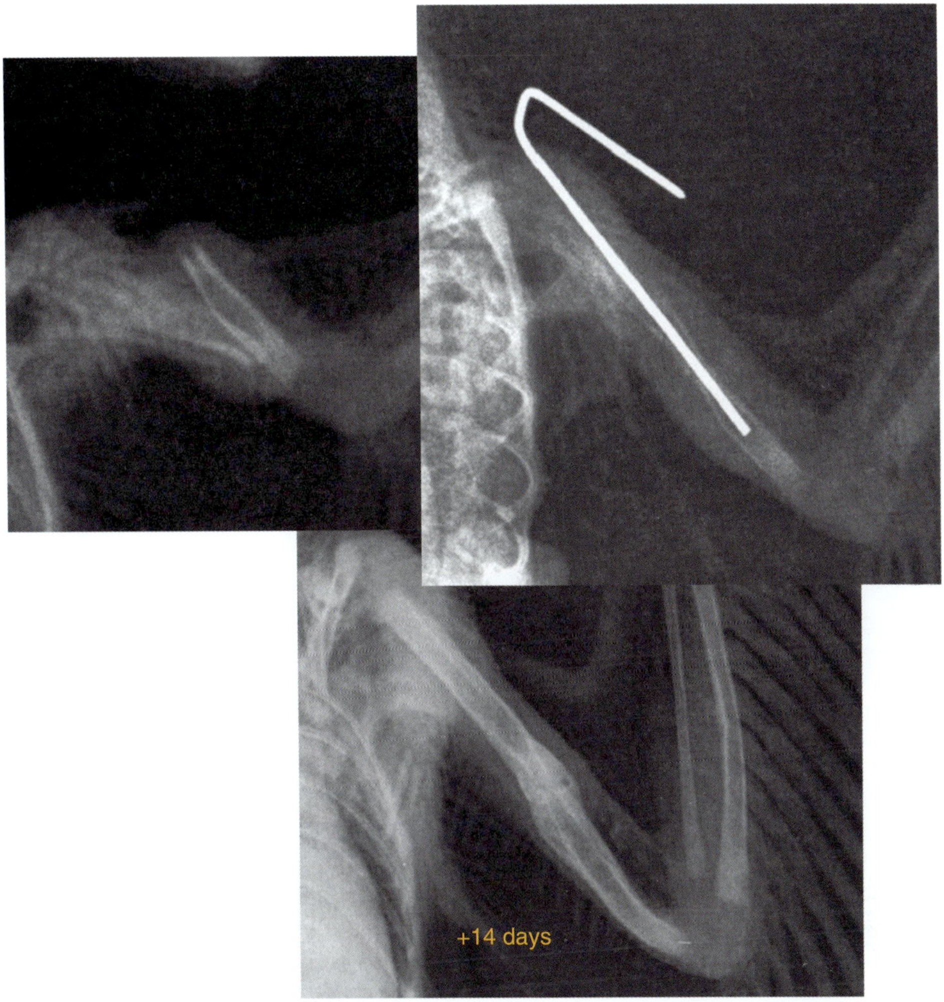

Fig. 10.48. A fractured humerus in an 8-day-old barred owl. The fracture was repaired with a small IM pin exiting at the shoulder. The pin was removed 7 days later. The fracture was completely healed after 14 days and the bird eventually flew perfectly.

The Healing Process

The bone healing process in juvenile and adult birds is very rapid when compared to the typical mammal. Usually, there will be marked radiographical evidence of healing within 2–3 weeks in an adult and in less than 7–10 days in a juvenile (Figs 10.48–10.51).

Implants are generally removed when the fracture is stable on palpation *and* there is radiographic evidence of bone healing. This is typically around 5 weeks for an adult bird. Primary bone healing does not occur in birds so you must see evidence of a callus on the radiograph before the fracture can be considered to be healing.

Complications

Osteomyelitis

Bone infections are surprisingly uncommon despite the fact that many fractures involve open

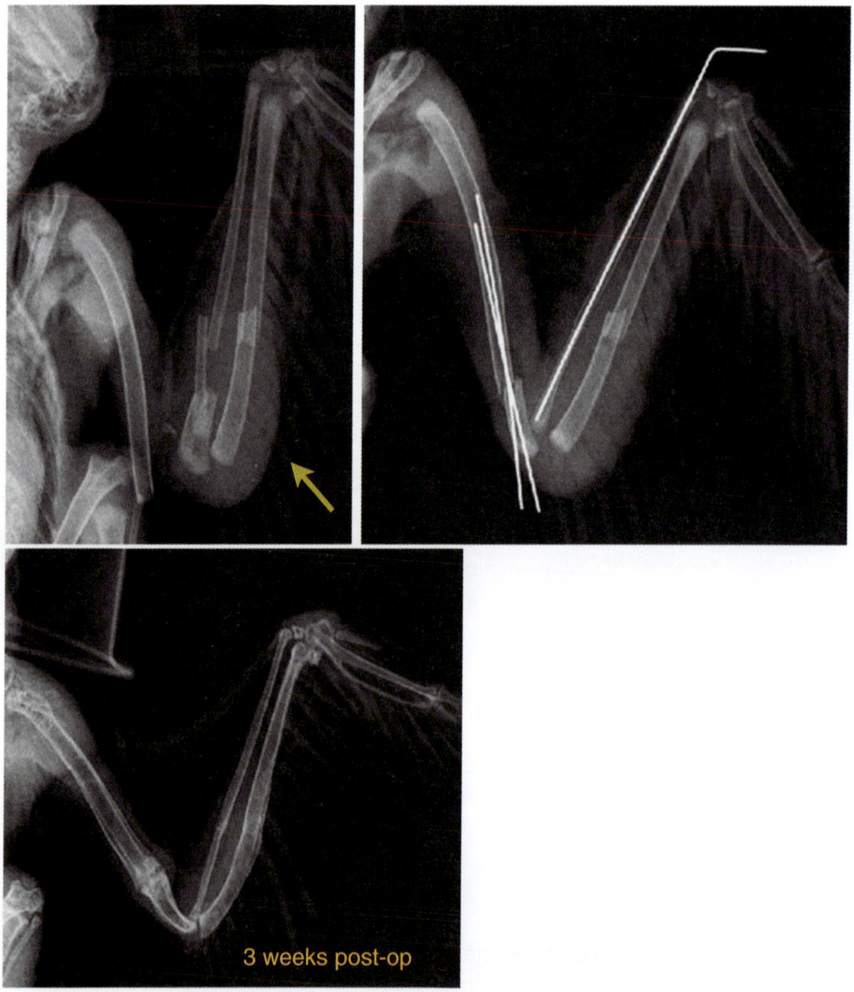

Fig. 10.49. Multiple fractures in a young owl. The radius and humerus were repaired with IM pins. The ulna was not repaired since there was concern about traumatizing the developing elbow joint. As a result, PT was very difficult since there was a tendency for the ulna to bend when the elbow was extended. However, all the fractures healed well as seen in the radiograph taken 3 weeks later. Note the massive soft tissue swelling pre-operatively (arrowhead).

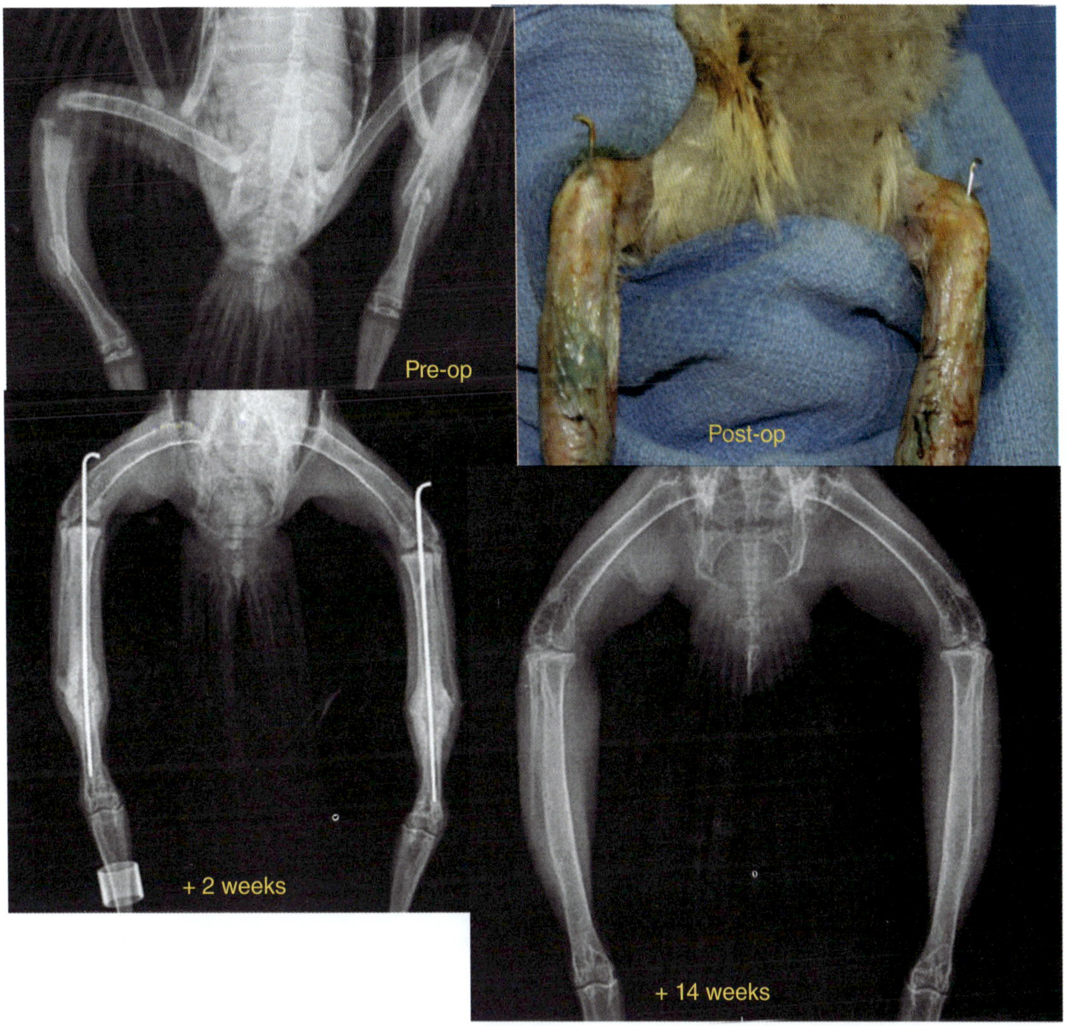

Fig. 10.50. Bilateral tibiotarsus fractures in a young red-shouldered hawk. They were both repaired with an IM pin exiting at the stifle joint. The legs were kept in hobbles for 8 days to prevent rotation and splay leg. The fractures were very stable with a large callus by 2 weeks and the bird was fully weight bearing. The pins were removed at 17 days and the calluses had completely remodeled by 14 weeks.

wounds with exposed and contaminated bone. Careful debridement of necrotic tissue and debris as well as copious flushing and the use of systemic antibiotics are keys to minimizing this problem.

Signs of osteomyelitis include bloody drainage from the incision or from the pin tracts. Additionally, fuzzy, indistinct areas of periosteal change on radiographs may be present but these can be difficult to differentiate from the normal healing process. Another more classic radiographic finding of osteomyelitis is the production of bony spicules or "fingers" around the infected site (Fig. 10.52).

Raptor Tip

Enrofloxacin and clindamycin BID is an excellent choice for osteomyelitis.

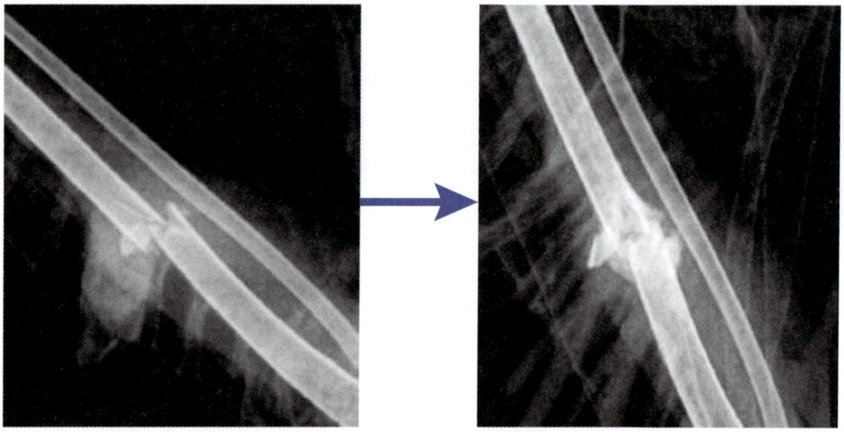

Fig. 10.51. An ulna fracture in an adult has significant bridging callus formation after only 2 weeks.

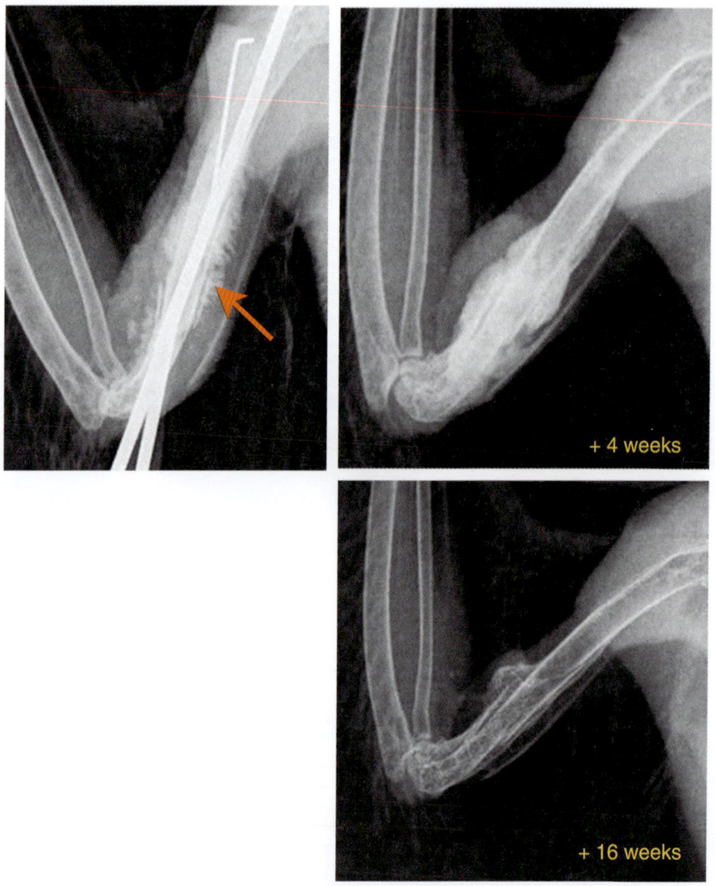

Fig. 10.52. Osteomyelitis in a post-op humerus fracture in a great-horned owl. The pin tracts and incision were draining, and the limb was very swollen and firm prior to treatment with clindamycin. The callus became smooth and less reactive after several weeks of treatment and the bird regained full flight. The fracture was healed and the bone was remodeled after 16 weeks. The arrow points to bony "spicules", which are indicative of active osteomyelitis.

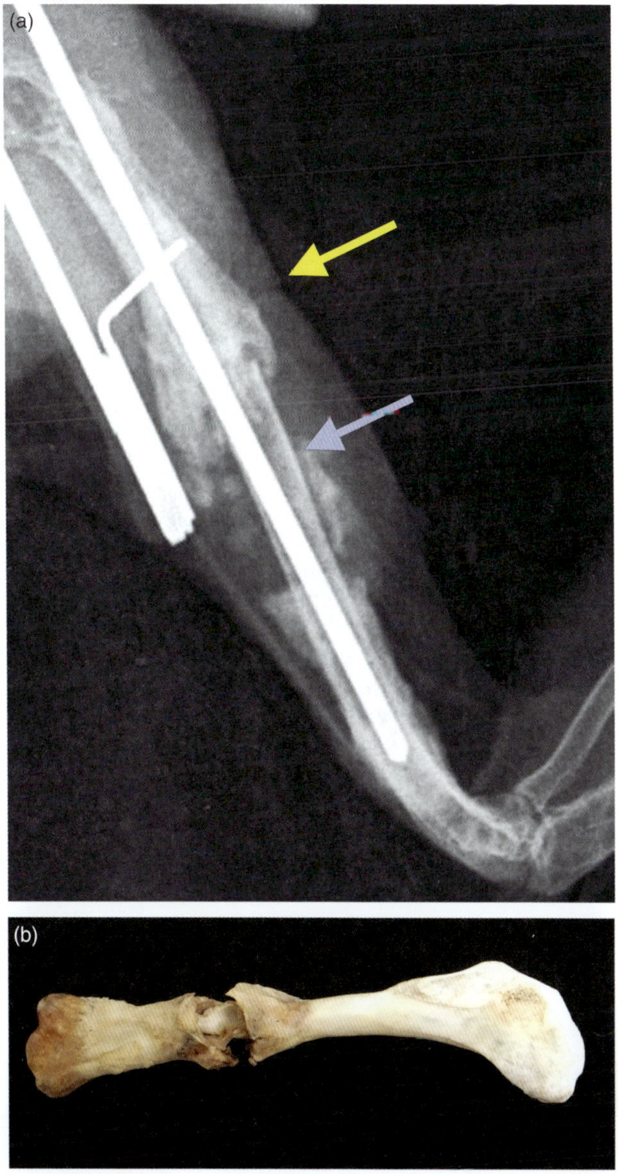

Fig. 10.53. (a) Non-union in the humerus of a barred owl. The central third of the diaphysis was exposed and off-color prior to surgery. It turned out to be non-viable (blue arrow) but the callus from the proximal segment is attempting to bridge over the fracture (yellow arrow). (b) A similar non-union with the sequestrum visible inside a cavity formed by the bridging callus.

Treatment includes the use of the appropriate systemic antibiotic based on culture and sensitivity, if available. Clindamycin is an excellent choice when in doubt because it has superior penetration into bone. All patients at risk of osteomyelitis should be started on clindamycin immediately upon admission. In addition to systemic antibiotics, opening an infected incision to debride and flush the affected area can be very helpful. This treatment may need to be repeated several times and all necrotic bone fragments should be removed.

Non-unions

Non-unions typically occur secondary to osteomyelitis, from inadequate fixation, or from a compromised blood supply (especially in metacarpal fractures) (Figs 10.53 and 10.54). Clearly, the best way to avoid this complication is to eliminate these risk factors. However, once a non-union has occurred, treatment can be attempted, but the prognosis should be considered very poor.

Depending on the fracture and the existing fixation, you may need to remove the implants and start over. Conversion of a non-union to a calcified bridge may not be possible but can be attempted by removing all fibrous scar tissue which has formed in the fracture gap. Use ronguers to freshen the bone ends and to produce a bleeding bone edge.

Poor ROM

Poor ROM usually results from not having done PT often enough or from not pushing the extension far enough. It can also result from fractures that did not achieve adequate surgical stabilization and have therefore developed a large, proliferative callus. Always remember to repair fractures as soon as possible, attempt to get a very rigid fixation, and do PT early and often. It is easier to lose a ROM than it is to get it back, but do not be discouraged if you have a bad PT session. Sometimes just increasing the frequency is all that is required.

Conclusion

Orthopedics is a very satisfying part of raptor rehabilitation and it is an area where you can have a huge and immediate impact. However, it does take practice and the willingness to experiment and to push the envelope, but you must also be willing to make mistakes and occasionally fail.

Practice as much as possible with cadavers in order to work out the logistics of how and where to place pins, as well as the basics regarding simple things such as the correct approach and how to drape your patient in appropriately. It is best to become comfortable with the procedures on a cadaver before you have to worry about a live patient that is not doing well under anesthesia and has a surgical field obscured with blood.

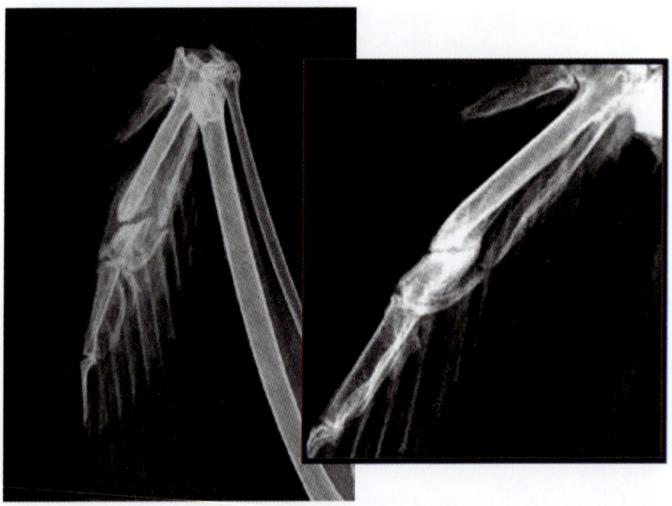

Fig. 10.54. This bird was admitted with an old non-union fracture of the metacarpal bone. There was no improvement for 8 weeks until IMEX TR Matrix was implanted in the fracture gap. Bone healing was slow but steady after that.

Bibliography

Ackermann, J. and Redig, P. (1997) Surgical repair of elbow luxation in raptors. *Journal of Avian Medicine and Surgery* 11(4), 247–254.

Bennett, K. (2008) Holistic treatment of osteoarthritis in psittacine birds. *Proceedings of the 29th Conference of the Association of Avian Veterinarians, Savannah, GA, USA*. Association of Avian Veterinarians, Teaneck, NJ, USA, pp. 49–52.

Burgdorf-Moisuk, A., Whittington, J.K., Bennett, R.A., McFadden, M., Mitchell, M. and O'Brien, R. (2011) Successful management of simple fractures of the femoral neck with femoral head and neck excision arthroplasty in two free-living avian species. *Journal of Avian Medicine and Surgery* 25(3), 210–215.

Chitty, L. (2008) *BSAVA Manual of Raptors, Pigeons and Passerine Birds*. BSAVA, Gloucester, UK.

Gjeltema, J.L., Degernes, L.A., Buckanoff, H.D. and Marcellin-Little, D.J. (2018) Evaluation of goniometry and electrogoniometry of carpus and elbow joints in the barred owl (*Strix varia*). *Journal of Avian Medicine and Surgery* 32(4), 267–278.

Langhofer, B. (2010) Clinical therapeutic options for the treatment of osteoarthritis in avian patients with case reports. *Proceedings of the 31st Conference of the Association of Avian Veterinarians, San Diego, CA, USA*. Association of Avian Veterinarians, Teaneck, NJ, USA, pp. 85–89.

Orosz, S.E., Ensley, P.K. and Haynes, C.J. (1992) *Avian Surgical Anatomy: Thoracic and Pelvic Limbs*. W.B. Saunders, Philadelphia, PA, USA.

Redig, P. (1993) *Medical Management of Birds of Prey*, 3rd edn. The Raptor Center, St. Paul, MN, USA.

Redig, P. (2009) Coracoid fracture management in raptors: assessment of the conservative approach. *Proceedings of the 30th Conference of the Association of Avian Veterinarians, Milwaukee, WI, USA*. Association of Avian Veterinarians, Teaneck, NJ, USA, p. 351.

Samour, J. (2008) *Avian Medicine*, 2nd edn. Mosby-Elsevier, Maryland Heights, MO, USA.

Scheelings, T.F. (2014) Coracoid fractures in wild birds: a comparison of surgical repair versus conservative treatment. *Journal of Avian Medicine and Surgery* 28(4), 304–308.

11 Endoscopy

Learning Objectives

1. Indications and uses for endoscopy.
2. The entry point and major internal landmarks.
3. Knowing what "normal" looks like.

The avian anatomy is well suited for endoscopic evaluation, due to the presence of a system of air sacs. Endoscopy is a valuable tool in the diagnosis and treatment of many disease processes since it allows direct access to various lesions in a relatively non-invasive manner (Fig. 11.1). Proper technique, however, can be challenging and practice with cadavers is recommended prior to working with actual patients.

Equipment

The proper equipment is key to success with endoscopy. A rigid endoscope is generally the most useful in avian medicine (Fig. 11.2). The length and diameter of the scope are the most important attributes to consider, but they can be at odds with one another. In general, longer scopes have a greater diameter, so a scope long enough to view the syrinx in a large bird may be too thick to enter the trachea in a small bird. Ideally, one would have access to a few different-sized scopes, but this may not be feasible.

Endoscopes with diameters of 2.5 to 3.0 mm and 13 cm in length offer the best compromise of length, diameter, and image quality. A scope with an integrated instrument channel can be very useful but the channel will increase the overall diameter of the scope.

Biopsy and grasping forceps are very useful. However, some of the very small instruments (around 1 mm in width) are too small to be practical and the biopsy samples are miniscule. Instruments closer to 2 mm in width are more clinically useful (Fig. 11.3).

A video camera and monitor are crucial since they allow the operator to remain in a comfortable, standing position while performing the procedure. Without the camera, the operator must view through the scope itself, and this means bending over and placing the head in the sterile field.

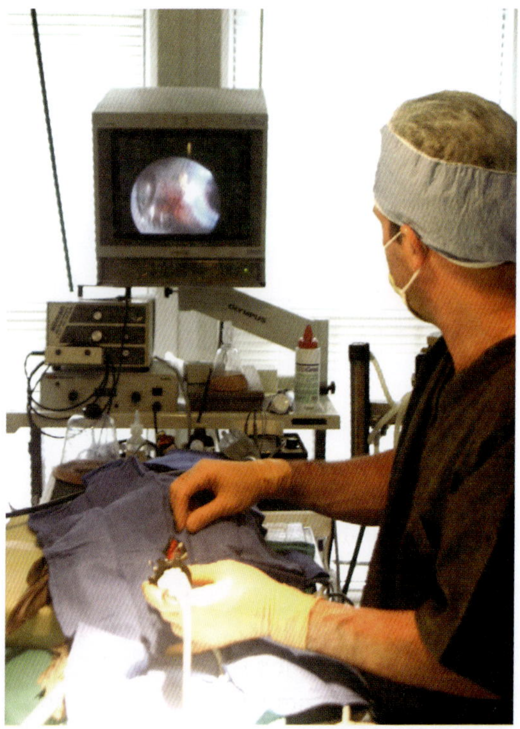

Fig. 11.1. Endoscopy is a valuable tool in avian medicine.

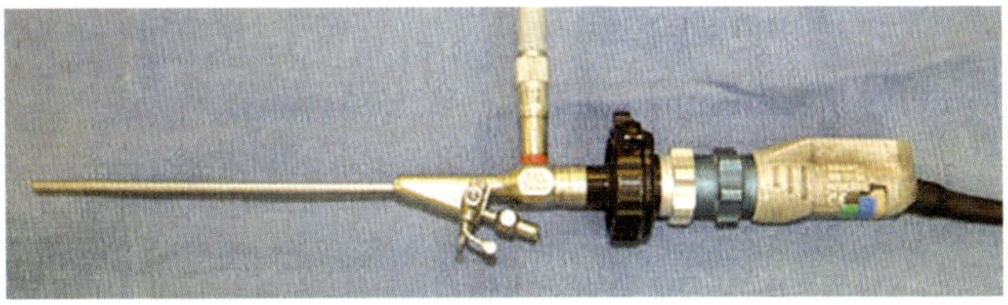

Fig. 11.2. A Storz 2.9 mm, 13 cm rigid scope (Storz, Tuttlingen, Germany) with an integrated 1 mm instrument channel and video camera is a good all-purpose combination.

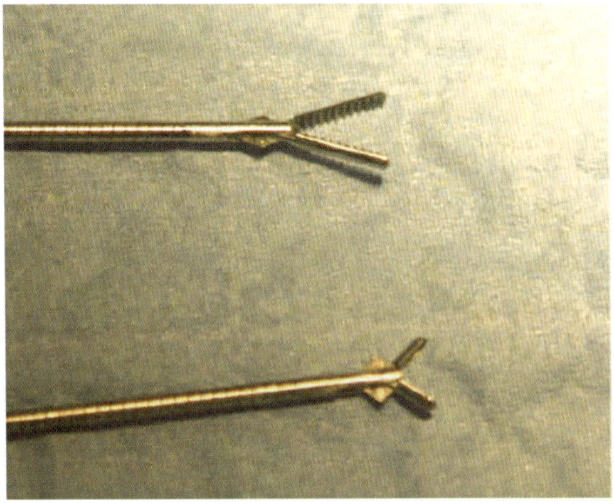

Fig. 11.3. Biopsy and grasping forceps.

Approaches

Left lateral approach

The left lateral/paralumbar approach is commonly used for endoscopy (Fig. 11.4). This approach is identical to the approach described previously for placing an air sac tube and for the left lateral celiotomy (see Figs 4.11 and 9.9). This approach is useful for most diagnostics as well as for determination of sex.

Make your approach as follows:

- The patient is anesthetized and placed in right lateral recumbency.
- Pull the wing dorsally and the left leg caudally.
- Surgically prepare and drape the paralumbar fossa. This area is mostly featherless so very little plucking is required.
- Make a 2–3 mm vertical skin incision just cranial to the thigh muscles and caudal to the last rib. The thigh muscles may need to be pushed caudally to get access to the body wall behind the last rib. The entry point should be approximately ⅓ of the distance from the hip to the knee.
- With a blunt instrument, such as a hemostat, penetrate the body wall and air sac. It is best to direct the instrument parallel to the body wall and the table top to avoid penetrating deeply. A "pop" will be heard and felt when successful.
- Insert the endoscope and always keep firm control on it by bracing the endoscope with your fingers as it passes through the body wall.
- The tip of the scope will be in either the caudal thoracic or the abdominal air sac, depending on your exact entry point.

Healthy air sacs are translucent with very few vessels present. An abnormal air sac can be opaque, hyper-vascular, and have inflammatory exudates, granulomatous masses, or fungal growths on the surface.

It is necessary to penetrate various air sac membranes with the tip of the scope in order to view the entire cavity (Figs 11.5–11.12). This damage does not seem to cause permanent harm.

When the exam is complete, the skin is closed with one or two sutures.

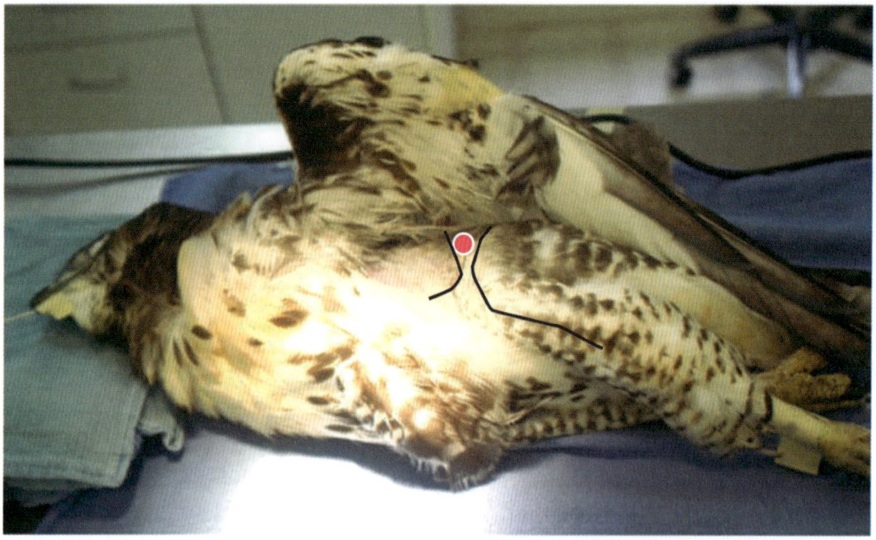

Fig. 11.4. Positioning for the left lateral approach with the leg and wing pulled back. The last rib and the cranial edge of the thigh are outlined. The entry point is highlighted with the red circle.

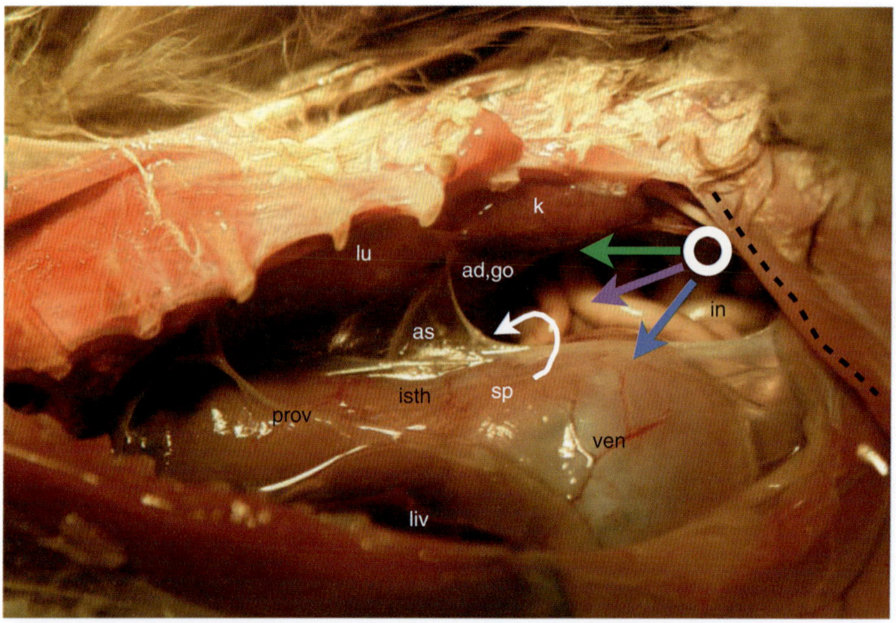

Fig. 11.5. A cutaway view of the coelomic cavity. The white circle is the entry point. The kidney (k), adrenal (ad) and gonads (go) are seen by pointing cranial-dorsally (green arrow). The lungs (lu) are further cranial but you may need to penetrate the air sac (as) membrane between the abdominal and caudal thoracic air sacs in order to see them. The spleen (sp) is located just ventral (purple and white arrow) to the adrenal gland and gonads and rests over the isthmus (isth) between the proventriculus (prov) and ventriculus (ven). The liver (liv) and heart are located cranial-ventrally (blue arrow) from the entry site. The intestines (in) are located just under the entry site. The cranial margin of the thigh muscles is indicated by the dotted line.

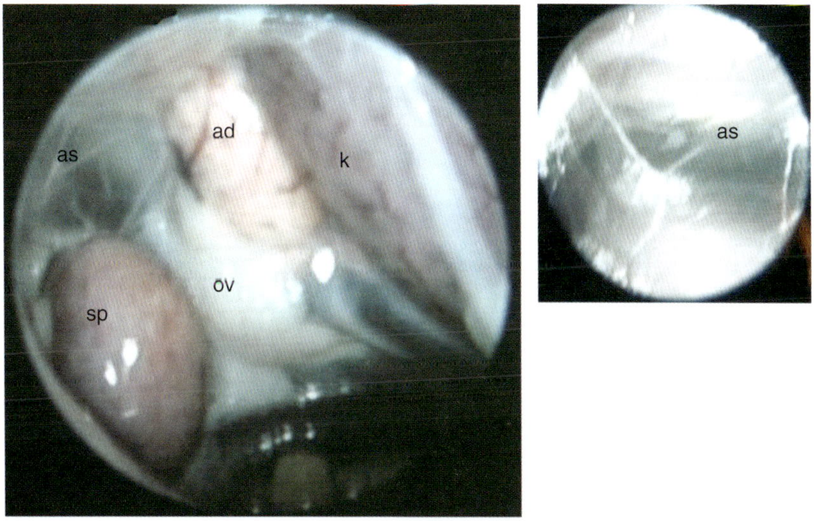

Fig. 11.6. The view directed dorsally, just after entry through body wall. The kidney (k), adrenal (ad), ovary (ov) triad, and spleen (sp) in a juvenile hawk. Note how translucent a healthy air sac (as) is.

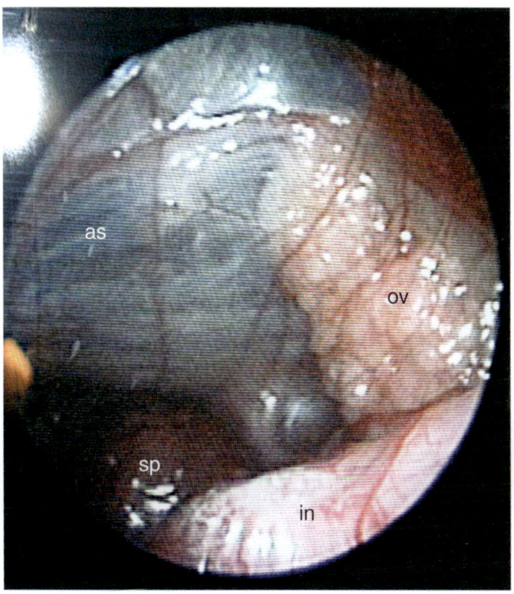

Fig. 11.7. The same view as in Fig. 11.6 in a bird with severe air sacculitis. Ovary (ov), spleen (sp), intestine (in). Note how opaque and hyper-vascular the air sac (as) is.

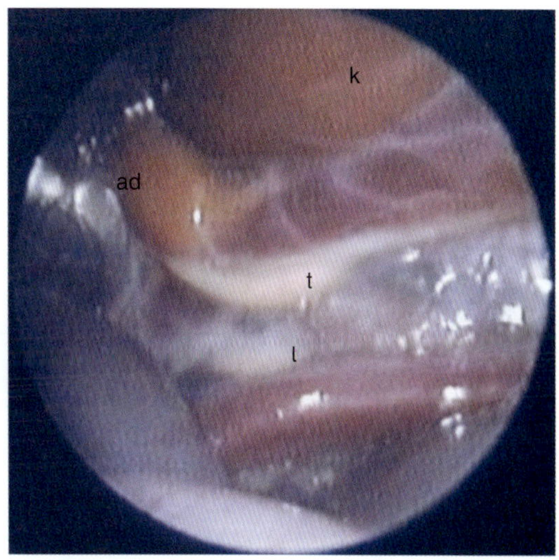

Fig. 11.8. The kidney (k), adrenal (ad), and testes (t).

Examination of the Trachea and Syrinx

Tracheoscopy is indicated in cases of dyspnea or a change in voice where a lesion is suspected in either the trachea or syrinx (Figs 11.13 and 11.14).

The bird is placed in ventral recumbency and the head and neck are extended so that the trachea is as straight as possible. For short procedures,

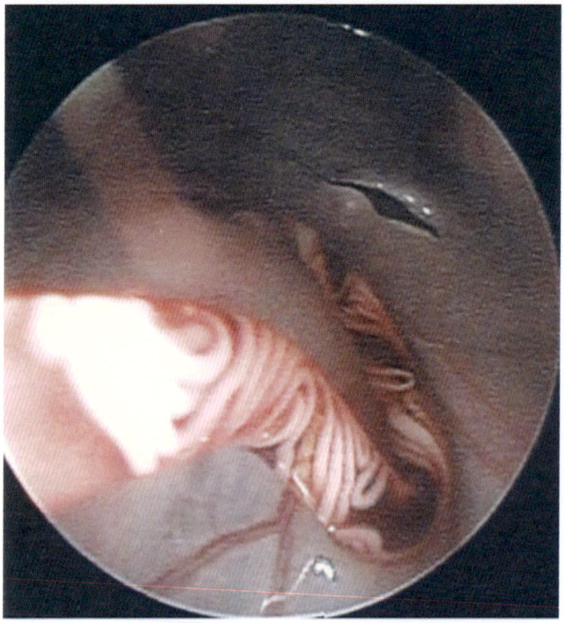

Fig. 11.9. A gapeworm (*Syngamus trachea*) is being removed endoscopically from the air sacs of a red-shouldered hawk.

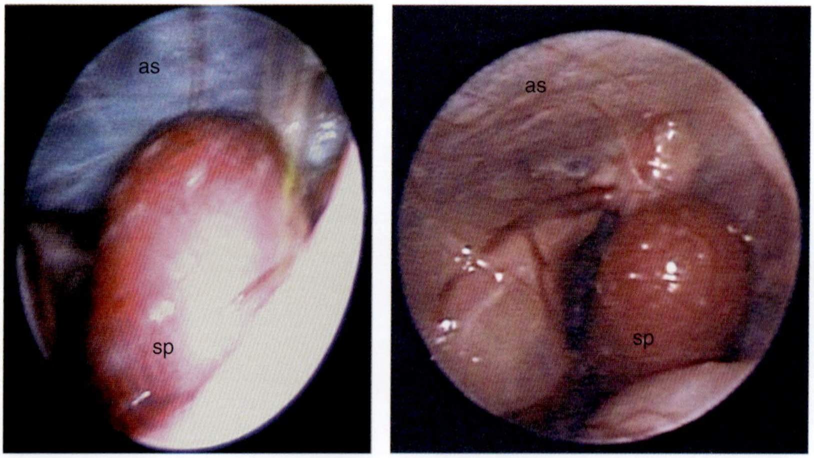

Fig. 11.10. The spleen (sp) with multifocal lesions on the surface. The air sac (as) behind the spleen is very opaque and inflamed.

the patient can be anesthetized via mask and the examination can be done quickly while the mask is removed. For longer procedures, anesthesia is maintained via an air sac tube (Chapter 4).

The scope diameter should not exceed ⅔ of the lumen of the trachea. The tracheal mucosa is very delicate so the scope should be advanced carefully down the trachea towards the syrinx.

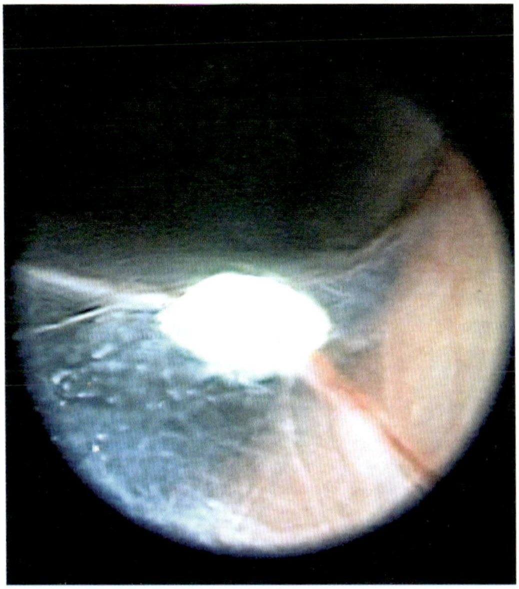

Fig. 11.11. A typical air sacculitis lesion. These lesions should be sampled for culture and/or cytology. This is most likely due to Aspergillosis.

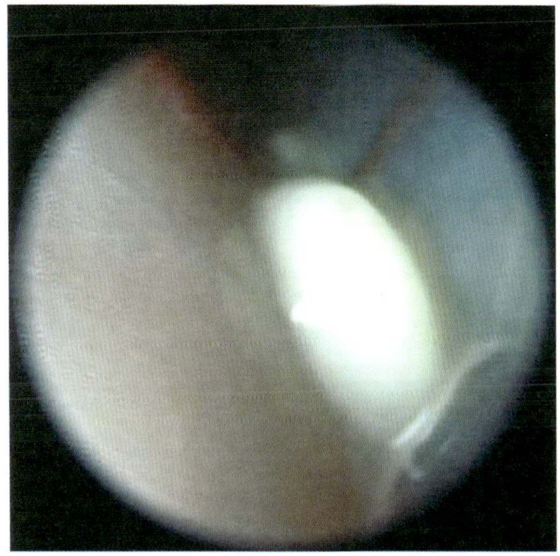

Fig. 11.12. A lesion on the serosal surface of the proventriculus.

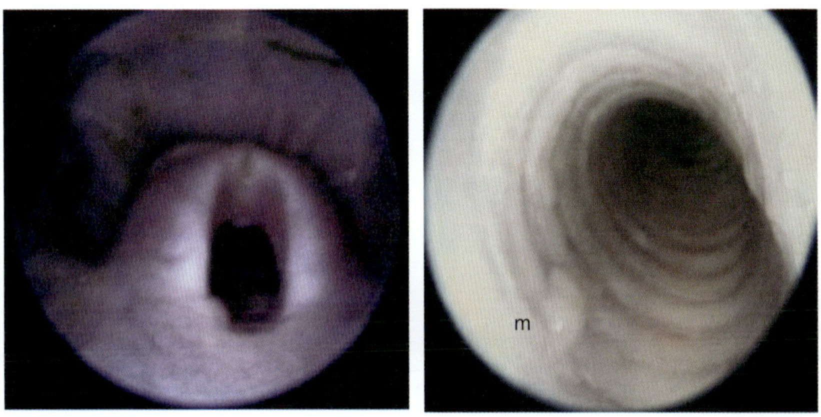

Fig. 11.13. Views of a normal glottis and tracheal lumen. A small amount of mucus (m) is not uncommon in the tracheal lumen.

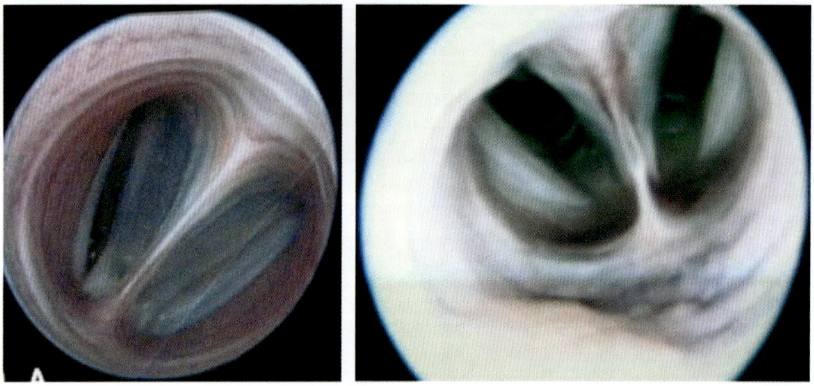

Fig. 11.14. View of a normal syrinx. The syrinx should be symmetrical and free from any obstructions.

Bibliography

Chitty, L. (2008) *BSAVA Manual of Raptors, Pigeons and Passerine Birds*. BSAVA, Gloucester, UK.

Harrison, G.J. and Lightfoot, T. (2006) *Clinical Avian Medicine*. Vols I & II. Spix Publishing, Palm Beach, FL, USA.

12 Caring for Nestlings and Hatchlings

Learning Objectives

1. The causes and avoidance of mal-imprinting.
2. Basic feeding protocols.
3. The typical developmental timeline.
4. Live-prey testing.
5. When to attempt to renest a hatchling.

Young nestling, hatchling, and fledgling-age birds are often admitted to rehabilitation facilities during the nesting season. Causes for admission include habitat destruction (e.g. tree cut down) as well as young birds being blown from the nest in a storm. These birds are often referred to as "orphans" but, in reality, the majority of these so-called "orphans" are healthy fledglings which were found by a member of the public and thought to be injured. They are essentially "kidnapped" and are best returned to their nest site (see "Renesting", below).

Orphan Season

The actual start and end of the orphan season varies with geography, weather, and species. In North Carolina, USA, orphan admissions usually begin in March or April, peak in May or June, and are usually over by July or August (Fig. 12.1). Most species have a typical timing for nest building, egg laying, hatching, and fledging (Chapter 3). Note that there is quite a bit of overlap, and barn owls are one species that reproduce throughout the year.

Identification of Species

It is important to correctly identify the species since this will affect how the birds are treated and

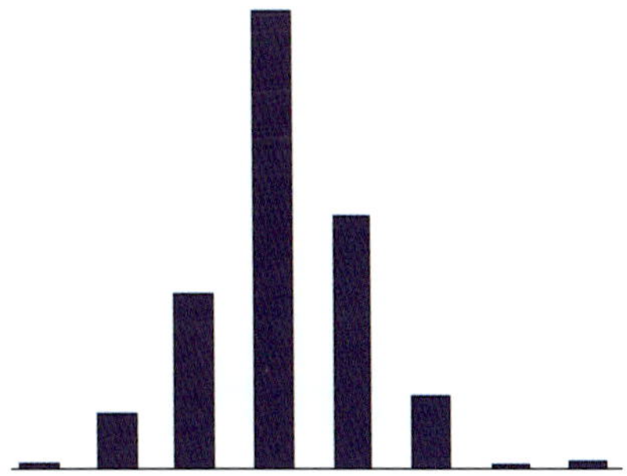

Fig. 12.1. Orphan admissions each month at Carolina Raptor Center in North Carolina, USA.

fed, and it will most certainly affect how the birds are grouped together. In most cases, young birds can be identified easily. The exceptions are young hawks, which can look very similar.

A large number of orphans are admitted at several weeks of age and are therefore quite large. To the untrained eye, they may not appear to be young birds, but the presence of remaining down and blood feathers should clue you in to their actual age (Figs 12.2–12.4).

Some identification tips:

- Great-horned owl: Largest owl, big eyes with yellow iris and black beak.
- Barred owl: Large eyes with dark iris and yellow beak.
- Eastern screech owl: Often mistaken for "baby" great-horned owl.
- Barn owl: Long ivory-colored beak and small, "beady", dark eyes. Sometimes mistaken for a vulture.
- American kestrel: Small hawk-like bird with dark, vertical bars below eyes, and brown iris.

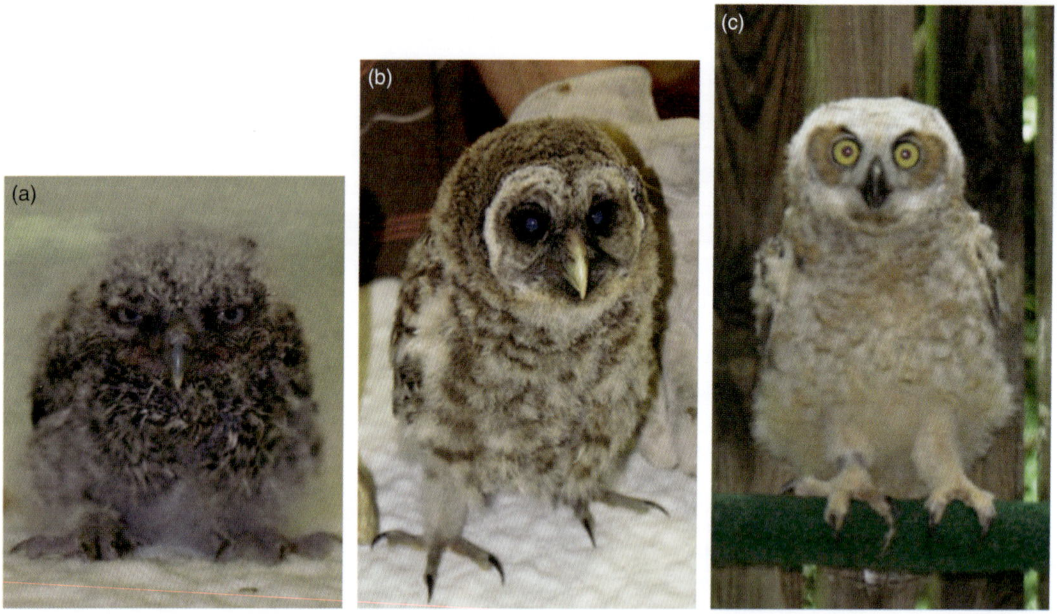

Fig. 12.2. Young owls: eastern screech owl (a), barred owl (b), great-horned owl (c). Note that the barred owl (b) has a dark iris.

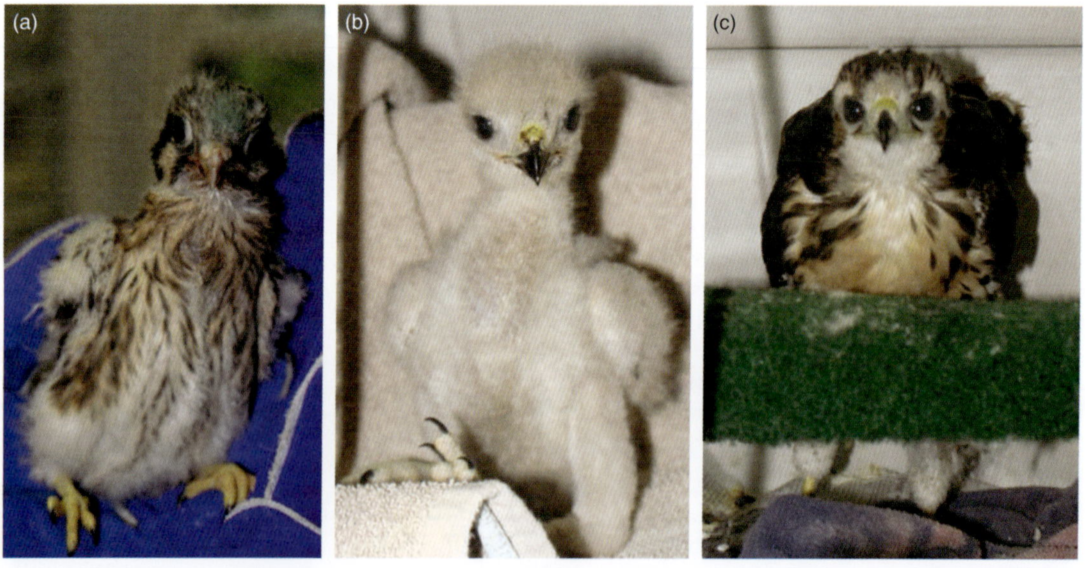

Fig. 12.3. Young American kestrel (a), a very young red-shouldered hawk (b), and a red-tailed hawk (c). Note that the kestrel (a) has a green mark on its head for easy identification.

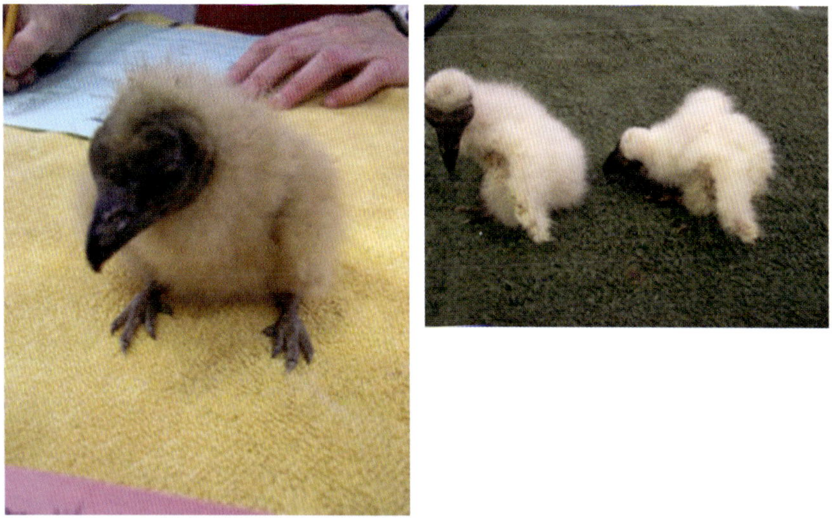

Fig. 12.4. Vulture hatchlings. Turkey vultures have white down (right) and black vultures have tan down (left).

- Cooper's hawk: Digit 3 is long with plantar protuberance (Fig. 13.23).
- Red-shouldered hawk: Very vocal; small yellow feet. Look for tan "windows" on dorsal side of the outer four primaries (Fig. 13.20).
- Broad-winged hawk: Similar to red-shouldered hawk, but not vocal and smaller feet.
- Red-tailed hawk: Similar to red-shouldered hawk, but not nearly as vocal and feet are much larger.
- Black vulture: Tan down and dark beak.
- Turkey vulture: Very similar to black vulture but with white down.

Most juvenile hawks have a gray/tan iris.

Handling

Hatchlings are extremely delicate since their bones, joints, and feathers are all forming simultaneously. *Young birds should never be grabbed by the legs*. Always use a body grab from behind, with the wings carefully folded up against the body (Fig. 12.5). Because of the significant risk of accidental injury, it is safest to carry, transport, and weigh young birds in a box (Fig. 12.6).

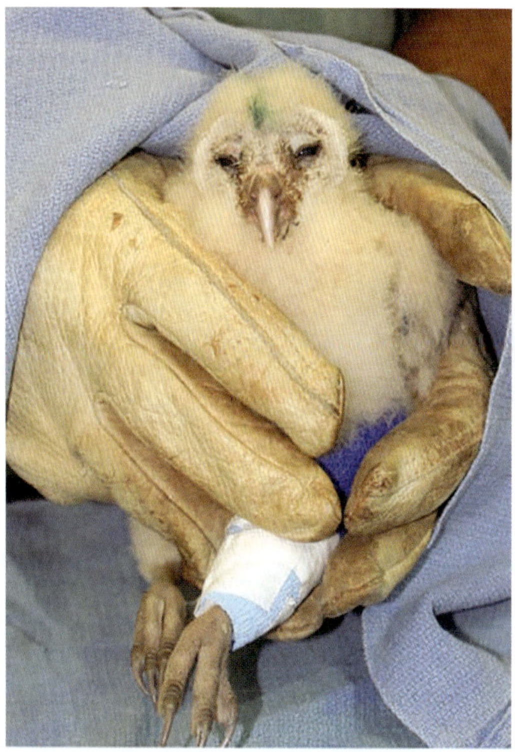

Fig. 12.5. Hatchling barn owl.

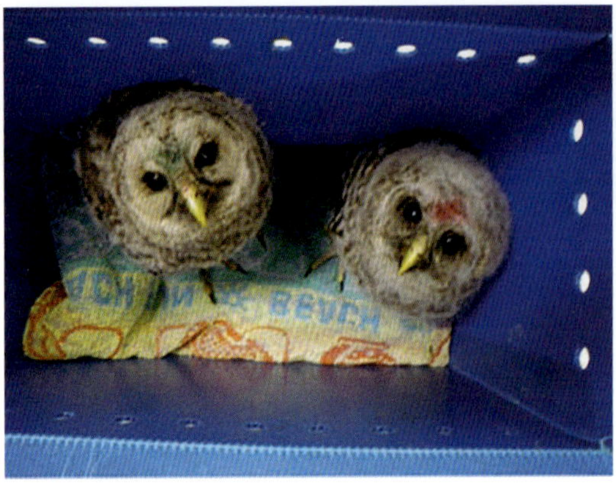

Fig. 12.6. Two barred owl juveniles being transported in a carrier. Note the color markings on their foreheads.

Generally, more than one hatchling can be placed in a box together as space allows. The exception is barn owls as these birds are very "footy" and they will grab each other with their talons and cause serious injury. They should always be transported separately.

> **Raptor Tip**
>
> Barn owls should always be transported in separate boxes.

Physical Exam

Examination of nestling/juvenile birds is challenging. They are extremely delicate since their bones are growing and their flight feathers may be completely in blood. Birds of this age are typically examined in a sitting/vertical position as it is dangerous to place them on their backs. The exam should be brief but thorough and should include the following:

- Palpate all long bones for fractures and joints for luxations or swelling.
- Examine both eyes, including the posterior chambers. The lenses of young birds are often somewhat cloudy with a bluish tint. This is normal and should resolve as they develop. However, juvenile-onset cataracts do occur and should be ruled out if in doubt.
- Examine both ear canals as it is not uncommon to find warble infestations.
- Look carefully for maggots or fly eggs, particularly around the vent, base of the tail feathers, and around the elbows.
- Check the body condition score. Young birds always seem a bit thin because their muscles have not fully developed. For this reason, a keel score of 2 out of 5 is probably normal.

Habituation and Imprinting

Young birds gain a great deal of crucial knowledge in the first 4 weeks of life through a process of imprinting. This is a critical time window and, when raised naturally with normal visual and auditory cues, they learn what species they are, what to look for in a nest site, what to eat, and how to find an appropriate mate. In effect, they imprint on their parents, siblings, and surroundings. This is an irreversible process that, under normal/natural conditions, serves them well throughout their lives.

In a rehabilitation situation, imprinting still occurs, but the sensory stimulation received will not be appropriate unless concerted efforts are made to provide the correct cues. If the correct cues are not provided, a baby can easily become imprinted on humans and will look to humans for companionship, as food sources, and possibly even as mates. This process is irreversible and birds in this state are not releasable. Inappropriate imprinting is guaranteed to happen when the appropriate measures are not taken within the crucial developmental time window. Vultures are particularly prone to imprinting and this often occurs despite the best efforts to avoid it.

> **Signs of a mal-imprinted bird**
>
> - Food begging around people.
> - Lack of fear: will not flee when approached.
> - Lack of fear: can be overly aggressive.

Steps to take to avoid imprinting include:

- Replacing all healthy hatchlings back into their nest, if at all possible. As an alternative, they can be placed back into another nest of the same species (see "Renesting" below).

- Using a surrogate parent of the same species to raise them, if available.
- Never talk around young birds. They should be kept in a quiet space away from any human-derived sounds.
- Using a species-appropriate puppet (Fig. 12.7) when feeding. See Appendix H for tips on making your own feeding puppets.
- Using camouflage whenever feeding an orphan or cleaning its kennel. The camouflage should cover the face, body, arms, and hands (Fig. 12.8).

Once the birds have moved to an outdoor cage, always deliver food through a feeding hatch so they do not associate the delivery with humans. Varying the time of delivery is also important to avoid habituation.

Do not raise young birds on their own, if at all possible. Place in groups of the same species and similar size/weight, since this facilitates normal behavioral development. The size of the group should mimic the natural nesting situation. This depends on species but is generally from two to five birds. A colored mark (e.g. with a permanent marker) on the forehead (Fig. 12.5) or temporary metal ID bands on the tarsometatarsus are necessary in order to differentiate one bird from another.

Typical Orphan Protocol

There is no set protocol that fits all cases but here are some guidelines:

- When very young, hatchlings should be fed three or four times daily.
- In the peak growth phase, total daily intake of food should be approximately 20–25% of BW. Hatchlings require two to three times the amount required by an adult. See the Feeding Guide in Appendix A.
- Initially, use furless mouse cut up into small pieces.
- Tweezer-feed with a puppet and camouflage until self-feeding.
- Weigh every day until self-feeding, then gradually increase the interval between weighings.
- The weight should increase daily until the adult weight is reached (Fig. 12.9). If it decreases for more than a day or two, or if the bird refuses to tweezer-feed, begin force-feeding. Beware that force-feeding can be dangerous

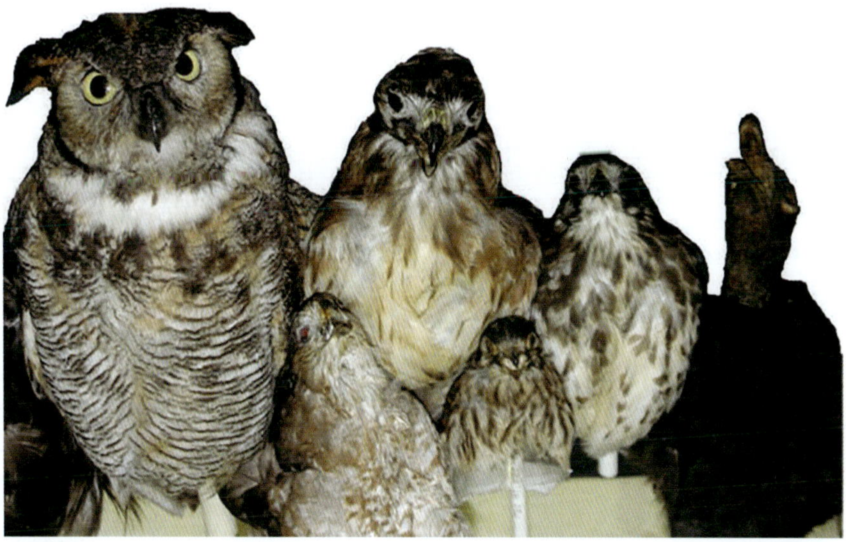

Fig. 12.7. Hand-made feeding puppets for many common species.

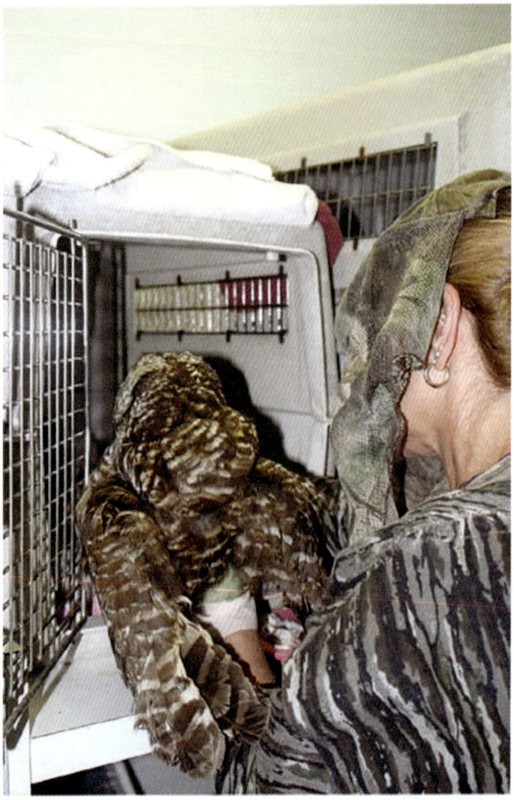

Fig. 12.8. A barred owl puppet and camouflage in use when feeding a neonate. The goal is to make the bird believe that an adult of the same species is providing the food.

since the jaw of a young bird is very fragile and fractures can occur.

- Placing young birds in groups of two or three (as they would be in the nest) is very helpful.
- The crop should be empty before tweezer-feedings. If it is not, skip a meal but monitor carefully, as this is not a normal finding. Remember that owls do not have a crop.
- Gradually wean off tweezer-feeding and begin leaving food in cage. The food must always be cut up into sizes appropriate for them to swallow. Remember that young birds are not able to tear up food until almost fully developed.
- Once self-feeding, feed enough so there are always some leftovers. Self-feeding should always be encouraged to reduce contact with human caretakers.
- Decrease to two meals per day, then decrease to one meal daily as the bird gets to full size and the feathers are fully developed.
- When the birds are self-feeding and doing well, they can be placed in relatively large groups in outside cages. If space is available in a cage, it is not a problem to house ten owls together in one cage, for example (Fig. 12.10). Hawks tend to be more stressed so they should not be housed in groups larger than five or six.

Timeline for Growth

This is adapted from a guide created by Mathias Engelmann (Staff member, Carolina Raptor Center):

Hatch to 7 days	Raptor hatchlings are altricial, meaning that they are weak, naked, and helpless. They are uncoordinated, their eyes are closed, they are unable to regulate body temperature, and they probably will not eat for the first 24 h. Feed small pieces of whole mouse without fur or large bones. Keep in a warm incubator set for approximately 85–90°F (29–32°C)
8–14 days	Eyes open and focusing on environment. The egg tooth should fall off, umbilicus should be healed. Birds are stronger but probably not able to hold head up very well yet. Start on diet of whole mice, cut into bite-sized pieces. They no longer require an incubator but cannot be exposed to large changes in temperature. House at room temperature unless with a foster parent
15–21 days	Eating large amounts but still require food to be cut into small pieces. Sitting on hock joints and fairly mobile

Continued

Continued

22–28 days	Depending on species, able to stand now (especially smaller birds such as the kestrel or screech owl). Able to regulate body temperature; primaries and tail feathers starting to emerge
29–35 days	Starting to lose some of the downy feathers; primaries and tail feathers ½" (12 mm) in length; good grip with feet. Can be moved outdoors if siblings or foster adult are available
36–42 days	Wings are flapping, short hops, losing down feathers. Juvenile plumage evident underneath. In the wild, many of the smaller species will start to fledge or "branch". Birds can be moved outdoors but cages may need to be modified to include low perches which are easily accessible
43–49 days	Most of down on wings has gone but remains on the body and head for several more weeks. Flying now. Can start to actively exercise and then begin "mouse school" except for the largest species (vultures and eagles). Can now eat whole food; no longer any need to cut food into smaller pieces

The table in Appendix F shows the normal weights for some typical North American species, listed at various ages. Note that the smaller species develop much more rapidly and fledge earlier (refer to Chapter 3).

Exercise and Live-prey School

Most young birds should reach full size and the flight feathers should be fully developed at approximately 6–8 weeks. Note that this will take longer in the larger species (vultures and eagles). At this time, the bird should be moved to a flight cage to begin exercise. The exercise period varies but should last at least 2–3 weeks. During this time, the exercise regimen should be gradually increased. Be sure not to overcrowd the flight cage, as collisions can lead to fractures in young birds whose bones are still relatively soft.

Once the birds have been exercised, they must be tested with live prey to demonstrate ability to recognize, kill, and consume prey. There are many protocols in use at different centers and they all have merit. The protocol in use at the Carolina Raptor Center is as follows:

- A large flight cage is used (see Table 15.2 for suggestions on cage size). The cage must have leaf litter on the ground to simulate a natural hunting environment and provide a place for prey to hide. This is the one case where organic bedding is used (see Chapter 15).
- Three or four fully developed and exercised birds are tested at once. Before beginning live prey, these birds should be fed a daily amount that is relatively close to the adult daily amount. Each bird is weighed and keel scored prior to the start of the test.
- For 7 days, they are provided a daily diet consisting of 50% dead food and 50% live prey. The live prey should simulate wild prey as closely as possible, so white mice are not an appropriate choice.
- After 3 days, the birds are weighed and keel scored again. It is not uncommon for them to have lost some weight at this first weighing, as they are learning how to hunt.
- The birds are weighed and keel scored again after the test is complete on the 7th day. A bird is considered to have passed if it did not lose more than 5% of its beginning BW.

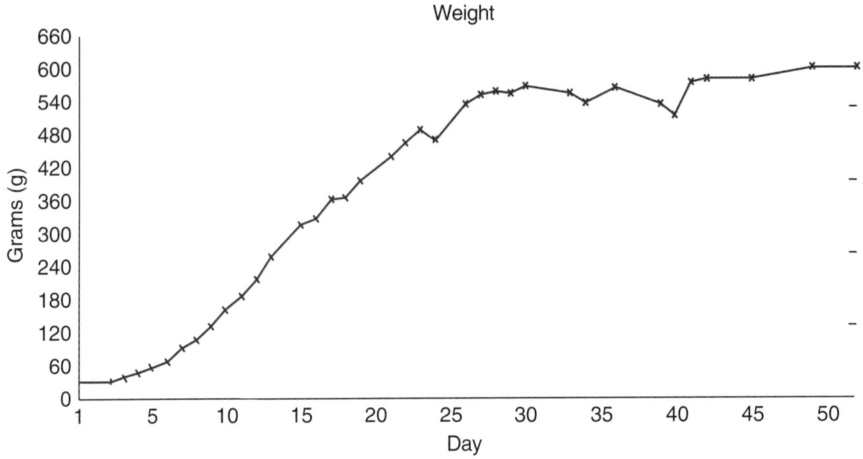

Fig. 12.9. Typical weight/growth chart for a red-shouldered hawk as displayed by the RaptorMed™ medical records software. There is a rapid weight gain for the first 3 weeks then the weight plateaus around the normal adult weight. The frequency of weighings decreases as the bird grows.

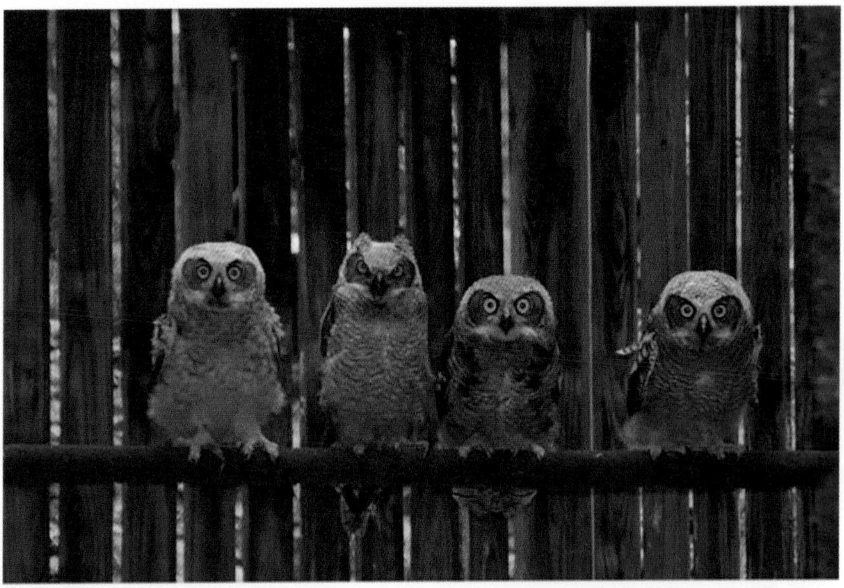

Fig. 12.10. Young owls do well in large groups of up to ten birds. Hawks should be kept in groups of five or six at most.

The majority of birds pass the first time through, but it is not uncommon for a few to have to be retested. It is very uncommon for a bird to fail for a second time. This protocol is by no means a perfect test for the following reasons:

- One bird may simply eat the dead food while its cage mates hunt live prey. Without witnessing the kills, it is hard to be sure. Testing birds in the smallest groups possible is always best. If in doubt, test a bird individually, and visually verify it can kill and consume prey.
- It is not clear if 7 days is long enough. The assumption is that if a bird is not eating it would lose much more than 5% of its weight in that time period.

- It is also not clear if a 5% drop is a valid cut-off. In reality, most birds that pass usually do not lose much at all, and many actually gain weight.
- Should the birds be tested on 100% live prey? The assumption is that these birds would be supplemented with dead food by their parents while they are learning to hunt. If this is true, then testing with a 50:50 mix seems to be appropriate.
- This test does not replicate or simulate actual hunting conditions in the wild.

Clearly, post-release tracking studies are needed to evaluate this protocol. Scott (2013) does seem to indicate that this process can be successful.

Eggs

It is not uncommon to receive unhatched eggs in cases where a nest is blown out of a tree or the tree was cut down. A detailed history is important to determine if the egg is still viable. Attempt to answer the following questions:

- Where and under what circumstances was the egg found?
- How many eggs were found?
- Was it warm when found and was it kept warm?
- How long has the egg been in the finder's possession?

Eggs can be candled (refer to color plates 29.14–29.18 in Joyner, 1994) to determine viability. Once received, all potentially viable eggs should be kept in an incubator that can control temperature and humidity. In addition, the incubator should have a mechanism to rock the eggs gently. If a rocker is not available, the eggs can be marked and then manually rotated several times each day.

The incubation period (Chapter 3) varies greatly with species. It can be difficult to tell exactly what type of egg you have but the size, shape, and color can provide some clues (Fig. 12.11).

The age of the egg will usually be unknown so incubation for the maximum period is required to give the egg the best chance of hatching.

For more detailed information on the incubation of eggs, refer to Chitty (2008).

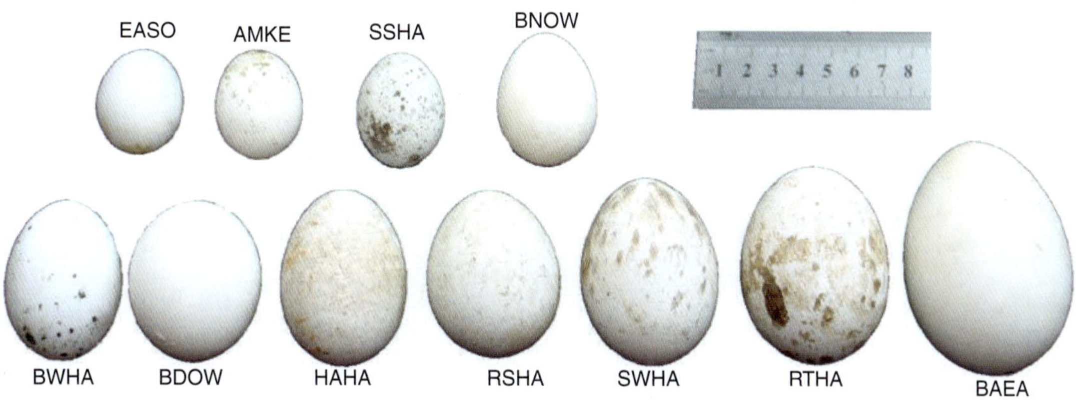

Fig. 12.11. Eggs of various raptors. Note how large the egg of the sharp-shinned hawk (average weight 150 g) is compared to the egg of the bald eagle (average weight 4500 g). EASO, eastern screech owl; AMKE, American kestrel; SSHA, sharp-shinned hawk; BNOW, barn owl; BWHA, broad-winged hawk; BDOW, barred owl; HAHA, Harris's hawk; RSHA, red-shouldered hawk; SWHA, Swainson's hawk; RTHA, red-tailed hawk; BAEA, bald eagle.

Renesting

Most juvenile raptors presented to rehabilitation centers are healthy nestling or hatchling-age birds. It is a normal part of development for these birds to spend some time on the ground as they learn to fly. The parents will feed them and will defend them during this vulnerable period. If their physical examination reveals no significant abnormalities, then they should be returned to the nest site immediately, if at all possible. Complications that may be expected include:

- The inability to find the nest.
- The presence of dogs, cats, crows, or other sources of danger (such as vehicle traffic) in the area.
- The inability to reach the nest.

Downy hatchlings and nestlings need to be returned to the nest with their parents as they cannot feed themselves or thermoregulate. Hatchlings and nestlings are either downy or may only have the beginnings of flight feathers and covert feathers visible. Examples include Figs 12.2a, 12.2b, 12.3a, 12.3b, and 12.4. Renesting these birds will require the help of a skilled

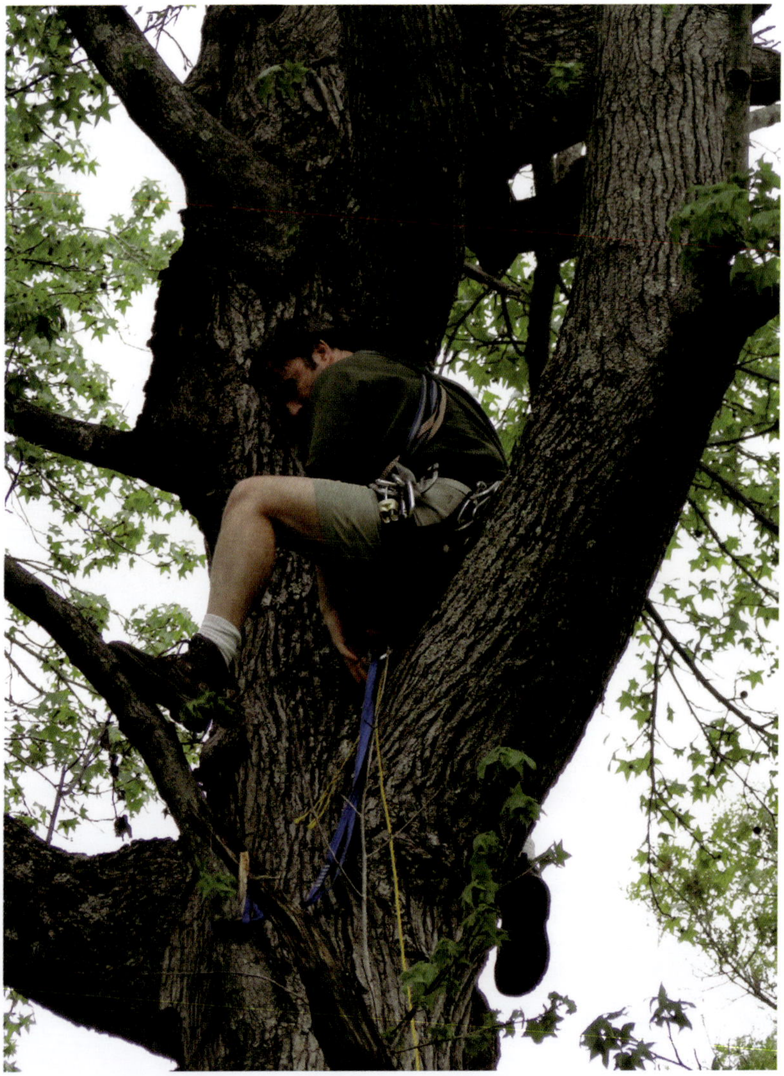

Fig. 12.12. Tree-climbing requires experience and the proper equipment. A local arborist is a great resource for renesting.

tree-climber or arborist (Fig. 12.12). If the nest cannot be reached, and the birds are old enough to thermoregulate, then an artificial nest can be used and secured in the tree as close to the original nest as possible. Artificial nests can be made from plastic buckets (with holes drilled in the bottom to allow them to drain), laundry baskets (Fig. 12.13), artificial wood platforms (Fig. 12.14), or they can be woven from branches, as shown in Fig. 12.15. Note that Cooper's hawks will not accept an artificial nest as well as other species. Sometimes the original nest is accessible but may require repair. This is particularly common with owls that nest in cavities. Be prepared with supplies to repair the nest such as bailing wire, hammer and nails, small pieces of wood, and sheets of artificial turf (Fig. 12.16).

Also note that nestlings can often be replaced into an entirely different nest. The foster parents will usually accept them as long as they are not overloaded (Fig. 12.17). In general, two or three chicks can be fed, but siblicide or parental rejection can occur if there is any type of stress or food shortage.

Branchers and fledglings can simply be placed back on a branch in the original or nearby tree. At this age, these birds will not stay in the nest even if you place them back in it. It is not uncommon for these birds to go back and forth between branches, the ground, and other structures such as fences. Note that branchers have pretty-well-developed flight feathers and coverts and can thermoregulate themselves. Examples include Figs 12.2c and 12.3c.

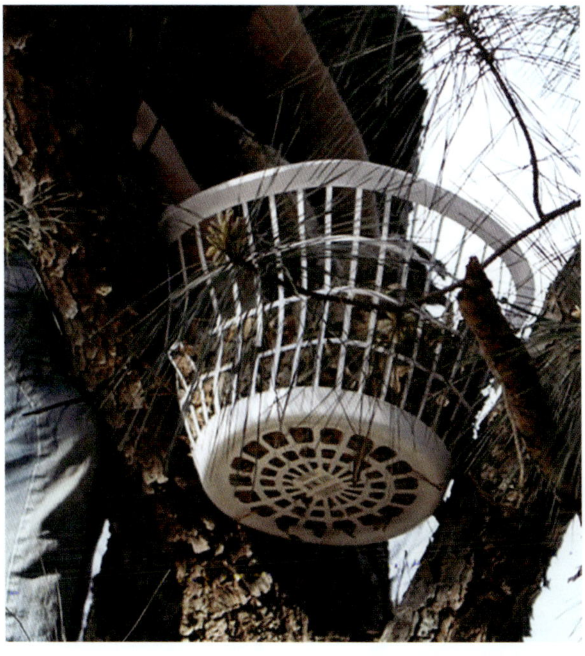

Fig. 12.13. A laundry basket filled with leaves and secured in a tree can make a very good temporary nest.

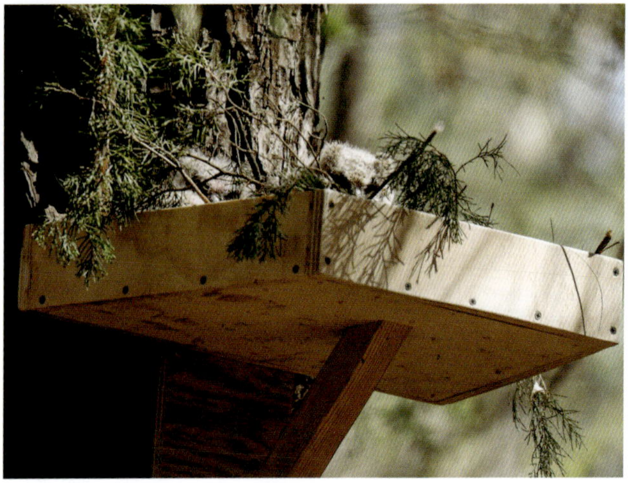

Fig. 12.14. An older nestling great-horned owl renested on an artificial platform near the original nest.

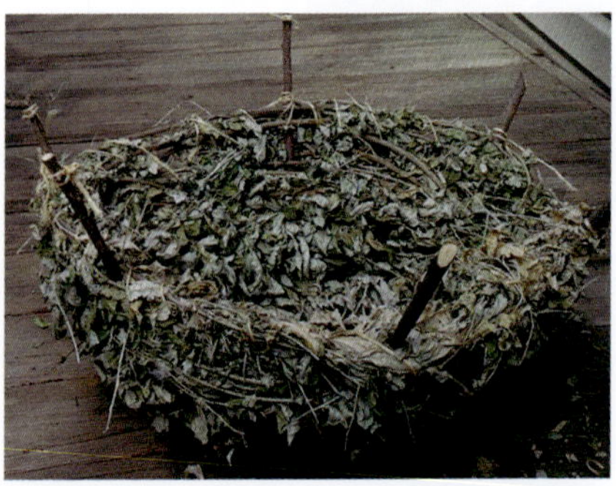

Fig. 12.15. An artificial nest woven from branches and vines. Refer to Appendix G for instructions on building a woven nest.

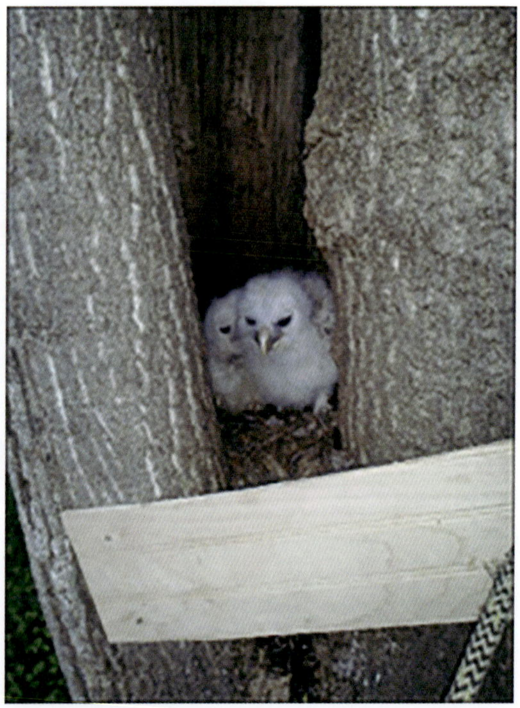

Fig. 12.16. This barred owl nest was repaired by nailing a board across the sloped, open side.

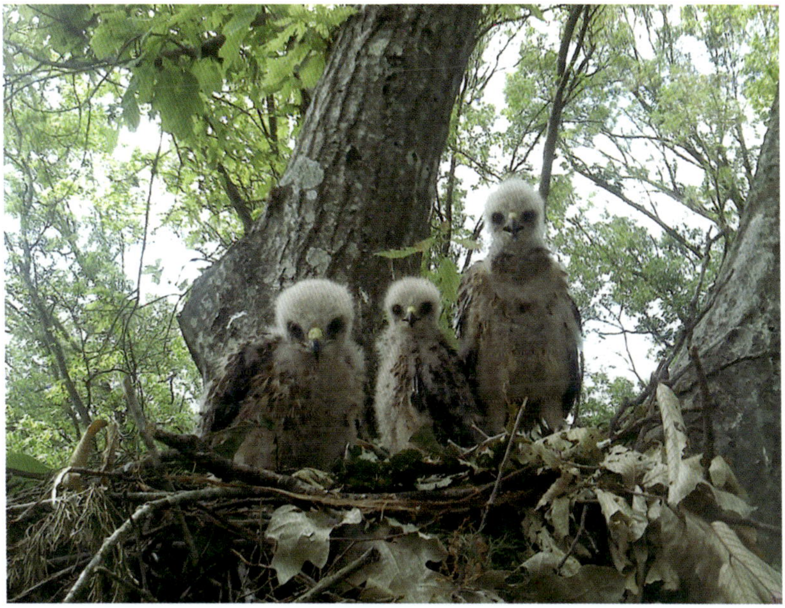

Fig. 12.17. A third red-shouldered hawk was added to an existing nest of two. This works well as long as the existing nestlings appear healthy and are not much larger than the newly added bird.

Decision Key: Rescue or Let it Be?

Is it injured?	If yes, then clearly it needs to be treated. Be sure to check for fly eggs and maggots and check the ears for warbles
Are there flies buzzing around it?	If yes, examine carefully for maggots and fly eggs. Renest right away otherwise
Is it a nestling?	If yes, then it needs to be returned to the original nest as soon as possible. The bird can be cared for for up to 48 h before returning to the nest. After that, the parent will abandon the nest unless there are other chicks still in it. If the original nest was destroyed, then an artificial nest can be placed as close as possible with the hope that the parents will relocate to the new nest
Is it a brancher?	If yes, then simply return to a branch in the original tree or nearby tree. Many owl species can climb very well and do not require a tree with many branches. In fact, barred owls can quite literally climb a vertical tree trunk with no branches. Hawks cannot climb so try to find a tree with many branches
Is it an eagle?	If yes, then it should always be examined carefully. Eagles are heavy and are often injured when they fall to the ground
Is it a vulture?	If yes, then leave them alone if at all possible, especially if a parent is present. Vultures are very easy to mal-imprint, so successfully raising and releasing them is very difficult

Continued

Continued

Are there dogs and cats around? Is the bird being mobbed by crows?	If the nest site is simply too dangerous to return the bird, you can take the bird into "protective custody" for a short period until it is able to fly or climb to a perch. As long as the parents are still at the nest site, you can return the bird
Don't see parents around?	True orphans are actually quite rare. If possible, stay quiet and keep a watch because the parents are likely close by. Placing the baby back in the nest or into a substitute nest nearby (if old enough) will lure the parents back. Note that a vulture's parents may be gone for several hours at a time and they typically nest on the ground or on a horizontal structure or building
Is the bird lying down and quiet?	This can be normal behavior for many young birds, especially hawks
Does the bird seem thin?	Young raptors often seem thin compared to an adult because their flight muscles have not developed yet. A body condition score of 2 or 2.5 out of 5 is normal

Bibliography

Arent, L. (2007) *Raptors in Captivity: Guidelines for Care and Management*. Hancock House Publishing, Surrey, BC, Canada.

Chitty, L. (2008) *BSAVA Manual of Raptors, Pigeons and Passerine Birds*. BSAVA, Gloucester, UK.

Joyner, K.L. (1994) Theriogenology. In: Ritchie, B.W., Harrison, G.J. and Harrison, L.R. (eds) *Avian Medicine: Principles and Application*. Wingers Publishing, Inc., Lake Worth, FL, USA, pp. 748–804.

Miller, A.G. (2007) *Calls of the Wild*. Alabama Wildlife Center, Birmingham, AL, USA. Available at: www.awrc.org (accessed February 2016).

Scott, D. (2013) A retrospective look at the survival of birds of prey released from a rehabilitation center in North Carolina. *Proceedings of the 2013 Association of Avian Veterinarians Conference, Jacksonville, FL, USA*. Association of Avian Veterinarians, Teaneck, NJ, USA, p. 359.

Sibley, D.A. (2001) *The Sibley Guide to Bird Life & Behavior*. Alfred A. Knopf, Inc., New York, NY, USA.

13 Feathers and Aging

Learning Objectives

1. Feather numbering and anatomy.
2. Determining age.
3. Imping feathers.

Feathers are an incredibly important part of avian anatomy. They are involved in several functions including:

- Flight.
- Insulation.
- Waterproofing.
- Courtship and mating.
- Camouflage.
- Sound level control (in owls).

Because of their importance, all attempts should be made to protect feathers. These include, but are not limited to:

- Proper handling (Chapter 1).
- Appropriate caging (Chapter 15).
- Use of tail wraps (Chapter 4).

Anatomy and Numbering

The feathers are arranged in tracts called pterylae. There are also several featherless areas or tracts called apterylae. One important featherless tract is over the jugular vein that allows easy access to this vein for blood collection.

The typical feather is composed of a shaft and vanes (Fig. 13.1). The shaft has two parts: the calamus and the rachis. The vane is composed of branches from the central rachis called barbs. In turn, the barbs have barbules, and the barbules have barbicels. The barbs, barbules, and barbicels intermesh to form a strong, unified sheet.

There are several types of feathers that vary in function and in construction:

- Contour feathers: these are the largest feathers and have the most typical appearance.
  - Remiges: the major wing flight feathers.
    - Primaries: these attach to the dorsal metacarpal and second phalange bones. There are ten of them numbered from the carpus outward (Fig. 13.2).

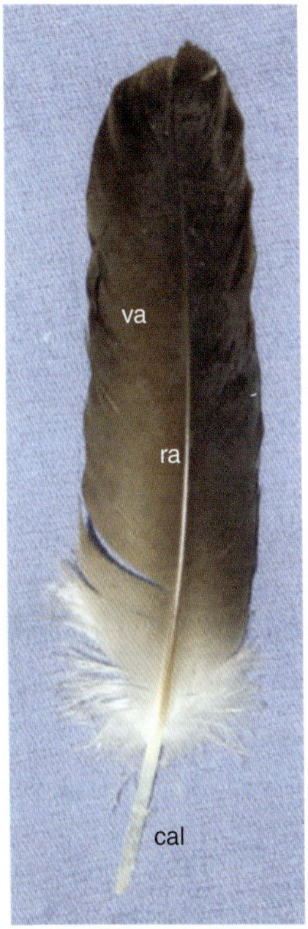

Fig. 13.1. Feather anatomy. The shaft is composed of the calamus (cal) and rachis (ra). The vanes (va) are composed of interlocking barbs, barbules, and barbicels.

- Secondaries: these attach to the dorsal ulna. They are numbered starting at the carpus inward toward the elbow. The exact number of secondaries varies with species, but typically there are a dozen or more.
  - Retrices: these are the tail feathers. There are six pairs numbered from the middle to the outer edge.
  - Coverts: these are smaller feathers that cover the roots of the remiges and retrices. There are usually several rows of coverts and they help create the overall body shape.
- Semiplumes: these are fluffy in appearance and are usually located along the margin of the feathered tracts.
- Filoplumes: these have a long calamus with a short tuft at the end. They are usually found near the follicle of each contour feather and are believed to provide sensory information regarding the orientation of the flight feathers.
- Bristles: these have a stiff, long rachis, and are located around the eyelids, nares, and mouth. They are believed to have a sensory role.
- Down: these are for insulation.

The follicles of the primary and secondary wing feathers are firmly embedded in the dorsal periosteum of the metacarpal/phalange bones and ulna, respectively. Pulling a damaged contour feather will therefore be painful and can cause permanent damage to the follicle. This should not be attempted without very good reason.

Some special details to be aware of:

- The outer primary feathers of owls have a series of bristles (Fig. 13.3) on the leading edge that assists in muffling their sound during flight.

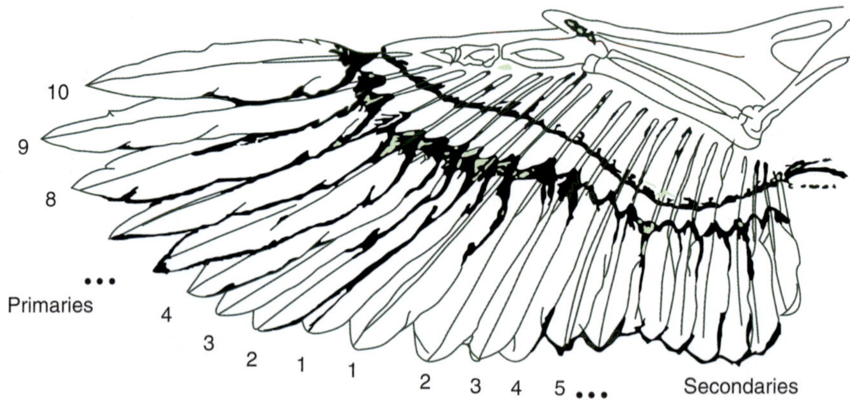

Fig. 13.2. Counting system for primary and secondary feathers. Drawing courtesy of Christina Hildreth.

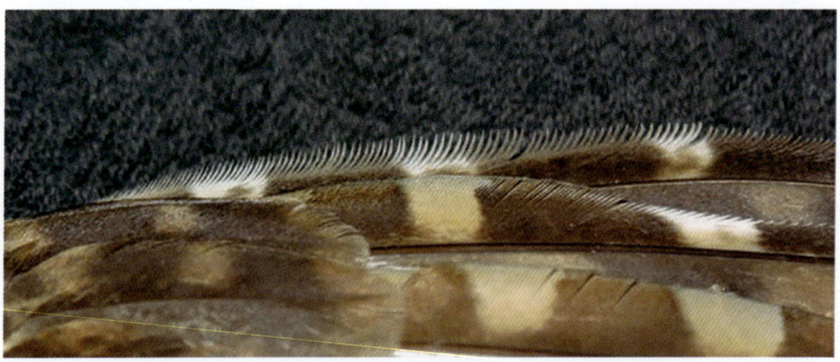

Fig. 13.3. Sound-reduction bristles on primary #10 in a barred owl.

- The first set of flight feathers can have a small tuft (Fig. 13.4) at the tip. This tuft generally wears off in the first few months but can be used to identify a bird's age as HY (see Table 13.1 below for age abbreviations used in the text).

Development

When a new feather develops, it expels the old one from the follicle in a process called molting. The new feather is sometimes called a pin feather or a blood feather as it is, quite literally, a keratin sheath filled with a bloody pulp (Fig. 13.5). At this stage, the feather is extremely fragile. Trauma can be painful; it can destroy the feather; and it can lead to extensive blood loss. As the feather develops within the sheath, the sheath begins to fall off or is preened away. This allows the feather to dry and fully expand its vanes.

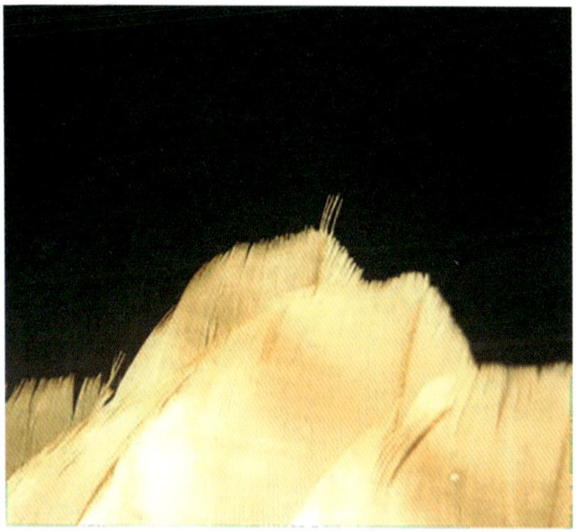

Fig. 13.4. Feather tuft in a HY bird.

Fault or stress bars are defects which are visible across the feather vanes and shaft. They are caused by any type of stress (such as illness or malnutrition) that occurs during the feather's development. Since the feather is weaker at these locations, parts of the feather may break off (as noted in Fig. 13.6). Most often, fault bars do not appear to cause a real problem, but in owls they could potentially cause flight noise if the damage is severe.

The Molting Process

A bird molts repeatedly throughout its life. Molting allows damaged feathers to be replaced and also allows a bird to display its breeding status.

The molting process typically occurs in the late spring and summer, after the breeding season. It is usually orderly and involves the symmetrical replacement of the wing feathers. The primaries usually molt from proximal to distal and the secondaries are molted from distal to proximal. The process is staggered and ensures

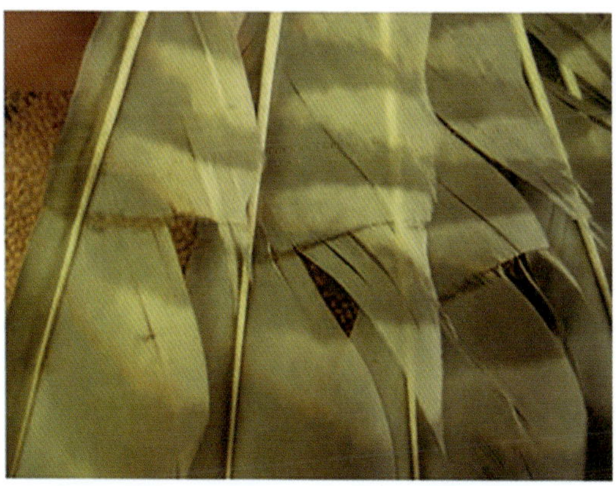

Fig. 13.5. Blood feathers in a 4-week-old bird.

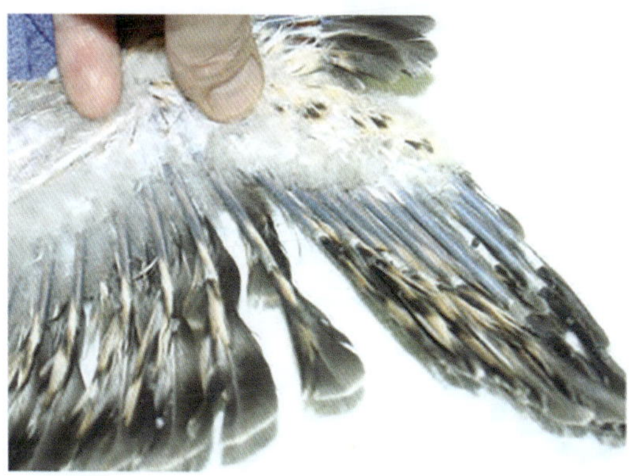

Fig. 13.6. Fault bars on multiple, adjacent feathers.

that large gaps are never present and that flight capability is not seriously impacted during the process. The tail feathers are also molted in a symmetrical, staggered fashion. However, there are some deviations from this since it is not uncommon, for example, for nesting barred owls to molt their entire tail all at once. Also, trauma to the area can induce a spontaneous molt of feathers in the area and it is not uncommon for several secondary remiges to molt after an ulna fracture.

Juveniles/nestling birds grow an entire set of feathers almost simultaneously, so all of their flight feathers will show very similar color and wear patterns. This will be the only time in their life that all flight feathers are uniform. In general, these juvenile feathers are weaker than future adult feathers and may have a different length/shape.

Not all feathers are molted each year and a bird will retain feathers from previous molts. This pattern is helpful when attempting to age a bird (see below).

The molt cycle is believed to be triggered by seasonal changes in day length. As a result, it is possible to manipulate the molt by artificially controlling the light cycle in a specially prepared molt chamber. Although the process is primarily triggered by the light cycle, it is very complex, and hormones (including thyroid hormone) undoubtedly play an important role.

The process of molting is energy- and resource-intensive, and birds undergoing a molt require a much higher plane of nutrition than normal. Malnourished birds going through a molt will likely grow feathers with defects known as fault bars (Fig. 13.6).

Feather Checks

When dealing with birds that have feather damage, it is important to accurately record the state of each feather. Recorded observations (Figs 13.7 and 13.8) will allow for an objective comparison over time and to judge whether the bird is improving or in need of some type of intervention.

Aging

This section is adapted from a guide created by Mathias Engelmann (Staff member, Carolina Raptor Center).

Birds are aged primarily by distinguishing characteristics of their feathers (Table 13.1). In some species, other clues such as eye color can also be helpful. Aging raptors is a very complicated process and the following guide is just a

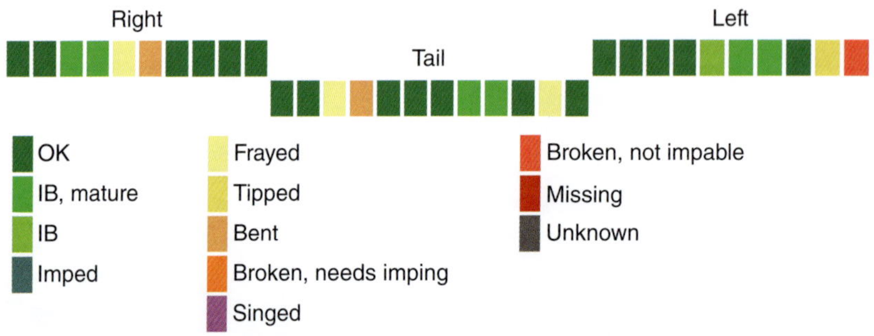

Fig. 13.7. A typical feather check entry displayed by the RaptorMed™ medical records software. As indicated, there are many "states" that a feather can be in. IB, in blood.

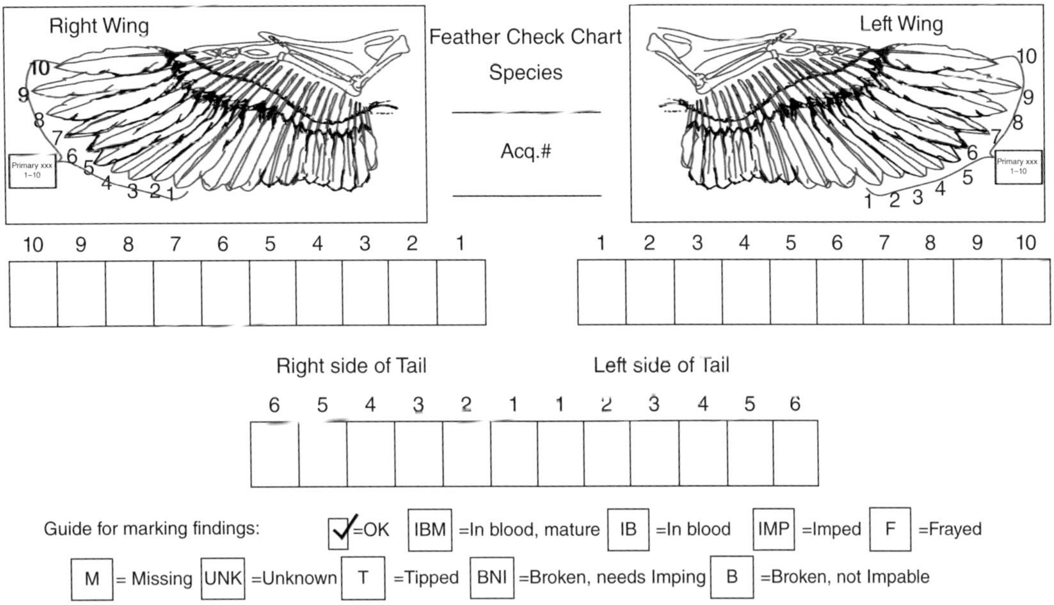

Fig. 13.8. This laminated card and an erasable pen make it easy to record feather checks in the field.

Table 13.1. Age classifications as specified by the Bird Banding Lab in the USA.

Abbreviation	Age
L	Local to nest. Hatchling, unable to sustain flight
HY	Hatch year
AHY	After hatch year
SY	Second year
ASY	After second year
TY	Third year
ATY	After third year
4Y	Fourth year
A4Y	After fourth year
...	

very brief introduction. The many publications by Peter Pyle should be consulted for a more complete description.

General rules and clues

In owls, ignore the tail. If using tail feathers for aging in a diurnal bird, ignore #1 and #6 since their color and pattern may be different from the other feathers.

Focus on the *dorsal* side of the primaries and secondaries when determining differences in coloration and wear pattern of tips or edges. Do not ignore the ventral side completely since there can be some helpful clues there as well. Sometimes color differences are more obvious on the feather shaft.

Primaries and secondaries are often longer in juveniles than in adults (Figs 13.9 and 13.19).

In young HY birds, feather tufts remain on the primaries and secondaries for several weeks or months, depending on wear (Fig. 13.4).

Downy feathers on the head can persist until late summer or early fall in a HY bird.

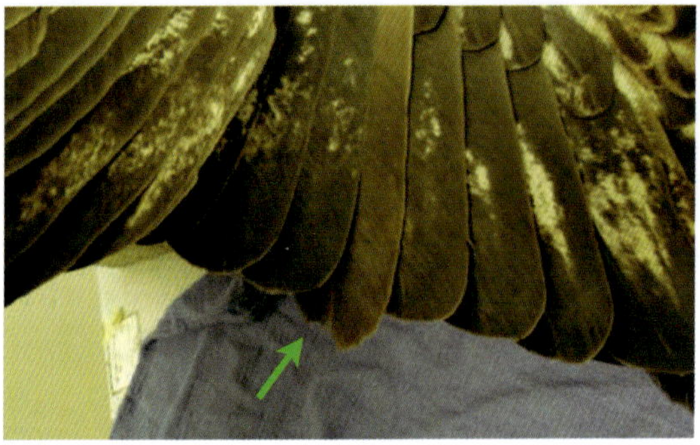

Fig. 13.9. This SY bald eagle has one retained juvenile secondary feather (arrow). Note that it is longer than the others and is also a different shade.

> **Box 13.1. Age determination**
>
> Determine whether juvenile and/or adult plumage is present using the general rules and the species-specific hints listed below; then use the season (Table 13.2) to determine the specific age.

All birds are assumed to have a birth/hatch date of 1 January and age by 1 year at the beginning of each new year.

At any one time, there can only be one age class of juvenile feathers present, but there can be multiple age classes of adult feathers. Therefore, if you see mixed feathers, you can eliminate HY as an age possibility.

The one exception to the above rule involves the fact that injuries can affect the next molt. At any time of year, if feathers are dropped due to injury, the next age class of feathers will be produced. So, for example, a HY red-tailed hawk could grow adult tail feathers in December of its hatching year if its juvenile tail feathers were injured and were molted prematurely (Fig. 13.22b).

In general, a brood patch is found in females only.

Fault bars may help in aging. For example, uniform fault bars across all or most of the primaries would indicate HY or SY. When the fault bars are across all feathers, they must all have grown simultaneously. This only occurs in a young bird when it is growing its first set of feathers. Conversely, it would be very unlikely that an adult would have replaced all primaries simultaneously.

Seasonality

The season impacts how the feathers are used to determine age, since a feather pattern in the spring may be interpreted entirely differently in the fall. Table 13.2 summarizes the important distinctions.

Species-specific aging

The following tips may help age the various species. In most cases, it is difficult to differentiate beyond the determination of juvenile versus adult. In some species, there are distinct markings which can be used to determine age.

In many birds, wear patterns and uniformity of color can be useful to determine age. Specifically, feathers that are all the same shade or are worn equally are likely from the first molt and would indicate that the bird is a juvenile. After the first molt (i.e. an adult), individual feathers are molted separately (instead of all at once) so you

Table 13.2. Seasonal age classifications[a].

Uniform juvenile feathers	
Fall	HY
Spring	SY (has not molted yet)
Mixed juvenile and adult feathers	
Fall	SY
Spring	TY
Uniform adult feathers	
Fall	AHY
Spring	ASY
Mixed adult feathers	
Fall	ASY
Spring	ATY

[a]See Table 13.1 for age abbreviations.

would expect slight variations in color and wear in an adult bird. It is rarely possible to accurately age these birds beyond calling them an adult.

The presence of single feathers in molt indicates an adult bird, since juvenile birds produce all the feathers in their first molt at once, not one at a time.

The color of the iris (Fig. 13.10) may be used to determine age in some hawks. In general, juvenile hawks have a tan-gray iris and this color changes as the bird develops. The resulting color varies with species. In the red-tailed hawk or red-shouldered hawk, for example, the iris will change from tan-gray in the juvenile to dark brown after 3–4 years. The brown coloration progresses from ventral to dorsal and it is not uncommon to have a bird (2–3 years old) with an iris that is half gray and half brown. In accipiters such as Cooper's hawks, the iris color progresses from pale gray to yellow to orange to red in the adult (Fig. 13.25).

Eastern screech owl

The primary covert feathers are either "notched" in juveniles or non-notched in adults (Fig. 13.11). The outer two coverts should be ignored and some birds have mixed coverts so their age cannot be reliably determined. In addition, the shape of the tip of primaries 7–10 can be either tapered or broad/truncate. See Pyle (1997a) for more details. Screech owls can come in several color morphs, but this cannot be used for aging (Fig. 13.12).

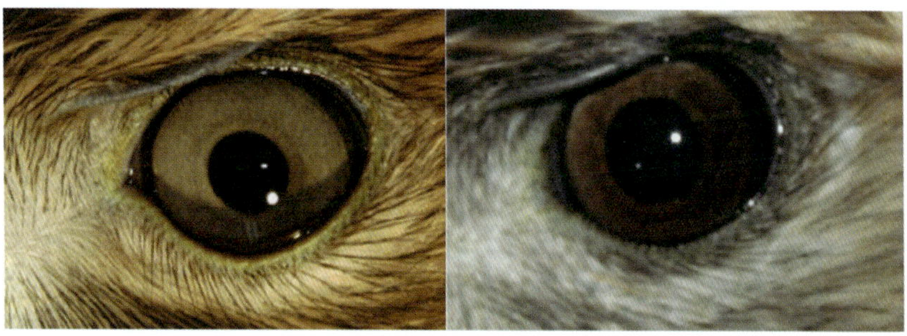

Fig. 13.10. Hawk eyes: juvenile hawks have a tan-gray iris (left) and adults have a dark brown iris (right).

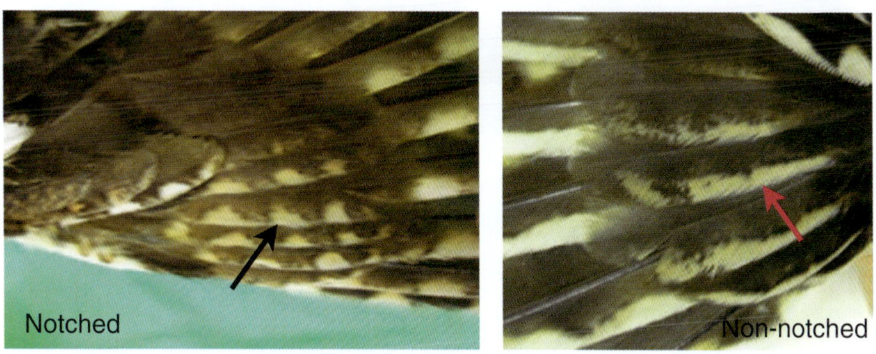

Fig. 13.11. Left: notched primary coverts in a juvenile eastern screech owl. Right: non-notched coverts in an adult.

Barred owl

The width of the *outermost three* bands on the dorsal side of the inner primaries and all secondaries is used to determine age (Fig. 13.13). Juvenile birds have narrow bands and adults have wide bands. Also, new feathers (in juveniles or adults) will have a pinkish hue on the ventral surface of the feathers. Adults may show evidence of multiple adult molts (Fig. 13.14).

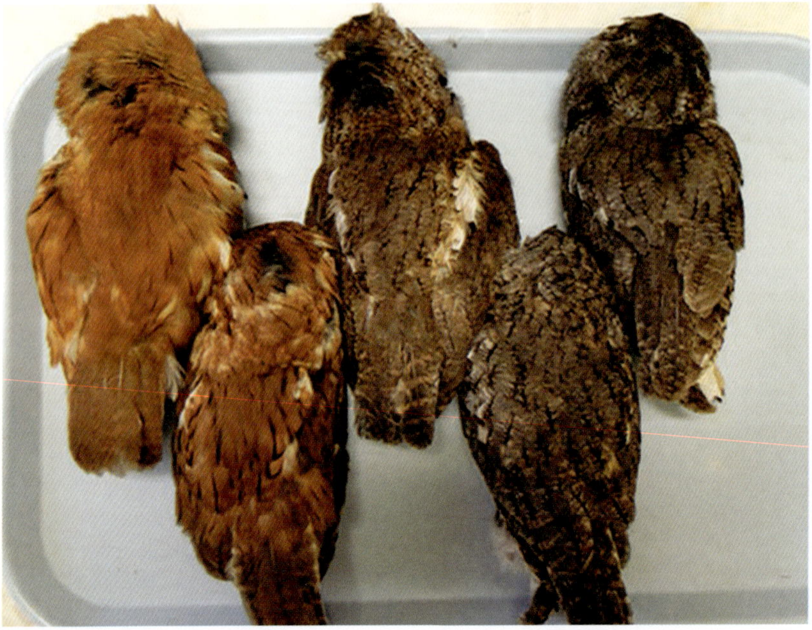

Fig. 13.12. Eastern screech owls can have multiple color phases from red to brown to gray. The color phase *cannot* be used to determine age.

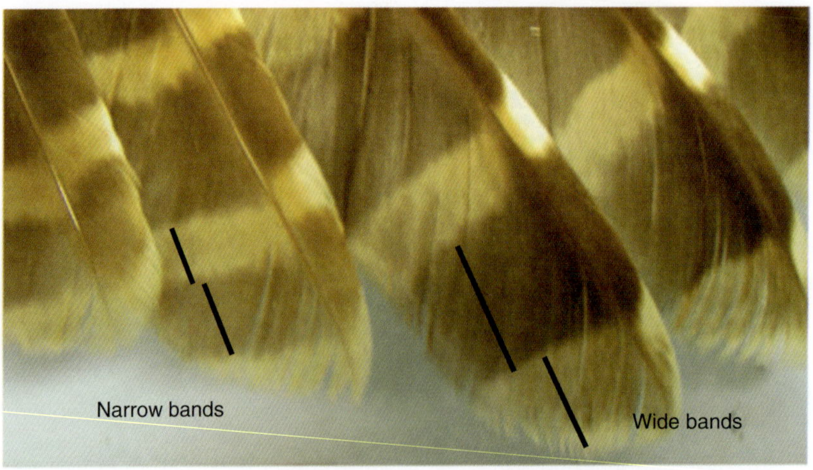

Fig. 13.13. A barred owl with juvenile and adult feathers. The two on the left are juvenile feathers with narrow bands. The two on the right are adult feathers with wide bands. The band width is indicated by the black bars.

Great-horned owl

There are no simple markings to look for but the uniformity (or lack of) in color, wear, and length of the primaries and secondaries can be used to determine age (Fig. 13.15). Sometimes the color of the feather shafts themselves can offer the best clues. Refer to Pyle for a detailed aging guide.

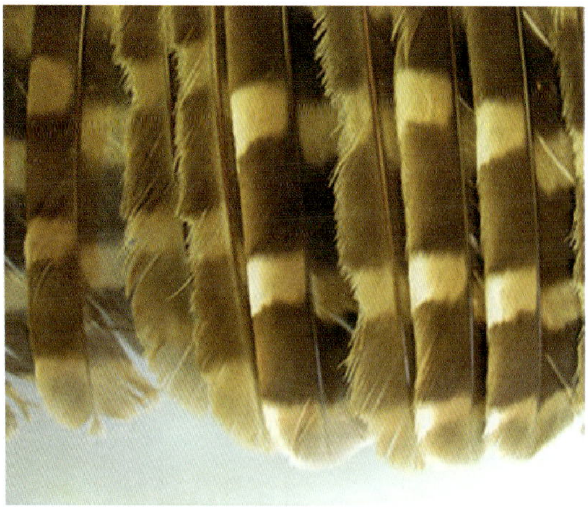

Fig. 13.14. A barred owl mixed adult feathers. Notice the wide bands and the difference in color and wear.

Barn owl

The feather markings used to age barn owls are complicated and often inconclusive. This is complicated by the fact that barn owls can have young at any time during the year. Refer to Pyle (1997a) for details. However, the uniformity (or lack of) in color, wear, and length of the primaries and secondaries can be used to determine age.

Although not an officially recognized method, the feather patterns may be used to determine the sex. Males have a very light facial disk and mostly white belly. Females have a darker facial disk and the belly is often butterscotch in color with many small spots (Fig. 13.16).

Broad-winged hawk

The adult tail has distinct dark and wide/broad white bands and the juvenile tail has bands that are less distinct. The adult tail has *two or three* visible bands. The chest pattern is also

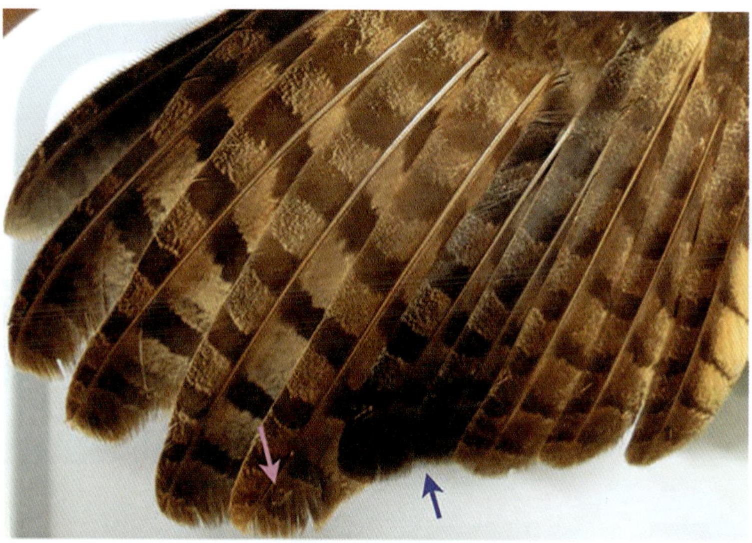

Fig. 13.15. This great-horned owl wing has multiple shades of primary flight feathers. The blue arrow is pointing to two newer, darker feathers. They are also somewhat shorter, indicating that they are still growing. The pink arrow is pointing to a feather tip which shows more wear, indicating that it is an older feather. This presentation shows evidence of multiple molts and would be aged as ASY in the spring or AHY in the fall.

quite different between juvenile and adult birds (Fig. 13.17). The iris color changes from tan-gray in the juvenile to dark brown in the adult (Fig. 13.10).

Red-shouldered hawk

The red-shouldered hawk has tail markings similar to the broad-winged hawk. The adult tail has distinct dark and narrow white bands and the

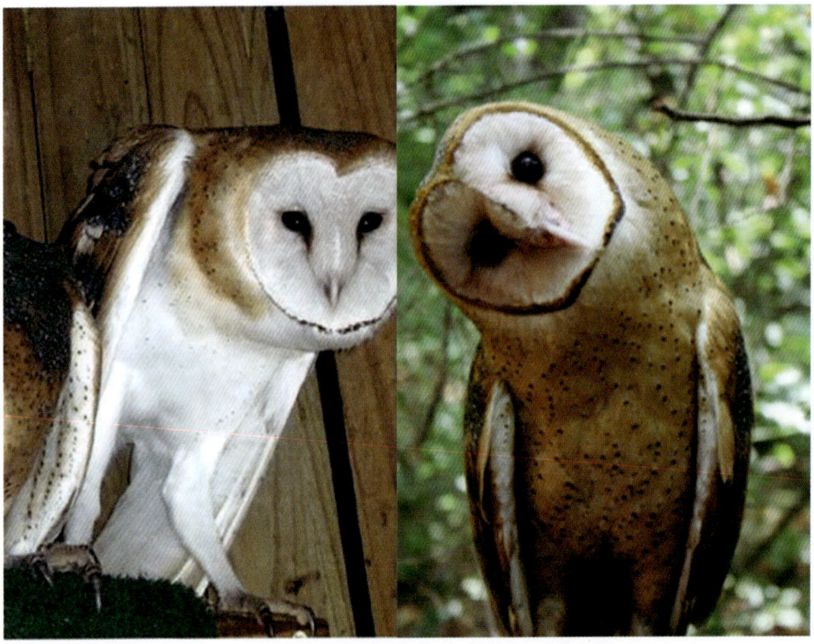

Fig. 13.16. Barn owl sex can usually be determined based on plumage. The male is on the left and the female is on the right.

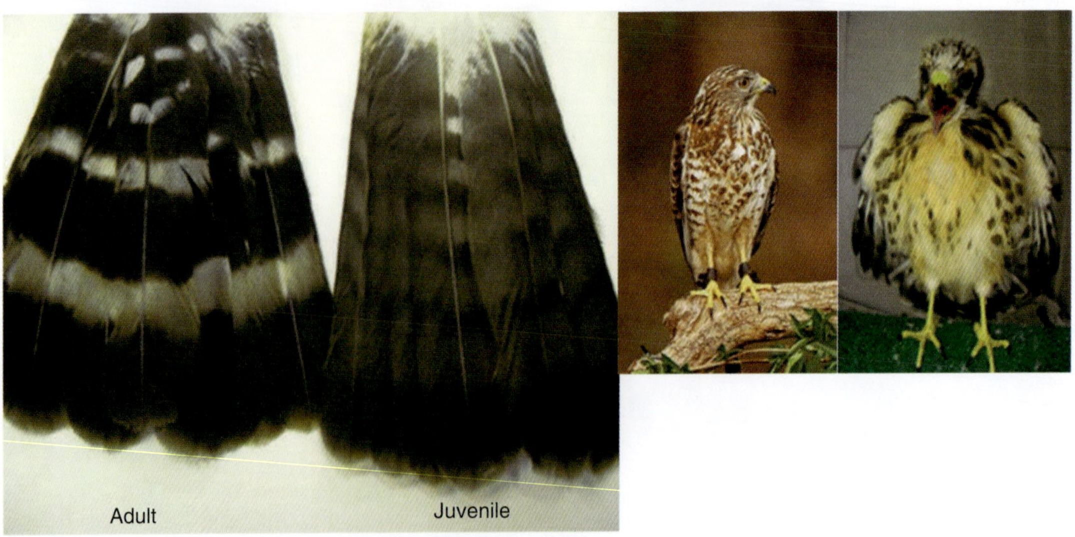

Fig. 13.17. Broad-winged hawk: the adult is on the left and the juvenile is on the right.

juvenile tail has bands that are less distinct. The adult tail has *four* or more bands (instead of *two or three* in the broad-winged hawk). Red-shouldered hawks also have colored "windows" on the dorsal side of their primaries (Fig. 13.20). The chest pattern is quite different between juvenile and adult birds (Fig. 13.18) and can vary greatly in adults as well (Fig. 13.21). The iris color changes from tan-gray in the juvenile to dark brown in the adult (Fig. 13.10).

Red-tailed hawk

Juvenile and adults have distinctly different tails (Fig. 13.22). The juvenile tail has 10–12 dark brown bands. The adult tail begins to molt to the classic rust-colored shade in the second year. The iris color changes from tan-gray in the juvenile to dark brown in the adult (Fig. 13.10). The coloration and patterns on the chest are extremely variable and cannot be used for aging purposes.

Cooper's hawk

Cooper's hawks can be easily identified by the pronounced protuberance on the plantar surface of the third digit (Fig. 13.23). Juveniles have *vertical* brown stripes or blotches on the chest and adults have brown *horizontal* bars. The feathers on the back are brown in a juvenile and gray in an adult (Fig. 13.24). The iris will change from gray in the juvenile, to yellow in HY/SY, to orange, and then to a dark ruby red in the adult (Fig. 13.25).

Sharp-shinned hawk

Similar patterns to the Cooper's hawk. Juveniles have *vertical* brown stripes or blotches on the

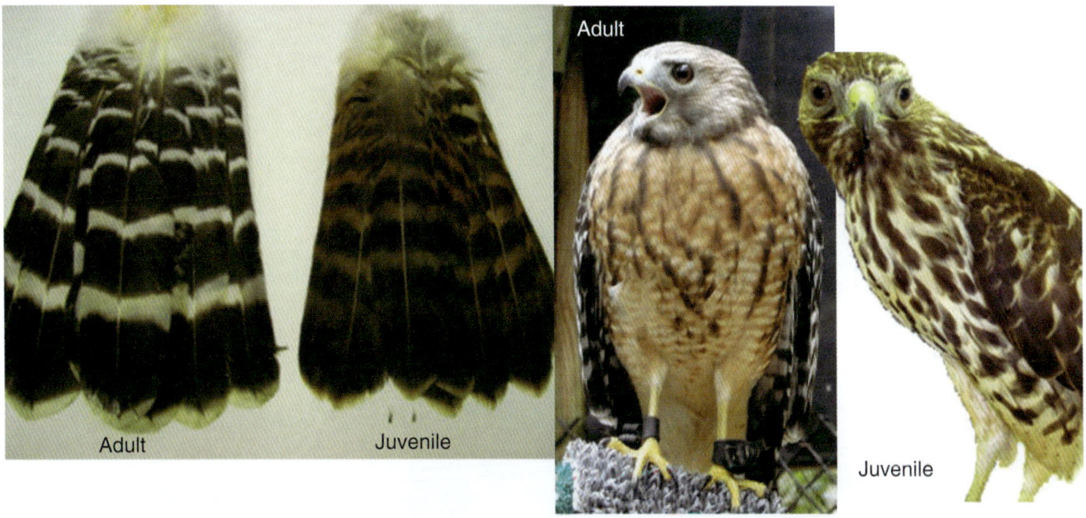

Fig. 13.18. Red-shouldered hawk: the adult is on the left and the juvenile is on the right.

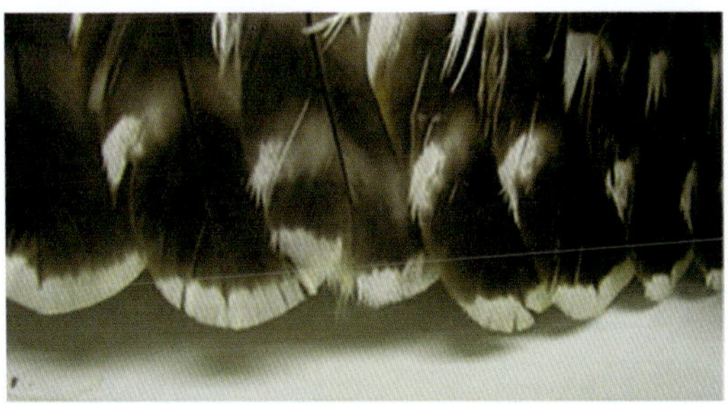

Fig. 13.19. Red-shouldered hawk adult with mixed primaries. Notice the subtle difference in length. This would indicate an age of ASY or ATY, depending on the season.

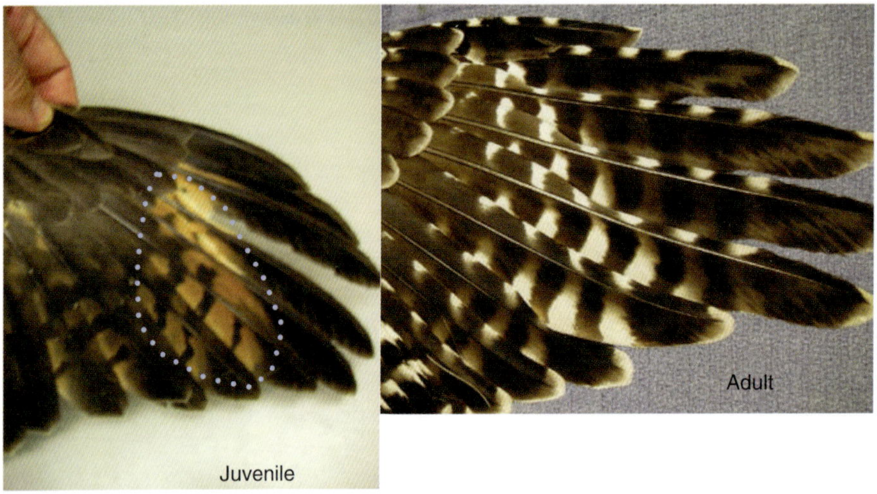

Fig. 13.20. One way to identify a red-shouldered hawk is to look for the "windows" on the dorsal side of the outer primaries. The juvenile's are an orange-gold shade while the adult's are white.

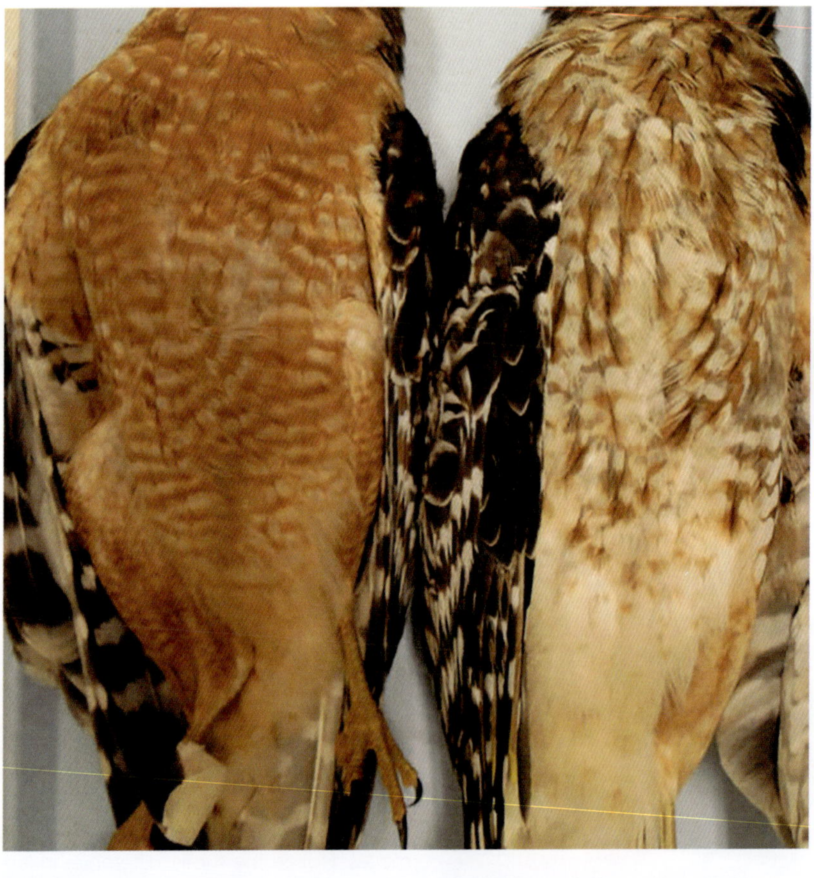

Fig. 13.21. Red-shouldered hawk adults can vary in appearance, especially on the chest.

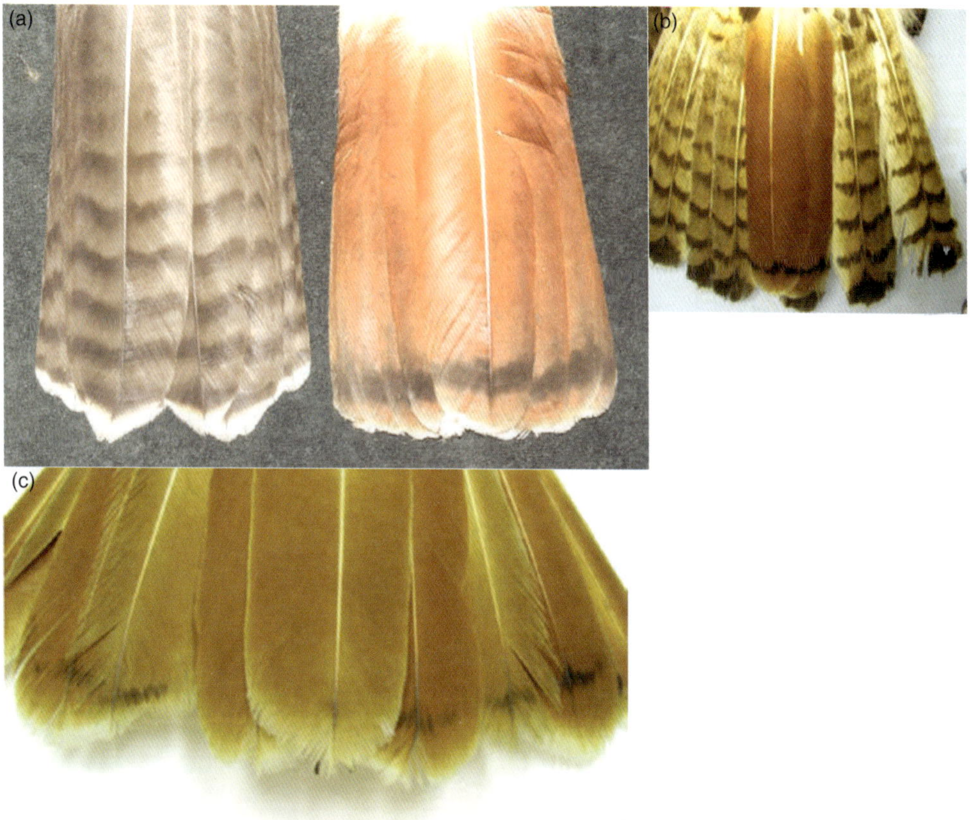

Fig. 13.22. Red-tailed hawk tail feathers. (a) Juvenile (left) and adult (right) tail feathers. (b) Mixed adult/juvenile tail. This pattern only occurs in SY birds. (c) A mixed adult tail. Notice the subtly different shades of red and the slight differences in length.

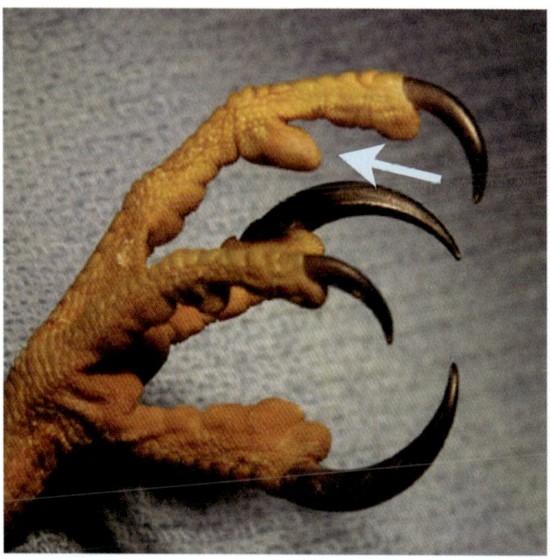

Fig. 13.23. The protuberance on the Cooper's hawk third digit.

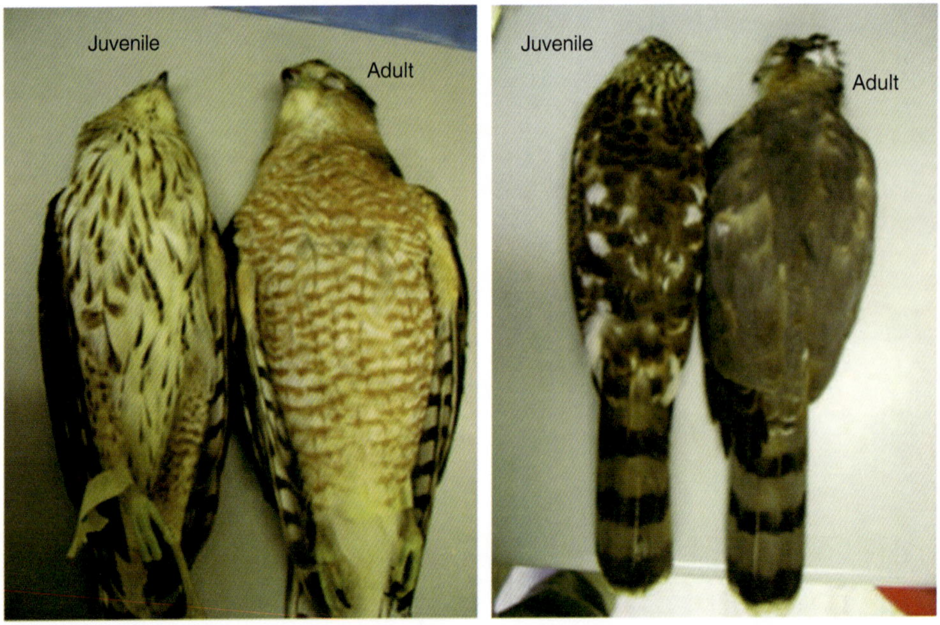

Fig. 13.24. Cooper's hawk feather patterns.

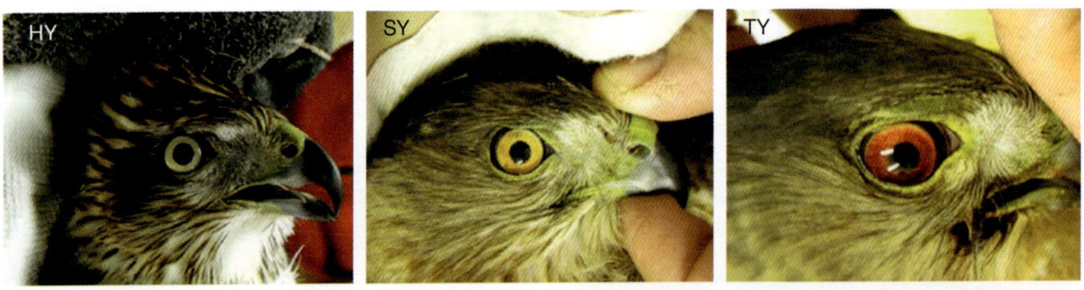

Fig. 13.25. Cooper's hawk iris color.

chest and adults have brown *horizontal* bars. Juveniles often have rufous edges on brown covert feathers on the rump. Adults have gray rump coverts without rufous edges (Fig. 13.26). The iris will change from gray/yellow in the juvenile to orange and then to a dark ruby red in the adult (Fig. 13.25).

Determining Sex in Accipiters

It can be very difficult to determine sex based on external physical traits. In general, female raptors are much larger than males and this difference is more pronounced in accipiters than in other species.

In Cooper's hawks and sharp-shinned hawks, the sex can be definitively determined based on weight and wing chord. However, these measurements cannot be used reliably in other species. The wing chord is measured from the carpus to the tip of the longest primary feather when the wing is folded up to the body in a natural position (Fig. 13.27; Table 13.3). It is important to measure the wing with the natural bow of the feathers intact since straightening or flattening them will lead to an inaccurate measurement. A ruler with a

Table 13.3. Wing chord measurements (in mm).

Species	Male	Female
Sharp-shinned hawk	<185	>185
Cooper's hawk	<247	>251

corner that can be hooked over the end of the carpal joint makes it easier to measure the wing chord accurately.

American kestrel

Aging kestrels is difficult but, as with most species, the uniformity (or lack of) in color, wear, and length of the primaries and secondaries can provide some clues. Kestrels are, however, sexually dimorphic so determination of sex is easy (Fig. 13.28).

Black vulture

The juvenile will have feathers on the upper neck and back of the head (Fig. 13.29). In the adult, the head and neck are bare (Fig. 13.32) and the skin is rough and "warty".

Turkey vulture

The juvenile has a gray head and gray/black beak (Fig. 13.30). The beak will start to turn ivory color and the face will become light red/pink during late HY, early SY (Fig. 13.31). The full adult (Fig. 13.32) will have an ivory beak and a bright red face with many light-colored "warts".

Osprey

The iris changes from orange in the juvenile to yellow in the adult. The HY bird also has light buff feather edges on the back and upper wing coverts (Fig. 13.33). Note that this species spends its second year in its southern migratory range so birds should not be seen in the north during this time.

Bald eagle

The beak is black and the head and tail are dark brown in juveniles. By approximately 5 years, the beak has turned yellow and the head and tail are white. The iris color changes from dark brown in the juvenile to yellow in the adult. These changes are gradual with intermediate stages present during the transition (Fig. 13.34).

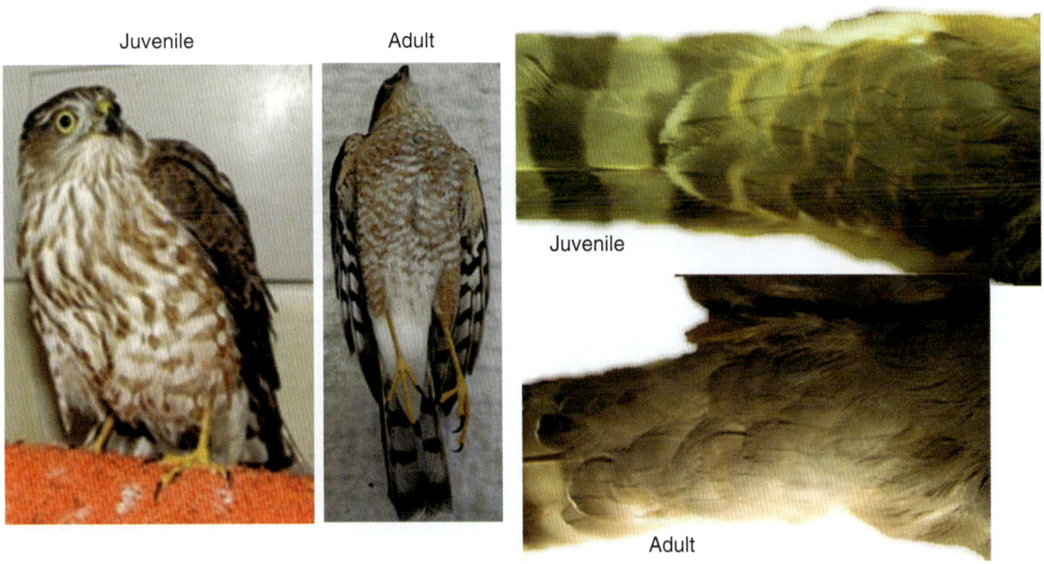

Fig. 13.26. Sharp-shinned hawk feather patterns.

Mississippi kite

The juvenile and adult have a dramatically different appearance, as shown in Fig. 13.35.

Peregrine falcon

The juvenile peregrine falcon has a tan chest with dark vertical streaks. The adult has a barred belly and legs, and the wings are a dark bluish-gray. Note that the coloration in the adult can vary quite a bit with geography (Fig. 13.36).

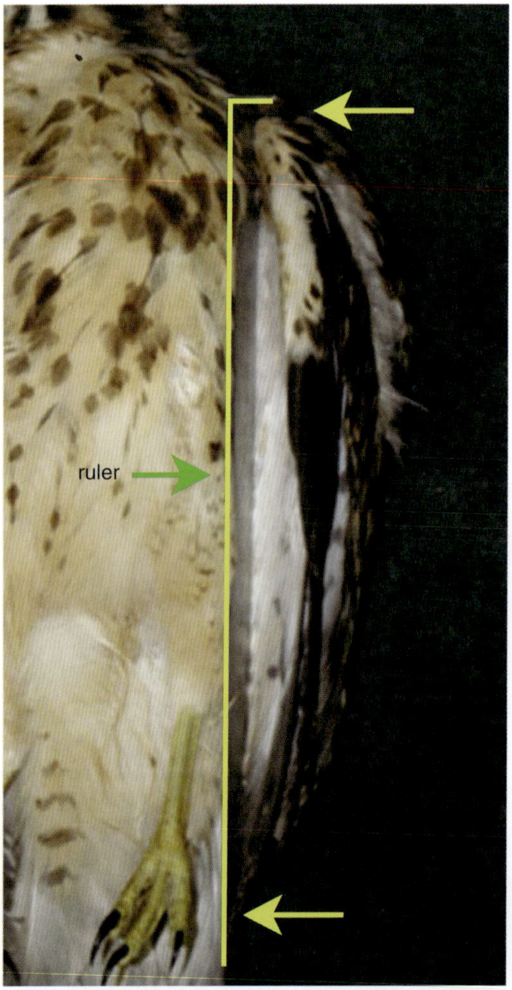

Fig. 13.27. Wing chord measurement. The yellow arrowheads indicate the extents of the wing chord. Note the normal bow of the wing is maintained while making the measurement.

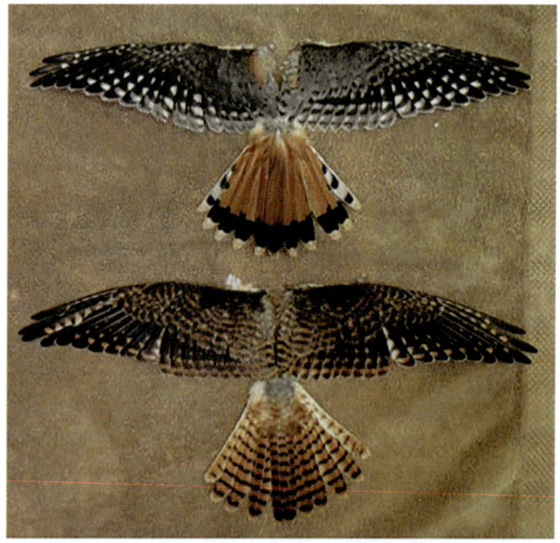

Fig. 13.28. Sexual dimorphism in American kestrels. Females (bottom) have dark brown upper wing coverts, the entire back is barred, and the tail has many stripes. Males (top) have gray upper wing coverts, the back is only partially barred, and the tail has few or no stripes.

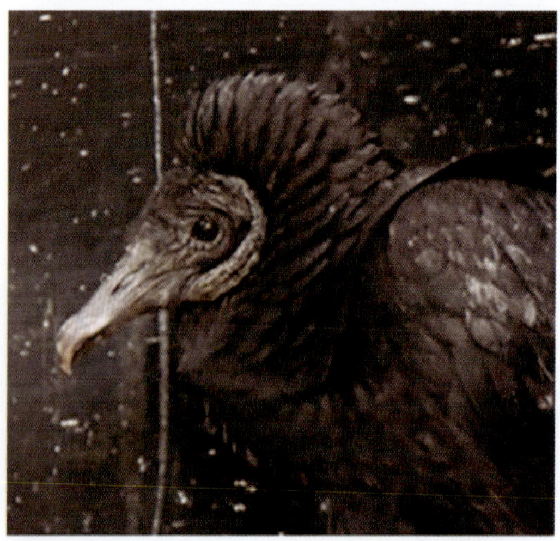

Fig. 13.29. The juvenile black vulture has feathers on the back of neck and the top of head.

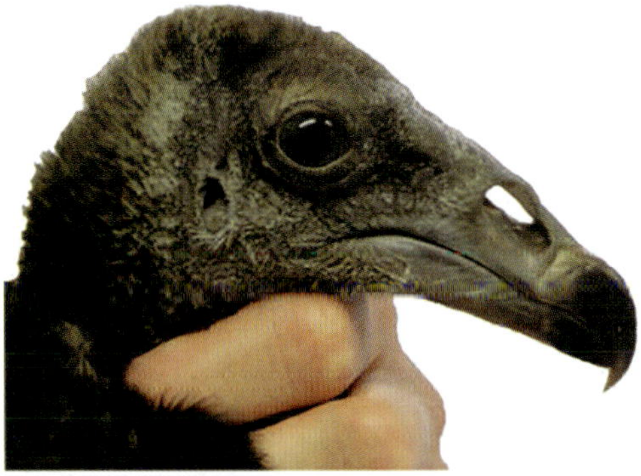

Fig. 13.30. A young HY turkey vulture has a gray head and black beak.

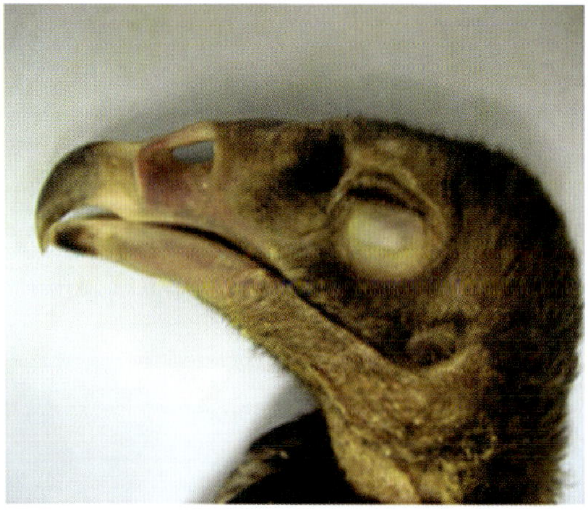

Fig. 13.31. This older HY/early SY turkey vulture is starting to get a red face and the beak is turning white.

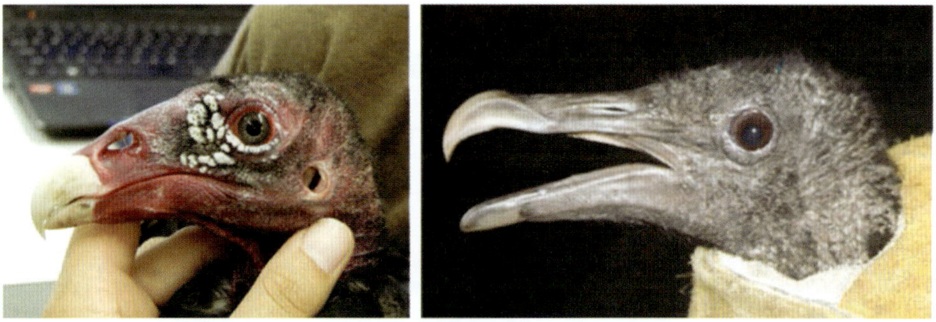

Fig. 13.32. Turkey vultures (left) have a shorter, stout beak, and large, open nares. Black vultures (right) have a longer, thinner beak, and the nares are thin slits. Note that the turkey vulture does not get the red head coloration or white beak until the second year.

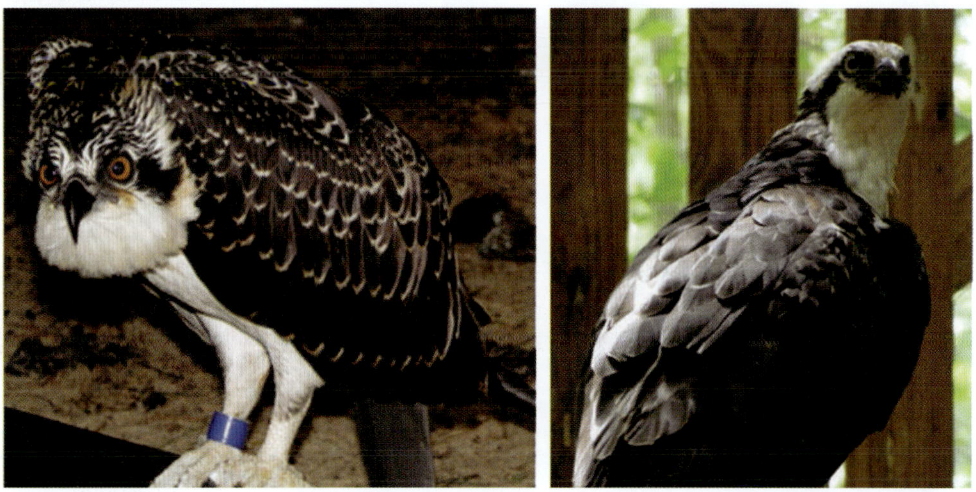

Fig. 13.33. The juvenile osprey (left) has the characteristic orange iris and light covert feather edges.

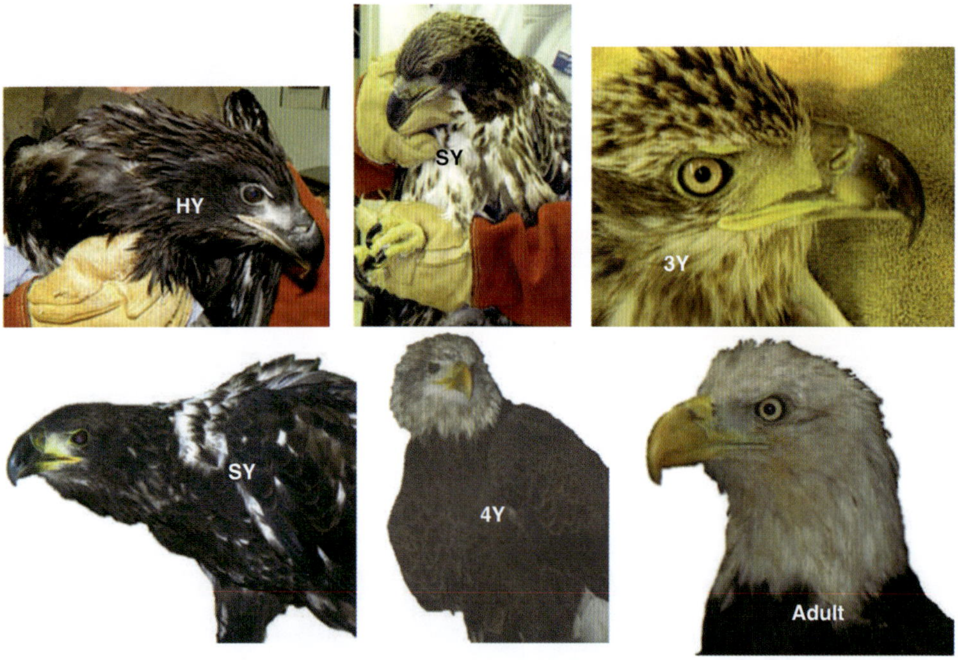

Fig. 13.34. Bald eagle. The HY and SY eagle has a black beak. The 4Y eagle has a yellow beak and a mottled white head. The mature adult has a full white head and tail. Note that it is not possible to reliably age an eagle after 5 years.

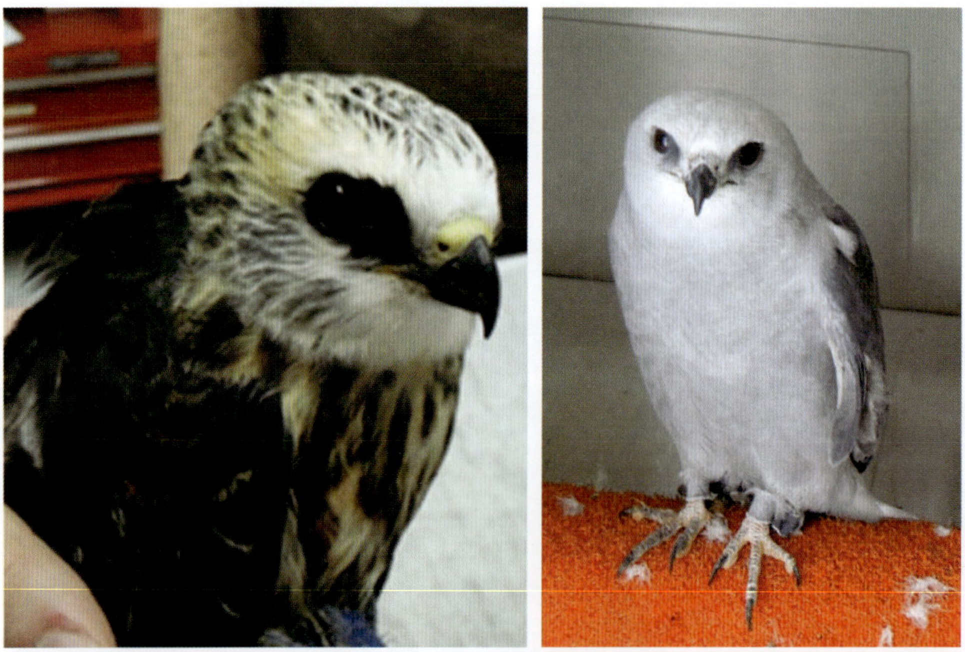

Fig. 13.35. The juvenile Mississippi kite has a tan chest with dark vertical stripes and dark wings. The adult has a light gray body, dark gray wings, and a light-colored head.

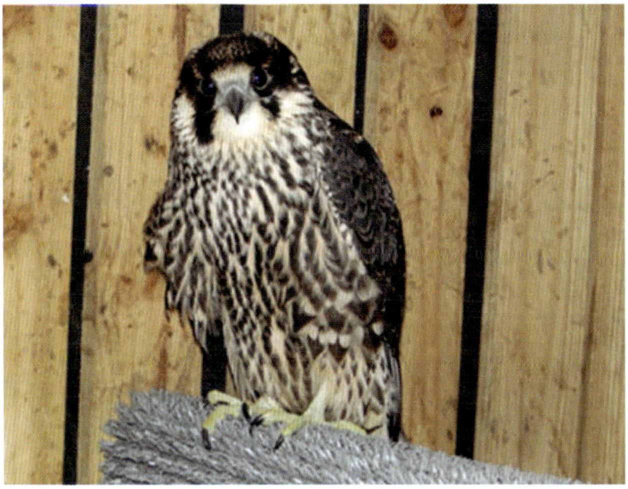

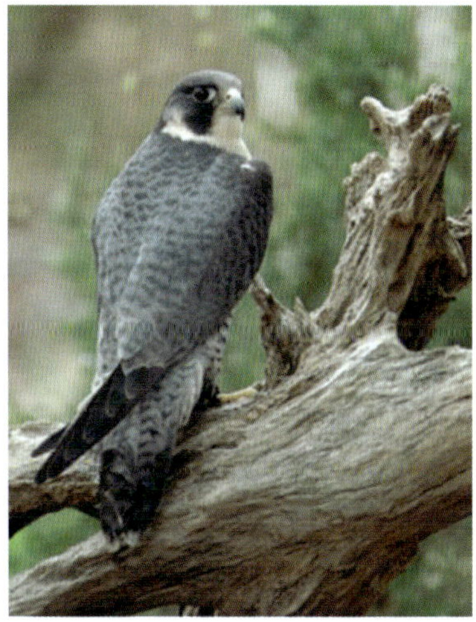

Fig. 13.36. The juvenile (left) and adult peregrine falcon.

Imping Feathers

Feather damage is a serious problem for any bird. Due to the molting cycle, it is possible that damaged feathers will not be naturally replaced during a normal molt for months or, in some cases, until the next molting season. In addition, when many feathers are broken and they do molt, there are often several blood feathers emerging at the same time. These fragile feathers are extremely vulnerable and can be re-broken before they have a chance to develop fully. Repairing or imping broken feathers is a very good option in these cases and may save months or even a year in captivity.

In order for a feather to be impable, there must be at least 1″ (2.5 cm) of intact feather shaft remaining and there should not be any longitudinal fissures in the shaft, which would severely weaken the union with the imped feather.

Supplies

The following supplies (Figs 13.37–13.39) should be available before proceeding:

- Feathers of the appropriate species, size, and age which are numbered and selected to match the broken feathers.
- Two-part, waterproof, 5-min epoxy.
- Small drill bits.
- Sharp scissors.
- 2″ × 2″ (5 cm × 5 cm) scrap paper squares.
- Feather shafts or bamboo rods to be used to splice the new feathers onto the old feather.

A large collection of feathers must be collected and stored. Specimens of each species and plumage configuration should be harvested whenever a bird dies or is euthanized. Wings are typically removed just proximal to the carpus and the tails are removed proximal to the base of the feather shafts. They are allowed to dry with the feathers fully spread out so that selecting and removing individual feathers is easy. Collecting feathers this way ensures they stay together in a group with the correct numbering and order preserved. Note that a special permit may be required to collect feathers for imping.

Technique

This procedure requires a good deal of time and firm restraint. To facilitate the process, light general anesthesia with isoflurane is helpful.

The technique is as follows:

- For each feather, select an appropriate match. It should be the correct size, plumage/age, curvature, and number. If the exact feather

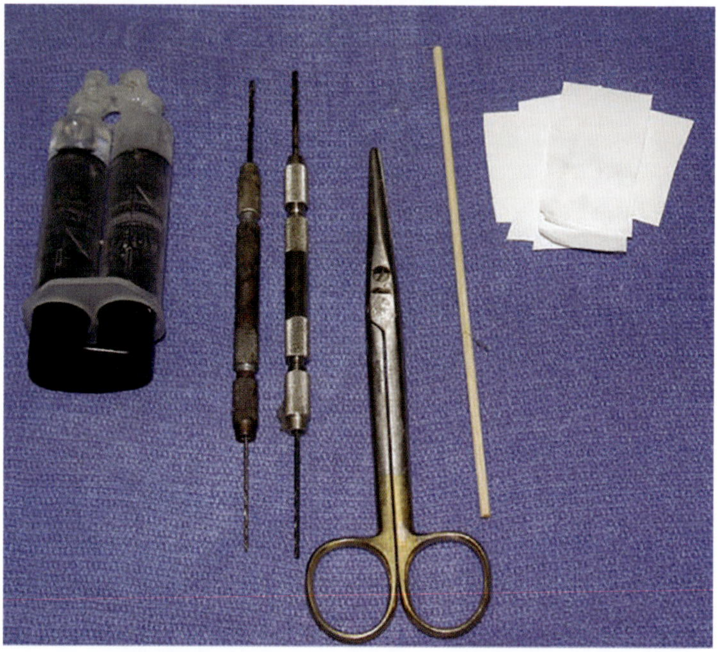

Fig. 13.37. Imping supplies needed include waterproof, 5-min epoxy, various sized drill bits, and sharp scissors.

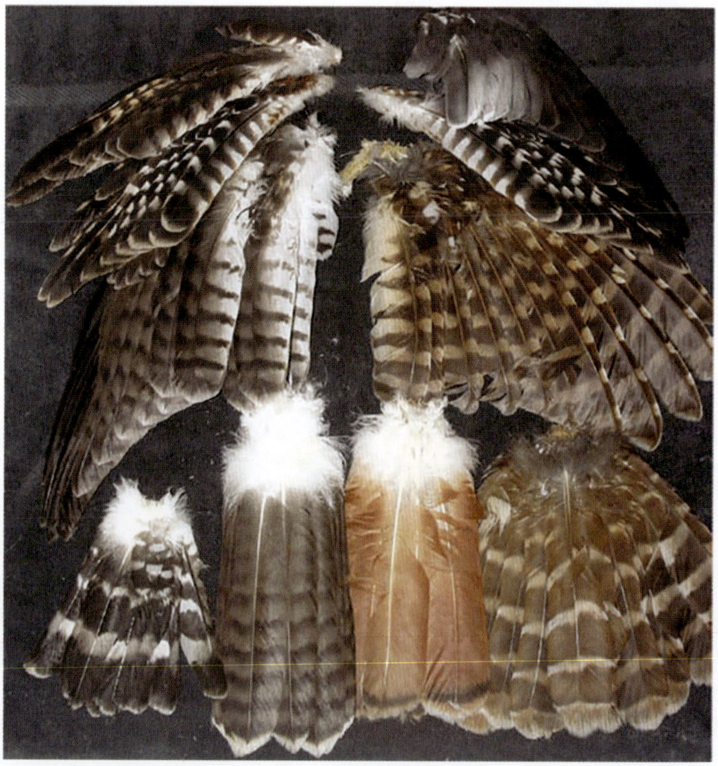

Fig. 13.38. Feathers are harvested as a group to preserve the ordering.

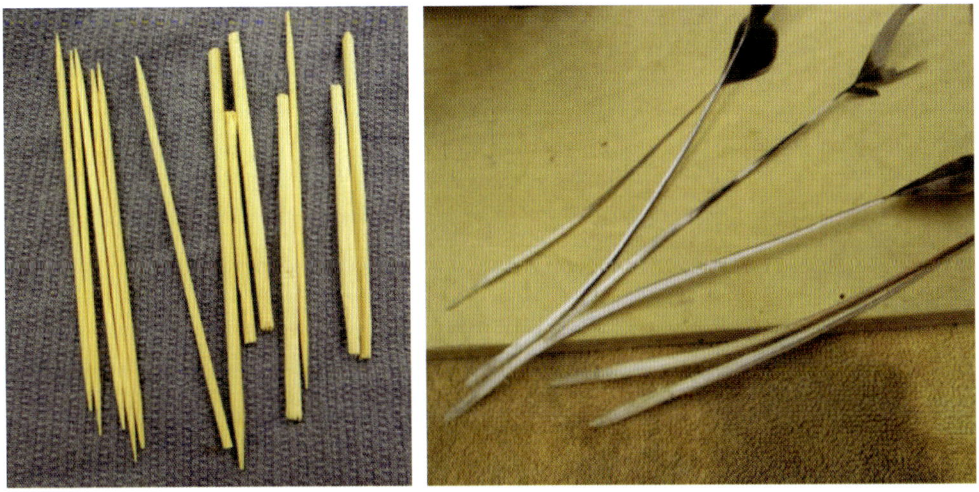

Fig. 13.39. Imping needles can be made with bamboo or with actual feather shafts (vanes already removed).

number is not available, you can sometimes use an adjacent feather.

- Trim the broken feather with sharp scissors to get a clean edge that is perpendicular to the shaft and is free from longitudinal fissures.
- With a drill bit, remove the debris from the center of the shaft.
- Hold the replacement feather up to the broken feather and cut it to the proper length.
- Remove the debris from the center of the shaft of the new feather.
- Create an "imping needle" to be used to splice the two feathers together (Figs 13.39 and 13.40):
    - Using the feather shaft from another feather works well since it already has the natural curvature and is lightweight, strong, and flexible.
    - Cut it from a section of feather that is distal, and therefore thinner, than the feathers to be spliced.
    - Remove all the feather vanes and whittle or trim it as needed so it fits snugly in both cut feather ends but be careful to not weaken the shaft when trimming. It should be long enough so that it extends approximately 1″ (2.5 cm) into the shafts of both feathers. Note that it is best to prepare several different-sized needles ahead of time and have them all ready to go before starting the process.
    - Small pieces of bamboo can also be used to form imping needles. Bamboo may be stronger than an actual feather but it takes time to whittle it down to the correct size.
- Dry-fit the new feather to the old using the newly prepared imping needle (Fig. 13.41).
- Prepare a new feather and needle for all other feathers to be imped. Make sure to keep them properly labeled since it is very important that each ends up in the correct location.
- Protect each feather by placing a small slip of paper around the shaft. This prevents the glue from spreading to the adjacent shafts. Once glue is applied, the paper should be shifted periodically to prevent adhesion to the feathers (Fig. 13.42).
- Mix the two-part epoxy to activate it.
- Glue each imping needle into the broken shaft and glue each new feather onto the needle. Be very careful to adjust the feather so that the length, curvature, and rotation of each feather match the adjacent feathers.
- Remember to periodically shift the position of the slips of paper to keep them from becoming attached to the feather shafts.
- Remove any excess glue and allow to dry.
- All done (Fig. 13.43)!

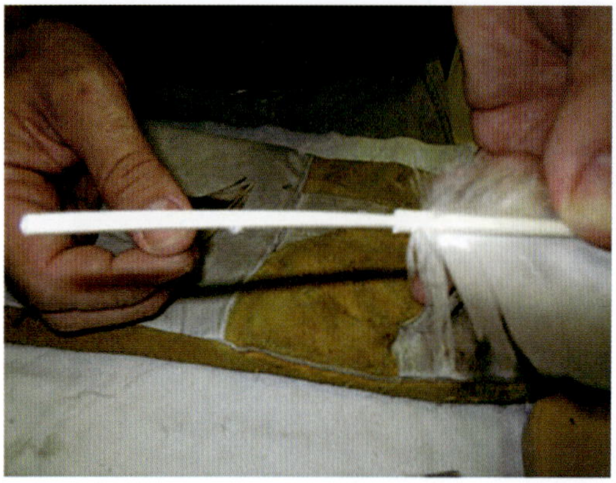

Fig. 13.40. The imping needle is trimmed and adjusted for a snug fit.

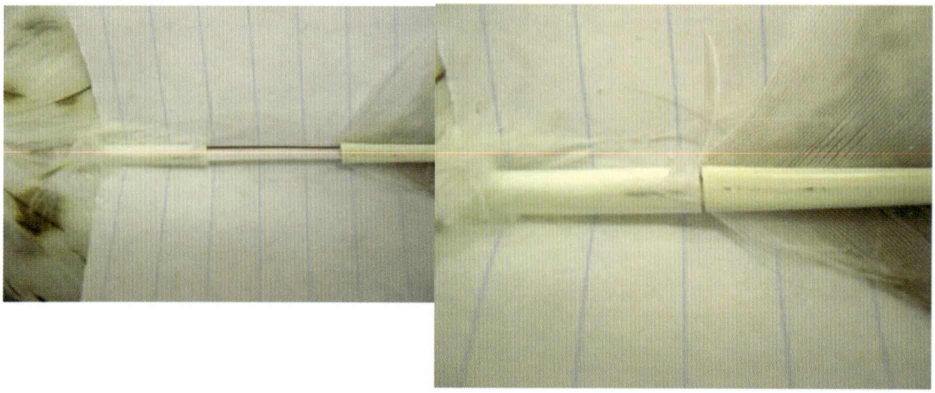

Fig. 13.41. The feathers are dry-fit together and aligned before gluing with epoxy.

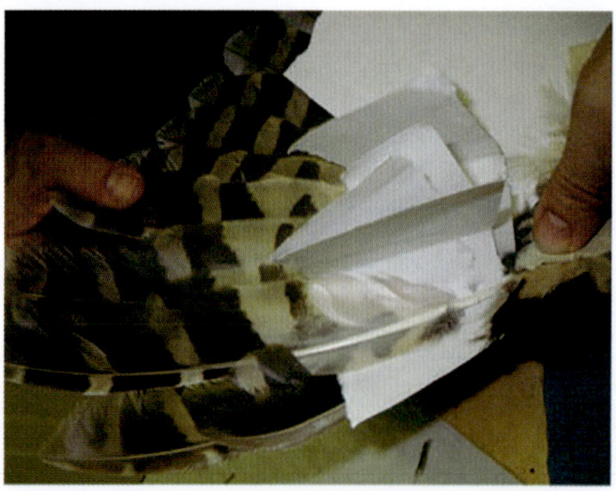

Fig. 13.42. A whole set of feathers are glued at once. Notice how the paper squares keep the epoxy from spreading onto adjacent feathers.

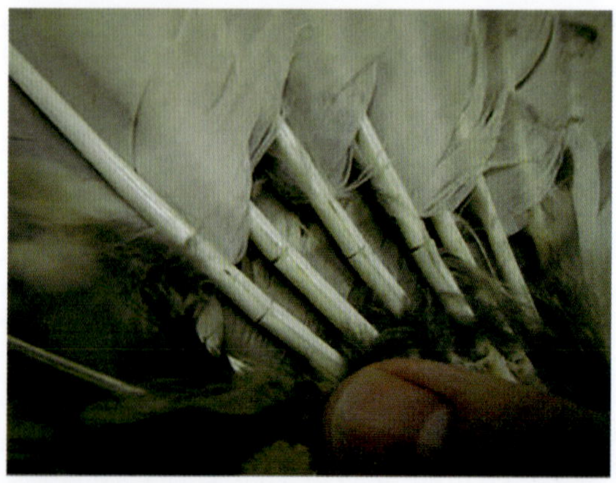

Fig. 13.43. All done! You can just barely see where the feathers are spliced together. A clean splice with no gaps or bumps is important, otherwise the bird may try to preen off the new feather.

It is best to observe the bird for 24 h to be sure the epoxy has bonded well. Note that a feather can usually only be imped once since it is very difficult or impossible to remove and then replace an imping needle from within a feather shaft after it has been glued in place. Because of this, the bird should be released quickly to avoid damaging the newly repaired feathers. Also, avoid placing these birds in a box for transport to a release site as the imped feathers can be easily broken. Typically, these birds should be carried by hand to a local site and released.

Bibliography

Arent, L. (2007) *Raptors in Captivity: Guidelines for Care and Management*. Hancock House Publishing, Surrey, BC, Canada.

The Birds of North America. Numbers 1 (1992), 52 (1993), 75 (1993), 107 (1994), 683 (2002). The Academy of Natural Sciences of Philadelphia, Philadelphia, PA, USA.

Johnsgard, P.A. (1988) *North American Owls: Biology and Natural History*. Smithsonian Institution Press, Washington, DC, USA.

Johnsgard, P.A. (1990) *Hawks, Eagles & Falcons of North America*. Smithsonian Institution Press, Washington, DC, USA.

Pyle, P. (1997a) *Flight-Feather Molt Patterns and Age in North American Owls*. American Birding Association, Colorado Springs, CO, USA.

Pyle, P. (1997b) *Identification Guide to North American Birds. Parts 1 & 2*. Slate Creek Press, Point Reyes, CA, USA.

Sibley, D.A. (2000) *The Sibley Guide to Birds*. Alfred A. Knopf, Inc., New York, NY, USA.

Sibley, D.A. (2001) *The Sibley Guide to Bird Life & Behavior*. Alfred A. Knopf, Inc., New York, NY, USA.

14 Clinical Pathology

Learning Objectives

1. What are normal values?
2. How to read a blood smear.
3. What do various abnormalities mean?

Hematology and the Complete Blood Count

Indications for a CBC

The complete blood count (CBC) is a valuable tool in avian medicine, can be run in-house with little cost, and the results are available in minutes. A CBC is useful:

- As part of a minimum database.
- To screen for disease.
- To monitor treatment.

PCV and TS

Packed cell volume (PCV) in a healthy bird is typically 40–50%. Dehydration can increase this value by 10 percentage points. Anemia and a low PCV commonly occur secondary to chronic disease and emaciation. Blood loss as a cause of anemia is very rare.

> **Raptor Tip**
>
> Normal PCV: 40–50%.
> Normal TS: 2.5–4.5 g/dl.

Total solids (TS) is measured on a refractometer. The typical range is from 2.5 to 4.5 g/dl in a healthy bird (much lower than the typical mammal). TS is increased by dehydration or inflammation and decreased for many reasons, but emaciation is the most common cause of hypoproteinemia in raptors.

Cell types

The standard cell types are present in birds, but there are some avian-specific differences which must be understood (Table 14.1). The most important difference is that every cell type, including erythrocytes and thrombocytes, is nucleated. The presence of nucleated cells makes reading a slide difficult and rules out the use of automated cell-counting systems.

In general, each cell type has a typical appearance. However, there are many commonly seen variations that must be recognized to accurately interpret a blood smear. Refer to Ritchie *et al.* (1994) for some great pictures of the developmental stages of all the cell lines.

Erythrocytes

The erythrocyte cell line follows a progression from the immature rubriblast and rubricyte to intermediate forms and finally develops into the typical mature oval RBC (Fig. 14.1). The level of immaturity or polychromasia, which roughly corresponds to the level of regenerative response (Fig. 14.2), can be measured by the polychromatophilic index (PI). The PI is subjective and ranges from 1 to 5 (Table 14.2).

The avian RBC is larger than the mammalian counterpart and the size ranges from 10 × 6 μm to 15 × 10 μm.

Table 14.1. Avian hematology cell types.

Cell	Function	Typical appearance
Erythrocyte	Oxygen transport	Elliptical, pinkish-orange cytoplasm with centrally located nucleus
Heterophil	Function similar to mammalian neutrophil. Typically the most common cell type in diurnal birds	Segmented nucleus. Cytoplasm packed with rod-shaped granules
Eosinophil	Function unclear. May be related to parasitic infections	Segmented nucleus. Cytoplasm packed with round/spherical granules
Lymphocyte	Immune response to antigenic stimulation	Mononuclear, dark, eccentric nucleus, small crescent of cytoplasm
Monocyte	Response to chronic, granulomatous infections as well as tissue trauma and wounds	Large, mononuclear, silver-gray cytoplasm with large bean-shaped nucleus
Thrombocyte	Clotting/hemostasis	Elliptical, dark nucleus, clear cytoplasm. May or may not be clumped
Basophil	Very rare, function unknown	Segmented nucleus. Cytoplasm packed with dark blue granules

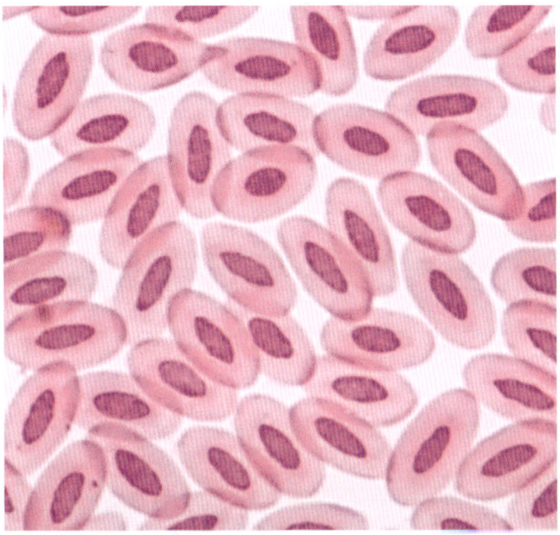

Fig. 14.1. Normal erythrocytes. Note the uniformity in size, color, and chromatin pattern. It is important to realize that rubriblasts and other immature forms can be easily mistaken for large lymphocytes and monocytes.

Raptor Tip

Elevated TS can sometimes be a much more sensitive indicator of infection than the white cell count.

Heterophils

Birds do not have neutrophils. Instead, they have heterophils, which perform a similar function (Fig. 14.3). Heterophils are usually the most common WBC type and the heterophil to lymphocyte (H:L) ratio is typically from 1.5:1 to 2:1. In owls, however, the H:L ratio can be reversed as it is not uncommon for them to have more lymphocytes than heterophils. The significance of this ratio is unclear.

The heterophil has a segmented nucleus and the cytoplasm is usually packed with rod-shaped granules. In fact, there may be so many granules that they cannot be distinguished individually. In these cases, it can be hard to tell an eosinophil with round granules from a heterophil with rod-shaped granules. The type of stain used will affect the color of the granules and this color difference can be used to help differentiate these cell types.

Atypical heterophil forms which are commonly seen include:

- Bands. These are immature forms with a less segmented, almost bean-shaped nucleus. Increased number of bands indicates a left-shift and may be the result of an overwhelming infection.
- "Degranulated". These cells have a cytoplasm filled with what look like clear vacuoles

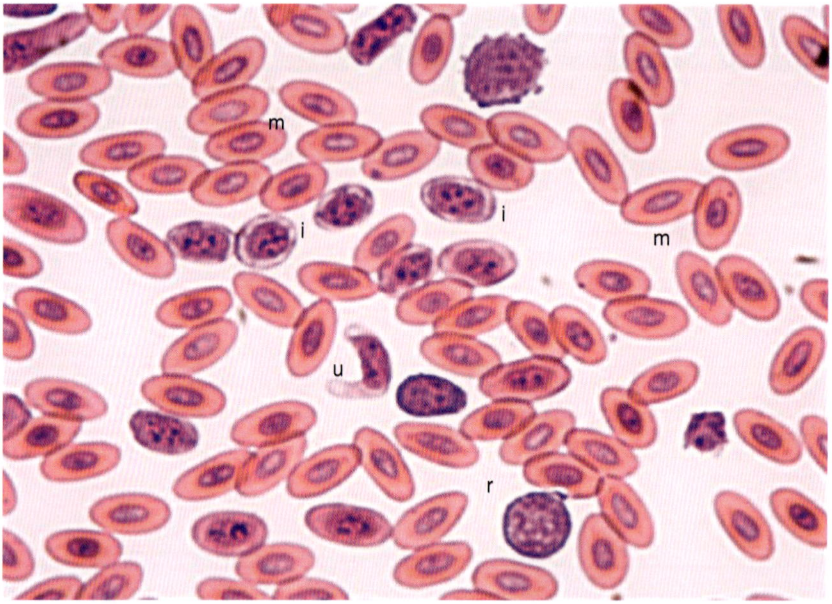

Fig. 14.2. Highly regenerative RBC population. Note the polychromasia and variations of the nuclei. Very immature forms such as rubriblasts and rubricytes (r) tend to be larger, more circular, and have intensely blue cytoplasm. Intermediate (i) forms start to become elliptical but the cytoplasm is light violet and the chromatin is clumped. Mature forms (m) have a fully elliptical shape and the cytoplasm is pink-orange in color. There are also some unusually shaped forms (u) of unknown significance in this smear.

Table 14.2. Interpretation of PI values. (Data from Pendl, 2006.)

PI	Interpretation
1	No immature forms seen. This is normal
2	At least some immature forms seen but less than 10% of cells are abnormal. This is a normal physiologic response to mild anemia
3	10–20% of cells are immature. This can be considered a normal response to anemia and is considered normal in young birds
4	20–50% of cells show immature forms. May also see some bizarre forms. This is either a severe degenerative response or potentially neoplastic
5	>50% of cells are affected. Many immature and bizarre forms. This is generally considered to be due to a neoplastic process or a severe degenerative response

(Fig. 14.4). The normal rod-shaped granules may be entirely absent. The cause for this anomaly is not known and may simply be a staining artifact. It is very important to differentiate these from toxic heterophils and to realize that this finding is not clinically significant.

- Toxics. These heterophils have an unusual appearance due to altered development in the bone marrow (Fig. 14.5). The most common changes are a foamy, vacuolated cytoplasm that may have a bluish coloration. In addition, the normal rod-shaped granules may be missing and there may be several small, dark-staining dots present in the cytoplasm. Toxic heterophils are associated with septicemia or a bacterial toxemia and can indicate a poor prognosis when present.

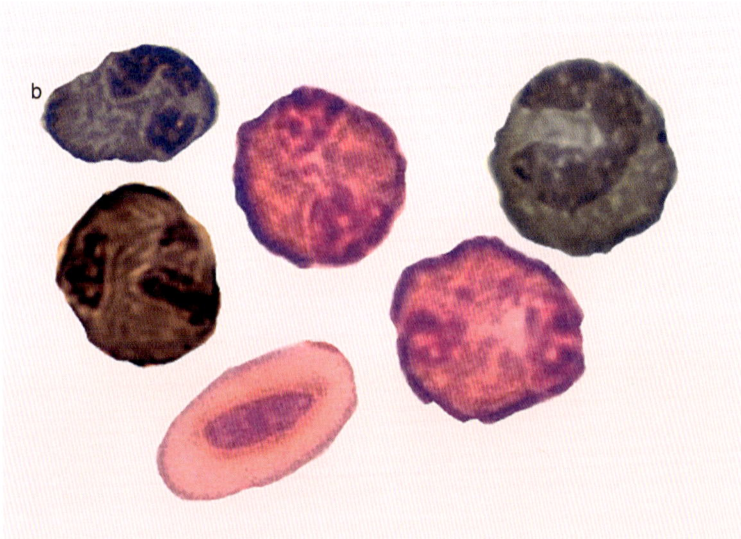

Fig. 14.3. Some examples of normal heterophils. An RBC is included for scale. The cytoplasm is so densely packed with rod-shaped granules that it can be difficult to identify individual granules. The cell marked with "b" is an immature band cell.

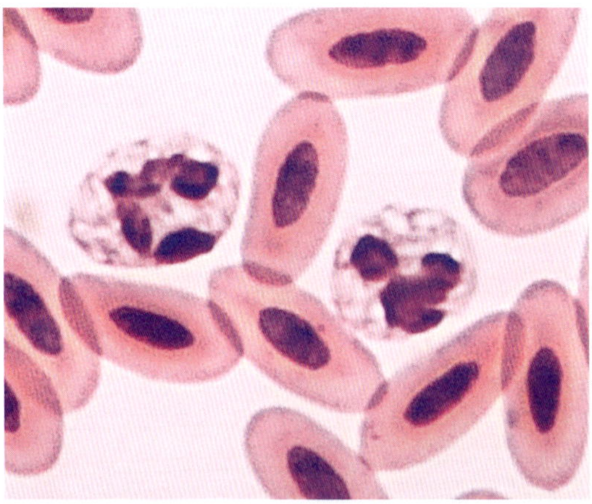

Fig. 14.4. Degranulated heterophils. Note the complete lack of rod-shaped granules and the cytoplasm is filled with what appear to be vacuoles. These are not toxic cells.

Eosinophils

The eosinophil has a segmented nucleus and the cytoplasm is packed with *round* granules. The size and color of the granules vary considerably with the species (Figs 14.6 and 14.7). When a DipQuick stain is used, hawk eosinophil granules are usually very small and bright red. In owls they are larger and can be purple or violet. The function of avian eosinophils is currently unknown.

Lymphocytes

Lymphocytes are mononuclear. They are typically round with a dark-staining, eccentrically located nucleus, and a very slim crescent of light-blue cytoplasm (Fig. 14.8). The nucleus may have a small indent on one side. Some common variations include:

- Large lymphocytes. These can have more cytoplasm and can look very much like monocytes (Fig. 14.12).
- Molded lymphocytes. These conform or mold around the surrounding RBCs (Fig. 14.9). This is an artifact formed during the staining process.
- Cytoplasmic blebs may be present projecting from the periphery. The significance of these is not clear but some references (Ritchie *et al.*, 1994) refer to them as degenerative.

Raptor Tip

Large lymphocytes can be difficult to differentiate from monocytes.

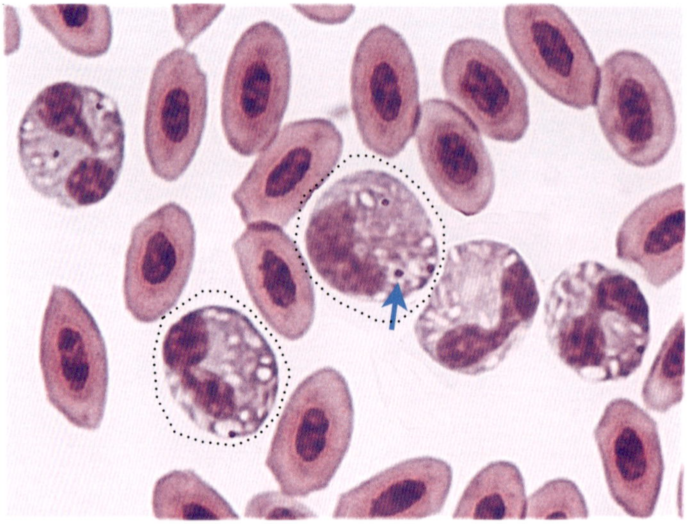

Fig. 14.5. Toxic heterophils (circled) with basophilic cytoplasm, vacuoles, and granule cores (blue arrow). The nuclei are not hyper-segmented, so these are considered toxic bands and indicate a poor prognosis. Note that the shape of the nucleus can make these look a little like monocytes.

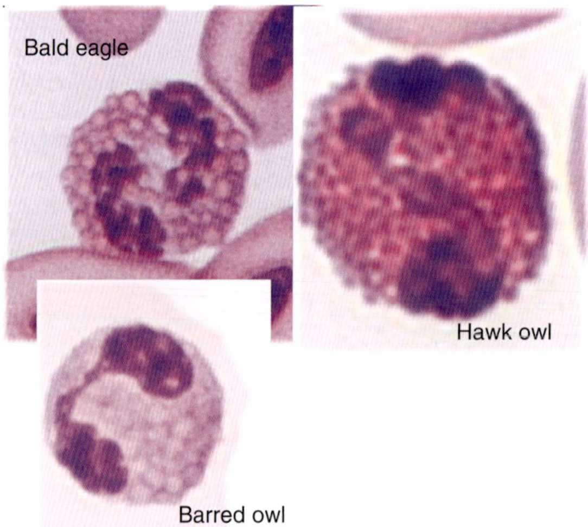

Fig. 14.6. Eosinophils.

Monocytes

Monocytes are usually big with a large amount of grayish-blue cytoplasm and a bean-shaped nucleus. Monocytes are variable in size and shape and can be very difficult to differentiate from a large lymphocyte. The classic monocyte (Fig. 14.10) has a "C-" or bean-shaped nucleus, but the size and shape of the nucleus is also highly variable (Figs 14.11 and 14.12). Monocytes are often associated with tissue trauma and chronic granulomatous infections such as Aspergillosis and *Mycobacterium*.

Thrombocytes

Thrombocytes may or may not be clumped. The actual shape can vary depending on the species, but they are typically elliptical with a dark nucleus

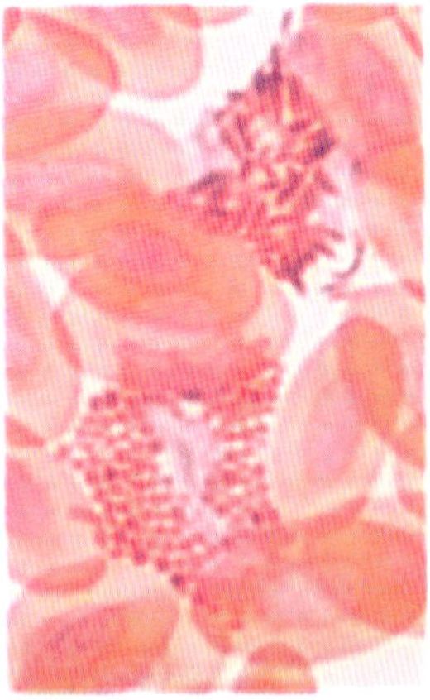

Fig. 14.7. Comparison of heterophil rod granules and eosinophil round granules.

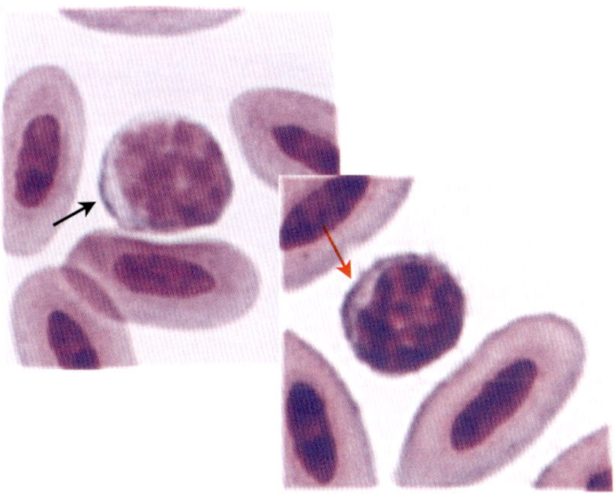

Fig. 14.8. Lymphocytes. Typical small lymphocytes with a thin crescent of light-blue cytoplasm (black arrow). Some can also have a small notch in the nucleus (red arrow).

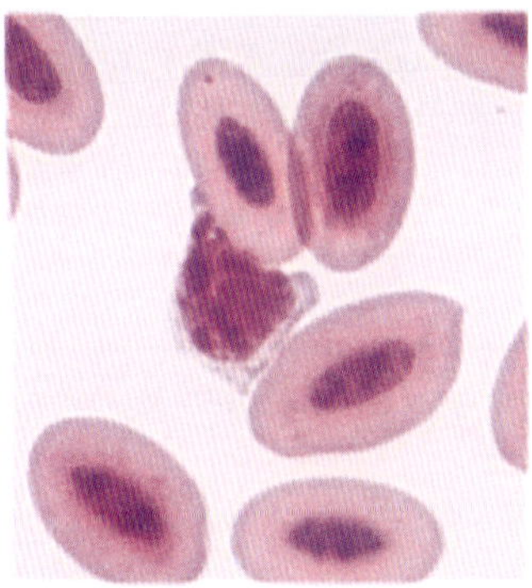

Fig. 14.9. Molded lymphocytes wrap around adjacent RBCs.

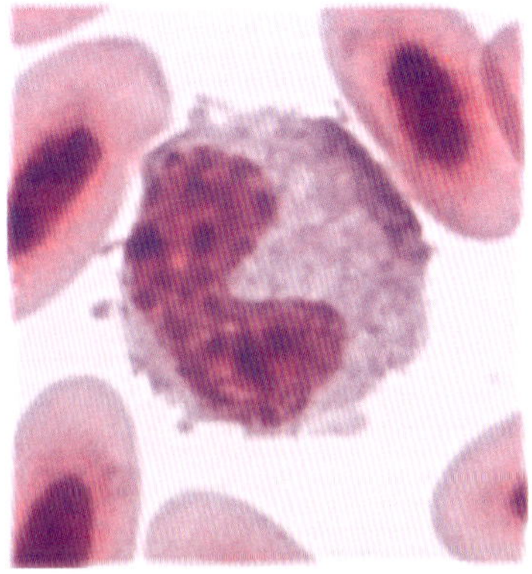

Fig. 14.10. A classic monocyte with the bean-shaped nucleus.

and clear cytoplasm (Fig. 14.13a). The less-elliptical forms (Fig. 14.13b) can be easily confused with small lymphocytes.

Hemoparasites

Refer to Chapter 6 for a complete description.

Making a smear

Reading a CBC requires that a good-quality blood smear be made so that there are areas with a thin monolayer of cells. To make a smear:

- Collect your sample with or without anticoagulant preloaded into the syringe. It is best to use a 25-gauge needle on a 1 ml syringe. Using a smaller needle can result in ruptured or damaged cells and a poor-quality smear (Fig. 14.14).
- Immediately place a small drop on the end of the slide.
- Place another slide at a 45° angle against the original slide.
- With very little pressure, pull it back to the blood drop.
- Allow the blood to spread out along the edge of the second slide.
- Again, with very little pressure, push the slide away and off the edge of the original slide. This should create a uniform, feathered edge (Figs 14.15 and 14.16).
- Label the slide with the patient ID, species, and date.

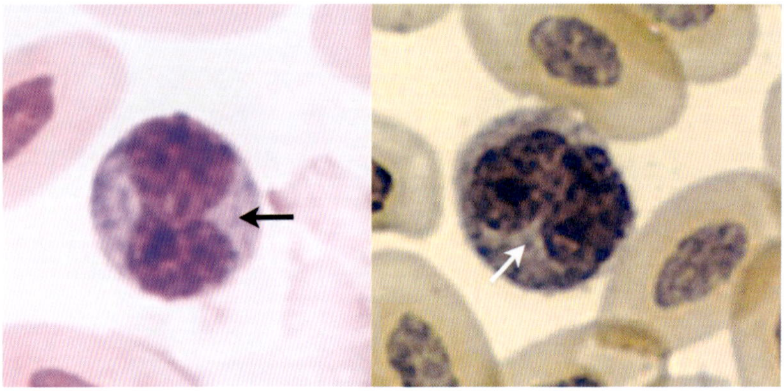

Fig. 14.11. Two monocytes with dumbbell or heart-shaped nuclei. Notice that the small notches (arrows) make these cells look like lymphocytes (Fig. 14.8) but the large amount of cytoplasm and their larger size indicate that these are monocytes.

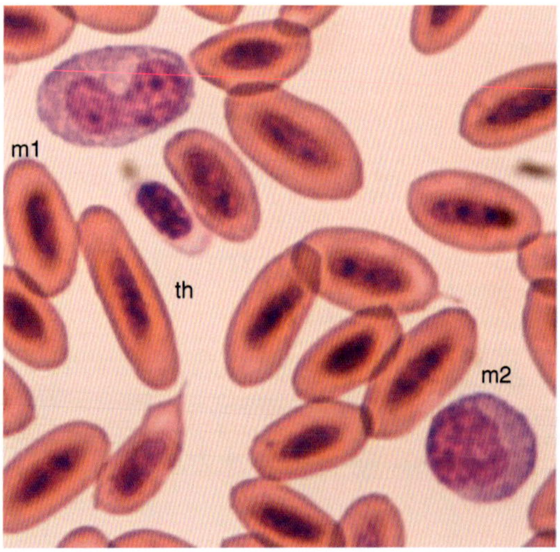

Fig. 14.12. A typical monocyte (m1) and another cell (m2) that is probably a monocyte but could easily be confused with a large lymphocyte. There is also a thrombocyte (th) present.

- Air dry and stain with a standard DipQuick stain (Fig. 14.17).

Determining an estimated CBC

Since all avian blood cells are nucleated, automated cell-counting machines will not work and the determination remains a manual process. However, with a little practice, a clinically relevant cell count and differential can be completed in under 5 min. To perform a CBC:

- Find a suitable monolayer area in the feathered edge by scanning around with the 10× objective (Fig. 14.18).
- Switch to 40× and count the number of white cells in 12 fields. Drop the high and low values and average the remaining ten. It is important to count fields from various parts of the slide and not concentrate on any one area.
- Multiply the average value by *2000*. This is your estimated total WBC count.
- Adjust the total count for the PCV. The formula is:

Adjusted count = Unadjusted count × PCV/45

- Switch to the 100× oil objective.
- Use a cell counter (Fig. 14.19) and count 100 WBCs to determine the differential. You should count four percentages (one each for heterophils, lymphocytes, eosinophils, and monocytes). Basophils are so rare that they are usually not counted.

Example 14.1

The estimated count is 20,000 and the PCV is 35.

Adjusted count = 20,000 × 35/45 = 15,500.

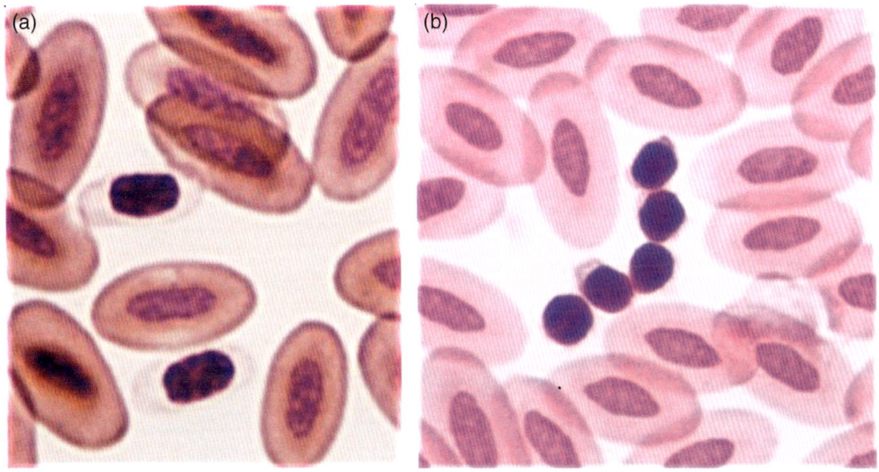

Fig. 14.13. Thrombocyte morphology varies between species. Some are more elliptical or elongated (a) and some are very round and almost look like small lymphocytes (b).

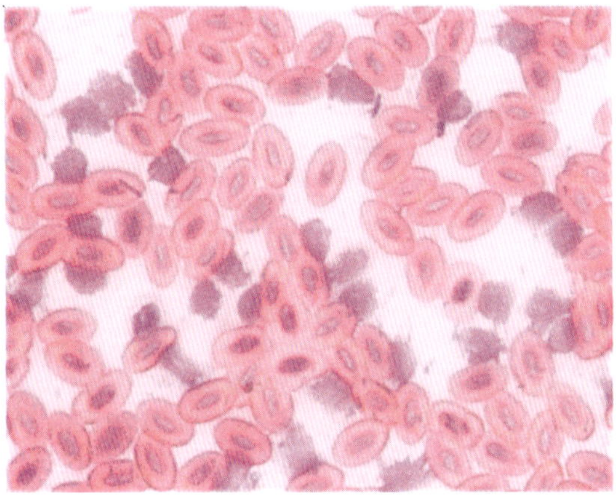

Fig. 14.14. A slide with too many smudged cells is not very useful. Smudged cells are caused by applying too much pressure when making your smear or by using too much suction when drawing the blood sample.

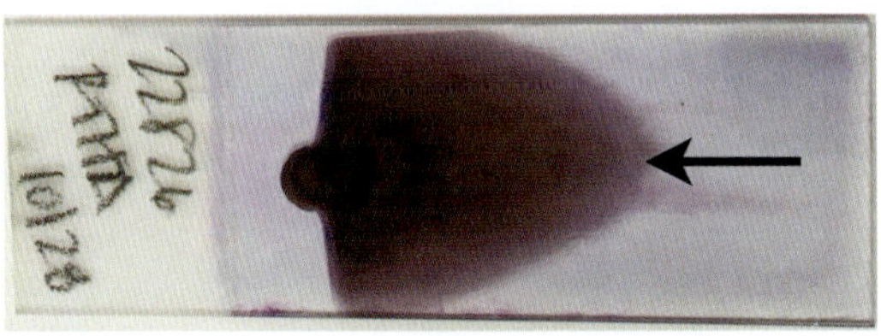

Fig. 14.15. A blood smear with a good feathered edge (arrow).

It is also important to get an estimate of the average number of thrombocytes per 100× field and to evaluate the appearance of the RBCs to determine the PI (Table 14.2). Also remember to look for hemoparasites.

Quick identification key

Most cells are relatively easy to identify using the keys in Fig. 14.20. However, there are some cells which fall into a "gray area" and are very difficult to differentiate with certainty. The following cases may be especially difficult:

- Large lymphocytes and monocytes with a round nucleus.
- Thrombocytes of certain species are more round than elliptical and can look like small lymphocytes. In general, thrombocytes tend to clump together and should always have some clear cytoplasm.
- Immature thrombocytes can have an eccentrically placed nucleus and can look like a small lymphocyte. They can still be differentiated since their cytoplasm is generally foamy and clear and lacks the bluish-gray color of a lymphocyte.
- Eosinophils and heterophils with tightly packed granules can be hard to differentiate from one another.
- Differentiating a "degranulated" heterophil (Fig. 14.4) from a "toxic" heterophil (Fig. 14.5) can be difficult. In general, look for the characteristic

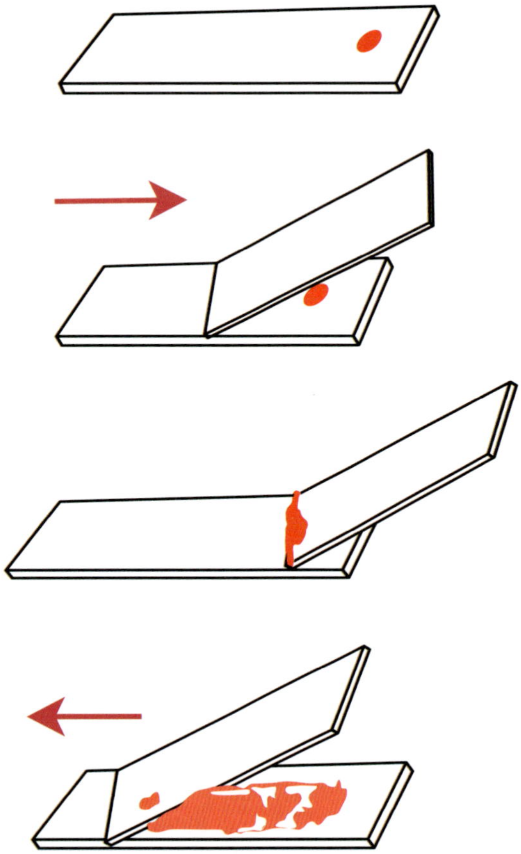

Fig. 14.16. Making a blood smear. Pull the slide toward the blood drop, then push the slide away.

blue cytoplasm, dark granules, and randomly placed vacuoles that are commonly seen in a toxic cell.

Normal values and interpretation

A review of the literature will reveal that so-called "normal" white cell count ranges and cell line percentages are not well defined for most raptor species. The published ranges for many species are wide and can vary by a factor of 2 or 3, and sometimes even more. In addition, the stressful conditions that most raptors are undoubtedly subjected to in a rehabilitation setting must have a significant effect on the white cell count.

For these reasons, it is difficult to clearly define what a normal white cell count is. However, here are some generalities which may be useful:

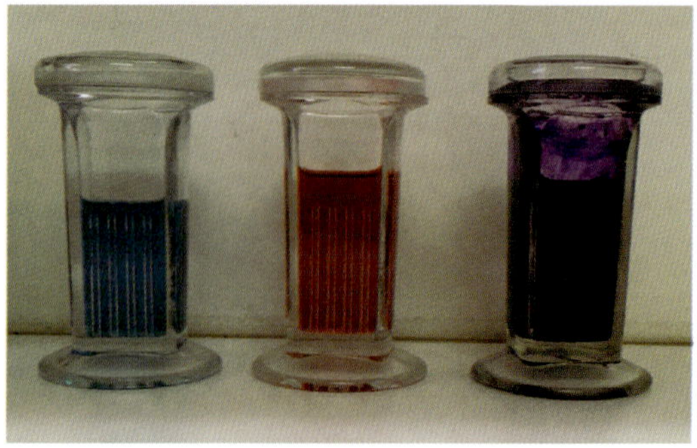

Fig. 14.17. Rapid differential stain kits (i.e. DipQuick) are quick and easy to use and they have good staining characteristics for hematology. From left to right: #1 is the fixative, #2 is the red stain, and #3 is the blue counterstain.

- A typical "normal" WBC count ranges from 8000 to 20,000.
- The stress response is not well understood in birds and can vary markedly with species. However, a leukocytosis/heterophilia is not uncommon and can easily lead to a total count of 25,000–30,000.
- Some species do not follow this general rule:
  - Normal great-horned owls routinely have WBC counts ranging from 20,000 to 30,000.
  - Falcons such as merlins routinely have very low total counts in the range of 2000–4000.
  - Vultures also seem to generate very high white counts (>65,000 is not uncommon).
- High or increasing monocyte counts are always a concern. An absolute monocyte count greater than 1500 in a juvenile red-tailed hawk is clinically significant and should alert you to the possibility of Aspergillosis.
- Always consider the cell morphology (PI, toxicity, left-shift) in addition to the absolute cell counts.
- Owls tend to have an inverted H:L ratio. That is, they can have more lymphocytes than heterophils. In addition, this ratio can be affected significantly by stress or an inflammatory response.
- The normal number of thrombocytes is 2–3 per 100× field.

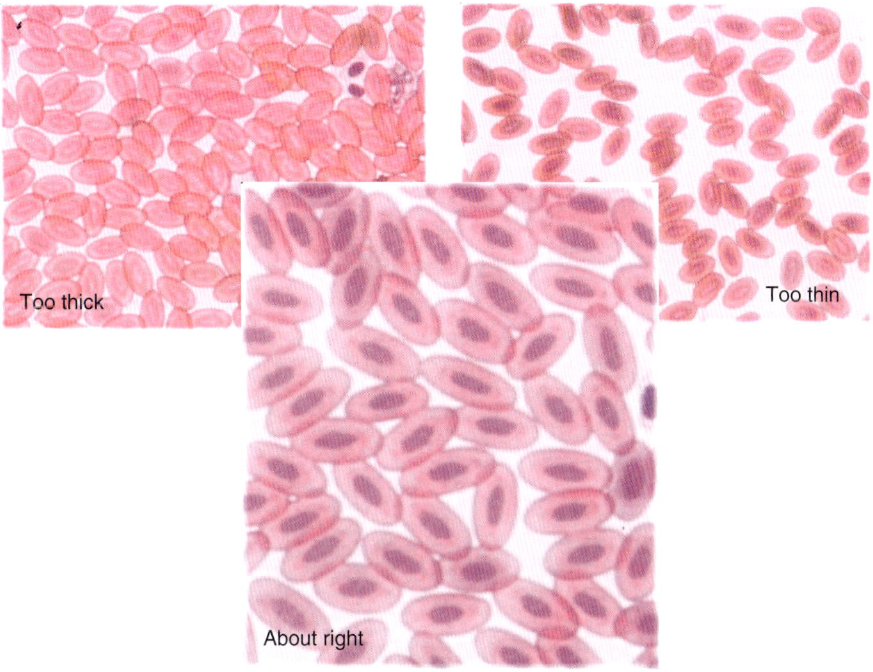

Fig. 14.18. The thickness of the smear is very important. Always evaluate cells in the feathered edge.

- Consider the overall smear as a whole. Do not get hung up on a few unidentifiable cells. Just call them "skipocytes" and move on.
- The estimated count method described above is not perfect but the results are clinically relevant once you get proficient at reading them. Being off by 10% or even 20% is not critical. Simply try to classify the white cell count as low, normal, high, or very high.
- Do not panic if you get a high white count in a clinically normal bird. Just recheck the CBC in 10–14 days.
- A single abnormal CBC may not be important. Serial CBCs and trends over time are much more useful.

Raptor Tip

Treat the bird, not the CBC. Recheck an abnormal CBC to look for trends.

Differentials for severe leukocytosis should include:

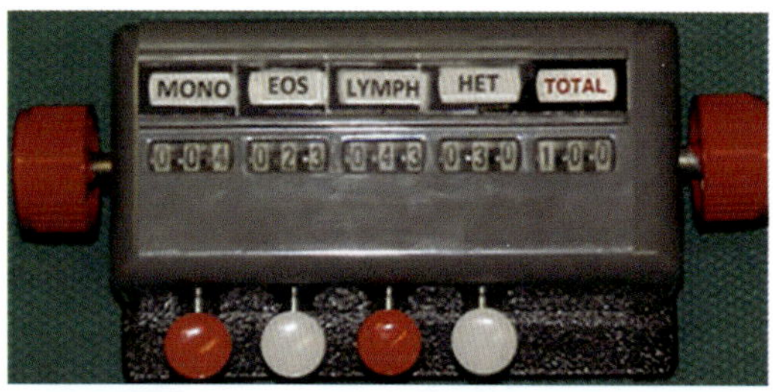

Fig. 14.19. A cell counter with four counters is adequate for avian CBCs.

- Aspergillosis.
- *Mycobacterium avium* complex (MAC).
- *Chlamydophila*: more of a worry in psittacines but studies (Hawkins, 2010) indicate that this may be an important clinical disease in raptors.

Biochemistries

Biochemistries are useful in avian medicine; however, as in mammals, they rarely point directly to a diagnosis. For in-house chemistries, the VetScan VS2® (Abaxis, Union City, CA, USA) machine is second to

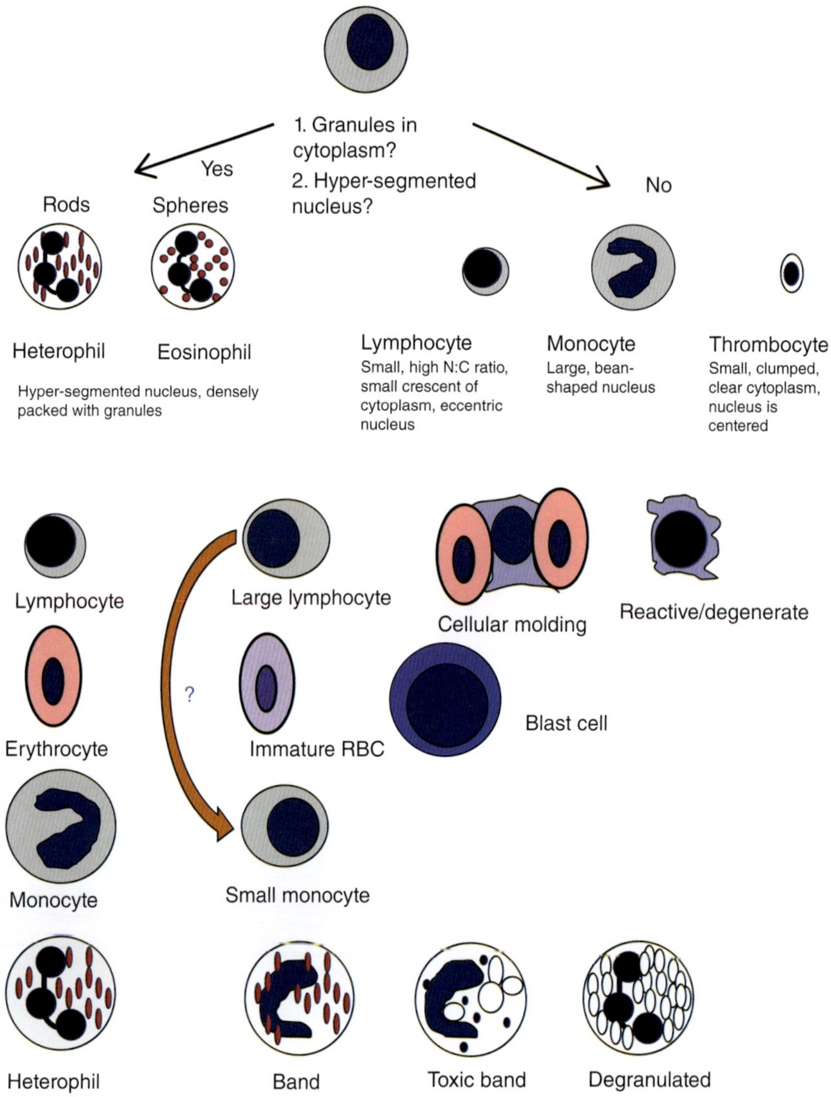

Fig. 14.20. Cell identification keys.

Table 14.3. Causes for changes in various cell lines.

Cell	Increase	Decrease
PCV	Dehydration	Chronic disease, emaciation, blood loss
Heterophil	Inflammation due to bacterial or fungal infection, stress/corticosteroids	Acute or overwhelming infection
Lymphocyte	Chronic antigenic stimulation, leukemia	Stress/corticosteroids
Monocyte	Chronic, granulomatous infections (Aspergillosis, *Mycobacterium*), tissue damage, stress/corticosteroids?	Not clinically relevant
Eosinophil	Parasitism? Hypersensitivity reaction?	Not clinically relevant

Table 14.4. Hematologic parameters in healthy individuals. Cell counts are ×10³ cells/µl. The values are presented as a mean with a standard deviation and/or a range. Some values are presented as a single mean. (The data presented are compiled and merged from several sources including Chitty, 2008; Black *et al.*, 2011; Szabo *et al.*, 2014.)

Species	PCV	WBC	Het	Lymph	Eos	Mono
Bald eagle	42 ± 5	17.7 ± 6.9 (6.4–26.6)	11.9 ± 4.9 (1.6–19.2)	4.5 ± 5.3 (1.0–21.5)	0.6 ± 0.8 (0.0–3.2)	0.8 ± 0.7 (0.0–2.3)
Barn owl	46.2 ± 4, 48	13.7 ± 2.7, 12.4	7.8 ± 2.0, 6.9	5.5 ± 1.9, 3.1	1.6	1.1
Barred owl	37 ± 6, 44	15.7 ± 5.8 (6.2–28.3), 16.5	8.4 ± 4.7, 4.7	4.9 ± 3.1, 9.6	1.0 ± 1.1, 2.1	1.4 ± 1.0, 2.5
Broad-winged hawk	36 ± 4 (31–45)	19.1 ± 7.1 (10.3–29.5)	10.3 ± 6.2 (2.5–26.0)	5.9 ± 4.1 (0.6–13.1)	1.7 ± 0.7 (0.3–2.6)	1.4 ± 1.5 (0.3–5.8)
Common buzzard	32–44	5–13	3.2–11	0.3–3.1	0.1–0.8	0.2–0.68
Cooper's hawk	40 ± 6	15.8 ± 7.4 (2.0–29.9)	9.7 ± 5.2 (1.7–19.1)	3.8 ± 3.2 (0.2–10.5)	1.1 ± 1.1	1.1 ± 1.1
Eastern screech owl	40 ± 7, 47	15.3 ± 6.7 (5.5–31.7), 15.2	8.1 ± 4.9 (1.5–26.0), 4.0	4.8 ± 2.6 (1.1–13.6), 6.0	1.4 ± 1.3, 2.8	1.1 ± 1.0, 2.3
Eurasian eagle owl	50	20.4	10.9	4.0	4.0	1.7
Ferruginous hawk	37–48	4.5–6.8	1.89–3.76	0.78–1.74	0.3–0.7	0.24–1.5
Golden eagle	31–53	6.2–17	4.5–15.2	0.75–3.37	0.1–0.6	0–0.63
Great gray owl	50	13.0	3.6	4.3	1.4	1.6
Great-horned owl	34 ± 4, 43	21.1 ± 8.6, 20.0	13.4 ± 6.2, 9.9	4.9 ± 3.3, 3.4	1.7 ± 1.8, 2.6	1.2 ± 1.1, 2.1
Gyrfalcon			2.31–8.85	0.48–2.36	0–0.68	0.03–0.9
Harris's hawk	40–55	4.8–10	2.3–6.71	0.6–2.36	0–0.75	0.2–1.49
Lanner falcon	37–53	3.5–11	1.65–8.8	1.1–5.13	0–0.2	0–0.9
Merlin	39–51	4–9.5	3.2–4.03	1.2–1.56	0–0.15	0–0.5
Northern eagle owl	36–52	3.5–12.1	2.2–9.23	1.5–5.07	0–0.48	0–0.48
Northern goshawk	43–53	4–11	3.5–6.97	1.38–1.93	0–0.65	0–0.1
Northern saw-whet owl	48	11.6	1.8	2.4	1.3	0.8

Continued

Table 14.4. Continued.

Species	PCV	WBC	Het	Lymph	Eos	Mono
Peregrine falcon	37–53	3.3–11	1.4–8.55	1.1–3.3	0–0.3	0.1–0.86
Red-tailed hawk	37 ± 5, 35–53	19.3 ± 7.5, 3.4–7.5	10.8 ± 4.8, 1.9–3.5	5.2 ± 3.0	2.0 ± 1.7 (0.0–8.7), 0.1–0.9	1.5 ± 1.2
Saker falcon	38–49	3.8–11.5	2.6–5.85	0.8–4.25	0–0.2	0–0.8
Short-eared owl	48	12.4	3.5	5.0	1.2	1.1
Snowy owl	49	10.2	4.5	3.3	0.8	0.9
Tawny eagle	37–47	5–9.5	3.58–6.45	0.51–2.72	0.3–2.1	0.2–1.07

Het, heterophil; Lymph, Lymphocyte; Eos, eosinophil; Mono, monocyte.

Table 14.5. Biochemical analytes.

Analyte	Normal range	Cause of increase	Cause of decrease
Albumin (Alb)	2.5–4.5 g/dl	Dehydration, inflammation	Emaciation, chronic disease, liver disease
Aspartate aminotransferase (AST)	<300 IU/l	Active liver disease and skeletal muscle	
Bile acids (BA)	<30 μmol/l	Liver disease	
Calcium (Ca^{2+})	9.5–10.0 mg/dl	Egg formation, osteosarcoma, granulomatous disease, hyperpara-thyroidism	Starvation, chronic egg laying
Creatine kinase (CK)	<1000 IU/l	Muscle damage including capture myopathy or from IM injections, Vitamin E/Se deficiency	
Globulins (Glob)		Dehydration, inflammation, egg formation	Neonatal, immunodeficiency, blood loss, protein-losing enteropathy
Glucose (Glu)	200–300 mg/dl	Stress, glucocorticoids, diabetes mellitus	Liver failure, starvation, septicemia
Potassium (K^+)	3.0–4.0 mmol/l	Renal disease, dehydration, diabetic ketoacidosis	Renal disease
Phosphorus (Phos)	2.0–4.0 mg/dl	Renal disease, egg formation (with increase in calcium), osteosarcoma	Starvation
Sodium (Na^+)	145–155 mmol/l	Renal disease, dehydration	
Total protein (TP)	2.5–4.5 g/dl	Dehydration: can increase up to 40% (Samour, 2008); inflammation or infection	Starvation, renal or intestinal loss, blood loss, liver disease
Uric acid (UA)	<15 mg/dl	Renal disease, post-prandial change (carnivores), dehydration	Liver failure, starvation

none. A full panel can be run with 0.3 ml of heparinized whole blood, the results are available in 15 min, and the machine requires little or no maintenance. The company has an "Avian/Reptile Panel", which includes BA.

Realize that there are fewer clinically useful analytes in avian medicine than there are for mammals. Table 14.5 summarizes the analytes of clinical relevance; and Table 14.6 lists some normal ranges for various raptor species.

EPH

Protein electrophoresis (EPH) can be very helpful in the diagnosis of many infectious diseases, as it attempts to evaluate the humoral immune response (Fig. 14.21). Utilization of EPH is important since changes in the proportions of the various protein components can be present in the absence of corresponding changes in the CBC or serum chemistry panel. The various protein components are:

- Pre-albumin: transport of metabolites.
- Albumin: transport of metabolites, maintenance of osmolarity.
- α Globulins: acute-phase protein including fibrinogen and serum amyloid A.
- β Globulins: carriers, acute-phase proteins, lipoproteins, complement. May have a twin peak.
- γ Globulins: immunoglobulins.

It is recommended that this test is run with serum rather than plasma, to eliminate interference with fibrinogen. Changes in the proportions of the various protein components can support the suspicion of an inflammatory process. In general, a decrease in the albumin:globulin (A:G) ratio may indicate an inflammatory process, since inflammation tends to increase globulins. However, any disease that decreases total albumin (such as liver failure, protein-losing enteropathy, or renal disease) will also decrease the A:G ratio. Some possible changes or patterns are:

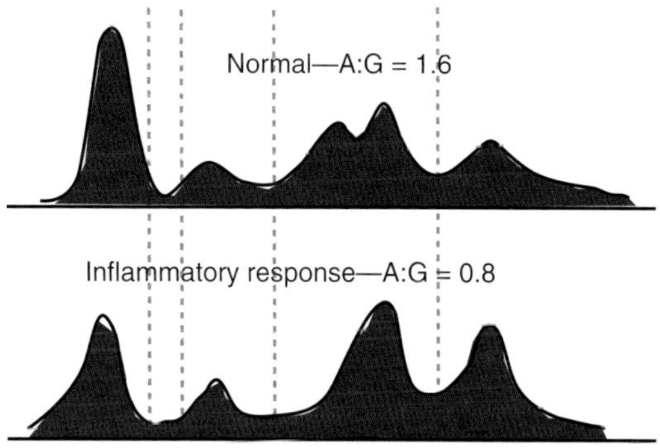

Fig. 14.21. Example electrophoresis (EPH). There can be a marked increase in β and/or γ globulins and the A:G ratio will decrease.

- Acute *Chlamydophila* infection: decreased albumin, increased β + γ.
- Chronic *Chlamydophila* infection: can be within normal limits or a mild increase in β.
- Hepatitis: decreased albumin with or without an inverted pre-albumin:albumin ratio, β, and γ increases with β–γ bridging.
- Acute nephritis: decreased albumin with moderate increases in β with or without increases in α_2.
- Malnutrition: decreased albumin and γ.
- Fungal infection: increased β + γ.
- Mycobacteriosis: increased β + γ.
- Heavy metal toxicities = variable, increased β.

Table 14.6a and b. Biochemical reference ranges for various species. The values are presented as a mean with a standard deviation and/or a range. Some values are presented as a single mean possibly with an *n* value in parentheses. (The data in these tables were compiled and merged from various sources including those listed in the Bibliography.)

Table 14.6a.

Species	AST (IU/l)[a]	CK (IU/l)	UA (mg/dl)[b]	BA (µmol/l)[c]	Glu (mg/dl)	Ca (mg/dl)	Phos (mg/dl)
Bald eagle	153–370, 210 (3)	383, 300 (3)	5–15, 8.9 (3)	12.3 (3)	325, 367 (3)	10.8, 11.0 (3)	3.03, 2.7 (3)
Barn owl	272 ± 43, 167 (90–303)	2228 ± 578, 895 (164–3084)	428 ± 102 (µmol/l), 692 (290–1044) (µmol/l)	43 ± 18, <35			

Continued

Table 14.6a. Continued.

Species	AST (IU/l)[a]	CK (IU/l)	UA (mg/dl)[b]	BA (µmol/l)[c]	Glu (mg/dl)	Ca (mg/dl)	Phos (mg/dl)
Barred owl	158–471	151–2434	88–1146 (µmol/l)	<35			
Common buzzard							
Cooper's hawk							
Eastern screech owl	76–452	4–864	171–1755 (µmol/l)	<35			
Eurasian eagle owl							
Golden eagle	95–210, 35–538, 133 (2)	498 (2)	5.3 (2)	<30 (2)	354 (2)	10.1 (2)	1.9–3.6, 3.0 (2)
Great gray owl	72–378	0–559	201–1334 (µmol/l)	<35			
Great-horned owl	287, 104–344, 179 (2), 44–314	977, 252–376, 481 (2), 233–1315	13.7, 8.5, 8.9 (2), 165–1192 (µmol/l)	8–54, 10.0 (2), <35	319, 347 (2)	10.2, 10.1 (2)	5.8(2)
Gyrfalcon	97, 149, 44–471, 44–471	402	13.93, 80–690 (µmol/l)				1.52
Harris's hawk	160–348	224–650	533–785 (µmol/l)				3.0–4.4
Kestrel	100–200						
Lanner falcon	30–118	350–650	318–709 (µmol/l)				
Merlin	50–125	521–807	174–800 (µmol/l)				
Northern eagle owl			475–832 (µmol/l)				
Northern goshawk	176–409	218–775, 218–775	511–854 (µmol/l)				
Northern saw-whet owl	248 (127–411)	377 (19–4299)	536 (157–752) (µmol/l)	50 (21–61)			
Peregrine falcon	50–105, 97–350, 35–327, 34–162	357–850, 120–442, 357–850, 120–442	4.5, 4.4–22.0, 170–1250 (µmol/l)	20–118, 55–69, 20–118, 5–69	198–288	9.7 ± 1.3, 8.4–10.3	2.3 ± 0.9, 2.4–6.5
Red-tailed hawk	110–392, 529 (1)	1124, 759 (1)	10.8, 8.1–17, 12.0 (1)	2.0 (1)	292–390, 352 (1)	10–12.8, 11.1 (1)	1.8–4.4, 1.8 (1)

Continued

Table 14.6a. Continued.

Species	AST (IU/l)[a]	CK (IU/l)	UA (mg/dl)[b]	BA (μmol/l)[c]	Glu (mg/dl)	Ca (mg/dl)	Phos (mg/dl)
Saker falcon	45–95, 40–358	355–651	320–785 (μmol/l), 110–1260 (μmol/l)	20–90			
Sharp-shinned hawk							
Short-eared owl	236 (179–511)	77 (0–2347)	565 (191–1631)	<35			
Snowy owl	262 (186–310)	213 (20–3246)	677 (306–1438) (μmol/l)	<35			
Tawny eagle	124–226		413–576 (μmol/l)				
Turkey vulture	25.7 (3)	339 (3)	10.8 (3)	3.3 (3)	246 (3)	9.6 (3)	2.9 (3)
White-tailed sea eagle							

[a]Affected by hemolysis.
[b]UA: to convert from mg/dl to μmol/l, multiply by 59.48.
[c]Values above 100 μmol/l are typical of liver disease.

Table 14.6b

Species	TP (g/dl)	Alb (g/dl)	Glob (g/dl)	A:G ratio[a]	K⁺ (mmol/l)	Na⁺ (mmol/l)
Bald eagle	3.0–4.1, 3.0 ± 0.7 (1.2–4.0)	2.6 (3)	1.6 (3)	1.0 ± 0.3, 1.62 (3)	3.0, 2.2 (3)	156, 145 (3)
Barn owl	3.2, 3.6 ± 0.53	2.4 (1.9–3.3)	1.3 (0.6–1.7)	1.5 ± 0.6, 1.95, 1.4 (0.7–1.6)	4.9 (3.2–8.7)	152 (134–165)
Barred owl	3.2–7.0	1.8–3.4	0.5–5.7	0.7 ± 0.3, 0.64, 0.5–0.8	2.9–6.8	145–165
Common buzzard	3.3–5.0	0.5–1.4				
Cooper's hawk	2.8 ± 0.9 (1.4–4.6)					
Eastern screech owl	3.0–5.4, 3.8 ± 0.8 (2.0–6.0)	2.6–5.3	0.0–0.9	1.6 ± 0.7, 0.6–1.9	1.0–6.7	140–165
Eurasian eagle owl	4.5					
Golden eagle	2.5–3.9, 3.9–6.3, 3.6 (2)	2.4 (2)	1.3 (2)	0.66, 1.8 (2)	4.2 (2)	152 (2)
Great gray owl	2.9–4.5, 4.6	2.1–4.0	0.1–1.8	0.6–1.9	2.9–5.4	140–164

Continued

Table 14.6b. Continued.

Species	TP (g/dl)	Alb (g/dl)	Glob (g/dl)	A:G ratio[a]	K^+ (mmol/l)	Na^+ (mmol/l)
Great-horned owl	4.3, 3.3–4.6, 3.3 ± 0.9 (2.0–5.3), 3.5–5.6	1.6, 3.1 (2), 2.0–3.5	2.52, 2.1–3.3, 0.6 (2), 0.5–2.5	0.7 ± 0.2, 0.71, 5.2 (2), 0.4–1.0	2.8, 4.5 (2), 3.0–6.7	156, 155 (2), 141–168
Gyrfalcon	2.8	0.66–1.68			1.9–4.9	
Harris' hawk	3.9–5.2, 3.1–4.57	1.39–1.7	2.1–2.94	1.4 ± 0.6, 0.46–0.55	0.8–2.3	155–171
Kestrel	2.5–3.4			1.34		
Lanner falcon	3.3–4.2	0.96–1.6	2.12–2.18	0.44–0.57	1–2.1	152–164
Merlin	2.7–5.4, 2.75–3.9	0.86–1.61	1.72–2.5	0.47–0.58	1–1.8	155–170
Northern eagle owl	3.01–3.45	1.11–1.35	1.87–2.24			
Northern goshawk	2.6–4.2	0.88–1.24	1.8–2.92	0.4–0.57		
Northern saw-whet owl	3.0 (2.7–3.7)	2.1 (1.9–2.7)	0.9 (0.4–1.5)	2.3 (1.3–6.5)	3.0 (2.6–3.6)	153 (129–155)
Peregrine falcon	2.6, 1.6–3.8, 2.5–4.0	0.8–1.3, 0.69–1.48, 1.27–2.24	1.6–2.83	0.4–0.6,	2.04, 1.6–3.2, 1.8–5.1	153–164, 152–168
Red-tailed hawk	3.3–4.5, 3.9–6.7, 3.4 ± 0.7 (2.0–5.0)	3.3 (1)	1.3 (1)	1.2 ± 0.3, 2.5 (1)	2.6–4.3, 2.5 (1)	157, 151 (1)
Saker falcon		0.9–1.23, 0.52–1.5	1.8–2.8	0.45–0.57	0.8–2.3, 1.6–4.7	154–161
Sharp-shinned hawk	2.4–3.2					
Short-eared owl	3.2 (2.4–4.5), 4.1	3.0 (2.6–4.6)	0.1 (0.0–0.6)	1.1 (0.8–1.4)	4.7 (3.4–6.6)	151 (145–157)
Snowy owl	3.8 (2.9–4.8), 4.8	3.4 (2.0–3.9)	0.3 (0.0–2.4)	0.8 (0.4–1.3)	4.5 (3.5–5.8)	156 (148–164)
Tawny eagle	2.9–4.14					
Turkey vulture	3.9 (3)	2.0 (3)	1.9 (3)	1.2 ± 0.4, 1.05 (3)	3.0 (3)	145 (3)
White-tailed sea eagle	2.8–4.5	1.11–1.35	2.53–2.84	0.44–0.55	1.5–3.1	153–157

[a]Many older references indicate that a normal ratio is less than 1.0 but this is inconsistent with findings from the University of Miami Avian and Wildlife Laboratory (www.pathology.med.miami.edu (accessed June 2020)), which shows ranges for various psittacines to be greater than 1.5. In addition, values measured at Carolina Raptor Center were also well above 1.0, and other publications (Tatum *et al.*, 2000; Cray *et al.*, 2009; Kummrow *et al.*, 2012) have reported much higher values.

Normal A:G ratios for many raptor species are not well documented, but this author believes a ratio of greater than 1.25 is to be expected in a healthy bird (see notes for Table 14.6). Note that while dehydration can increase TP, it should not affect the A:G ratio in an otherwise healthy animal.

Bibliography

Ammersbach, M., Beaufrère, H., Gionet Rollick, A. and Tully, T. (2015a) Laboratory blood analysis in Strigiformes—Part I: hematologic reference intervals and agreement between manual blood cell counting techniques. *Veterinary Clinical Pathology* 44(1), 94–108.

Ammersbach, M., Beaufrère, H., Gionet Rollick, A. and Tully T. (2015b) Laboratory blood analysis in Strigiformes—Part II: plasma biochemistry reference intervals and agreement between the Abaxis Vetscan V2 and the Roche Cobas c501. *Veterinary Clinical Pathology* 44(1), 128–140.

Black, P.A., McRuer, D.L. and Horne, L.A. (2011) Hematologic parameters in raptor species in a rehabilitation setting before release. *Journal of Avian Medicine and Surgery* 25(3), 192–198.

Campbell, T.W. and Ellis, C.K. (2007) *Avian and Exotic Animal Hematology and Cytology*. Blackwell Publishing, Ames, IA, USA.

Chitty, L. (2008) *BSAVA Manual of Raptors, Pigeons and Passerine Birds*. BSAVA, Gloucester, UK.

Cray, C., Reavill, D., Romagnano, A., Van Sant, F., Champagne, D., Stevenson, R., *et al.* (2009) Galactomannan assay and plasma protein electrophoresis findings in psittacine birds with aspergillosis. *Journal of Avian Medicine and Surgery* 23(2), 125–135.

Hawkins, M. (2010) Chlamydophila psittaci in wild raptors in northern California: 2000–2009. *Proceedings of the 31st Conference of the Association of Avian Veterinarians, San Diego, CA, USA*. Association of Avian Veterinarians, Teaneck, NJ, USA, p. 349.

Kummrow, M., Silvanose, C., Di Somma, A., Bailey, T.A. and Vorbrüggen, S. (2012) Serum protein electrophoresis by using high-resolution agarose gel in clinically healthy and Aspergillus species-infected falcons. *Journal of Avian Medicine and Surgery* 26(4), 213–220.

Maier, K., Fischer, D., Hartmann, A., Kershaw, O., Prenger-Berninghoff, E., Pendl, H., *et al.* (2015) Vertebral osteomyelitis and septic arthritis associated with *Staphylococcus hyicus* in a juvenile peregrine falcon (*Falco peregrinus*). *Journal of Avian Medicine and Surgery* 29(3), 216–223.

Pendl, H. (2006) Morphological changes in red blood cells of birds and reptiles and their interpretation. *Israel Journal of Veterinary Medicine* 61(1).

Ritchie, B.W., Harrison, G.J. and Harrison, L.R. (1994) *Avian Medicine: Principles and Application*. Wingers Publishing, Inc., Lake Worth, FL, USA.

Samour, J. (2008) *Avian Medicine*, 2nd edn. Mosby-Elsevier, Maryland Heights, MO, USA.

Szabo, Z., Klein, A. and Jakab, C. (2014) Hematologic and plasma biochemistry reference intervals of healthy adult barn owls (*Tyto alba*). *Avian Diseases* 58, 228–231.

Tatum, L.M., Zaias, J., Mealey, B.K., Cray, C. and Bossart, G.D. (2000) Protein electrophoresis as a diagnostic and prognostic tool in raptor medicine. *Journal of Zoo and Wildlife Medicine* 31(4), 497–502.

University of Miami (2015) *Interpretation of protein electrophoresis*. Available at: www.cpl.med.miami.edu/avian-and-wildlife/protein-electrophoresis (accessed October 2015).

15 Housing and Husbandry

Learning Objectives

1. Appropriate perching.
2. Basic cage construction details.
3. Minimum requirements for caging.
4. Resident bird husbandry basics.
5. Common husbandry problems.

Indoor Housing

In general, birds of prey do well in dog and cat carriers, as long as these are modified to include a perch (Fig. 15.1; Table 15.1). The appropriate-sized carrier should be provided so there is space above the bird's head when it is on the perch.

Outdoor Cage Construction

Cages of the appropriate construction and size are critical to the successful rehabilitation of raptors. Some construction factors to consider are discussed below.

Double doors

All cages with flighted birds must have a double-door system to prevent escapes and accidental release.

Predator proofing

Appropriate predator proofing must be incorporated into the construction and includes using materials of sufficient strength to keep predators out. It also must include a barrier to prevent predators from burrowing under the cage perimeter. Chain link fence secured on the ground around the perimeter for at least 2′ (0.6 m) is very effective (Fig. 15.3). Predator proofing should also be used wherever a perch meets the enclosure wall. This will prevent a predator from reaching in through a side wall.

Vertical slats

The walls should be made of vertical wood slats or other similar material. The important detail is that the openings are vertical and will not snag or

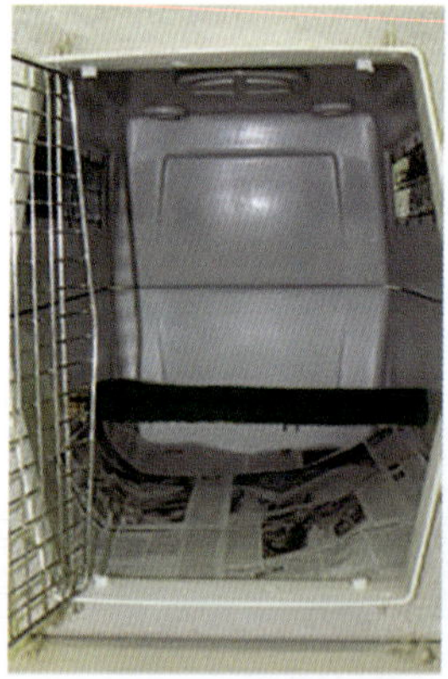

Fig. 15.1. A kennel modified with a perch.

Table 15.1. Kennel sizes for various species.

Species	Kennel size (L × W × H)
Kestrel, screech owl	18 × 12 × 15″, 45 × 30 × 38 cm
Broad-winged hawk, Cooper's hawk	24 × 17 × 18″, 60 × 45 × 45 cm
Red-shouldered hawk, barred owl	32 × 21 × 24″, 81 × 53 × 60 cm
Red-tailed hawk, great-horned owl	32 × 21 × 24″, 81 × 53 × 60 cm
Vulture	36 × 24 × 30″, 91 × 60 × 76 cm
Eagle	36 × 24 × 30″, 91 × 60 × 76 cm

catch the tail feathers if and when the bird grabs onto the walls (Fig. 15.2). The vertical slats also make it more difficult for the birds to cling to the walls. If chain link or any other mesh is used, the tail feathers will get caught and can be severely damaged. Note that chain link or mesh is an acceptable material to use for birds that are comfortable in their surroundings and are not prone to climbing and clinging to the walls. Birds in a permanent collection generally fall into this category but injured wild birds definitely do not.

Ventilation and light

It is critical that all cages have adequate ventilation and direct access to sunlight, as well as shaded areas.

Mosquito netting

In areas where mosquitoes or other biting insects are a problem, appropriately sized netting or mesh should be used. This netting should be attached to the *outside* of the slats so that the feathers cannot get caught in the fine mesh (Fig. 15.2).

Floor substrate

The substrate on the ground should be a *non-organic* material to decrease the risk of fungal diseases such as Aspergillosis. Smooth pea gravel ¼ to ½″ (5–15 mm) in diameter is ideal and easy on the feet. Gravel with jagged edges should never be used. The one exception to the "no-organic" rule is in cages used for live-prey testing. In these cages, it is important to provide natural ground cover such as leaf litter in order to provide hiding places for the mice and to ensure that the live-prey test is as realistic as possible.

Feeding hatches

These are important for juveniles so food can be provided without requiring entry into the cage. This is most crucial in young birds at risk of habituation or imprinting.

Perches

Perches of various sizes and textures should be provided. It is very important that birds are given

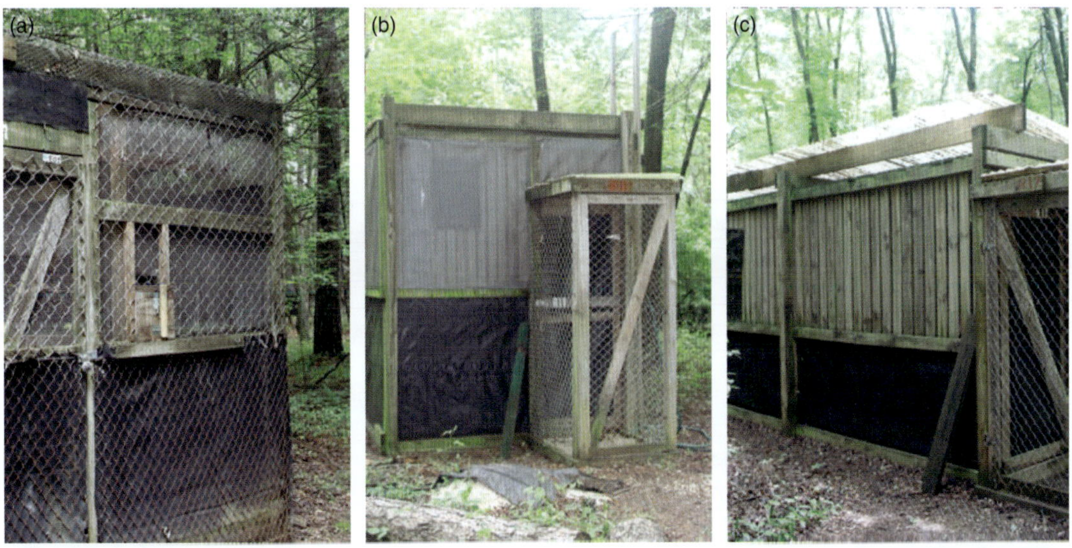

Fig. 15.2. (a) Chain link can lead to severe tail feather damage in birds prone to climbing on or clinging to the walls. Its use is not recommended on enclosure walls. (b) The double-door system. This cage also has mosquito mesh on the *outside* of the vertical slats. (c) The vertical slats allow tail feathers to slide freely without getting snagged and damaged.

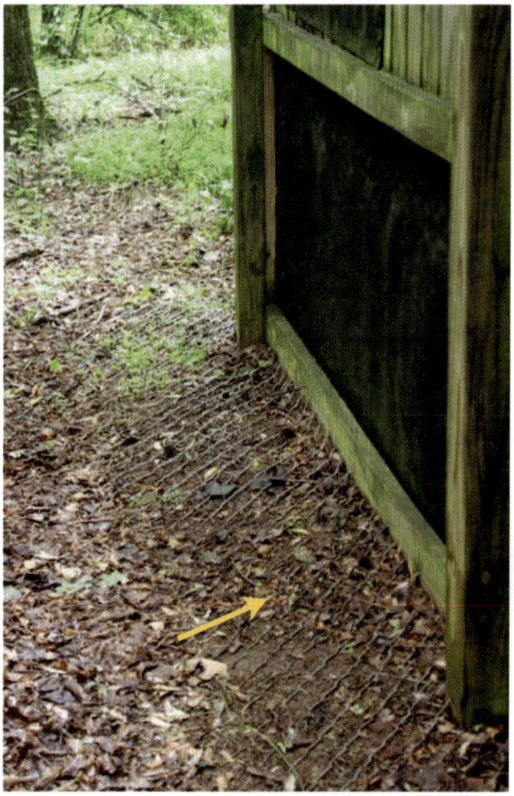

Fig. 15.3. Chain link predator proofing extends 2′ (0.6 m) out from the perimeter.

> **Raptor Tip**
>
> Only use inorganic materials such as smooth pea gravel for the ground substrate.

several different choices to minimize the risk of bumblefoot. Perches should be installed at various heights and provide enough space so that all the birds in the cage can find a comfortable place to perch without having to gather too closely together. In addition, floor-standing perches should be provided for birds that are unable to fly (Fig. 15.4). *With the exception of vultures, birds should never be forced to stand on the ground*. Perches can be made from the following:

- Natural branches and logs of variable sizes and textures. They are clearly the most natural but wear out and are difficult to clean or disinfect. It is usually best to simply replace them when dirty.
- Wood perches covered with green artificial turf or "daisy mat" (Fig. 15.5) material are excellent for providing good padding for the feet and are easy to clean. These perches, however, do not look very natural and this can be an issue in some display situations.
- Wood perches wrapped with sisal rope provide a good cushion and are more natural looking. Sisal rope dries out quickly and it stays relatively clean (Fig. 15.6). Cotton rope should not be used because it absorbs moisture and is impossible to clean.
- The ideal perch diameter is not always easy to specify since it depends on the type of covering that is added to the perch. In general, the perch should be of sufficient diameter so that the talons are not curled under too much or spread out too flat (Fig. 15.7). The key is to provide variety. If a perch is too small, bumblefoot tends to develop on the sole/center pads. If a perch is too large, bumblefoot tends to develop on the toes.
- Falcons nest on cliff faces and seem to do best with flat perches, but traditional, round perches should also be provided.

Water

All birds should have access to water, especially during the hot summer months. Although it is relatively uncommon for them to drink, they do enjoy bathing and preening. A large shallow pan or tub of water should be provided and the water should be changed regularly.

Size of cage

Cages should be sized appropriately for the species and for the planned use (Figs 15.8 and 15.9; Table 15.2). Overcrowding is always a concern and too many birds in a small space is guaranteed to result in accidents and in-flight collisions. Cages

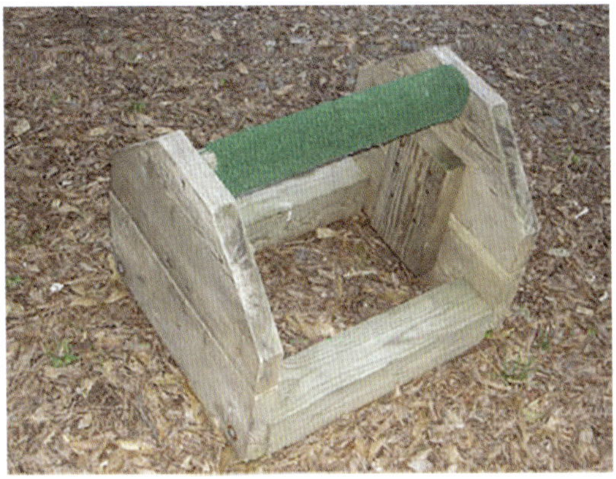

Fig. 15.4. A typical floor-standing perch.

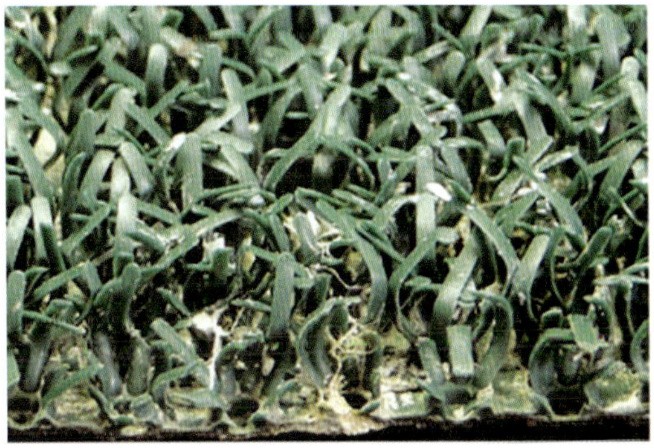

Fig. 15.5. Astroturf® (AstroTurf, LLC, Dalton, GA, USA)/ daisy mat is great for making perches.

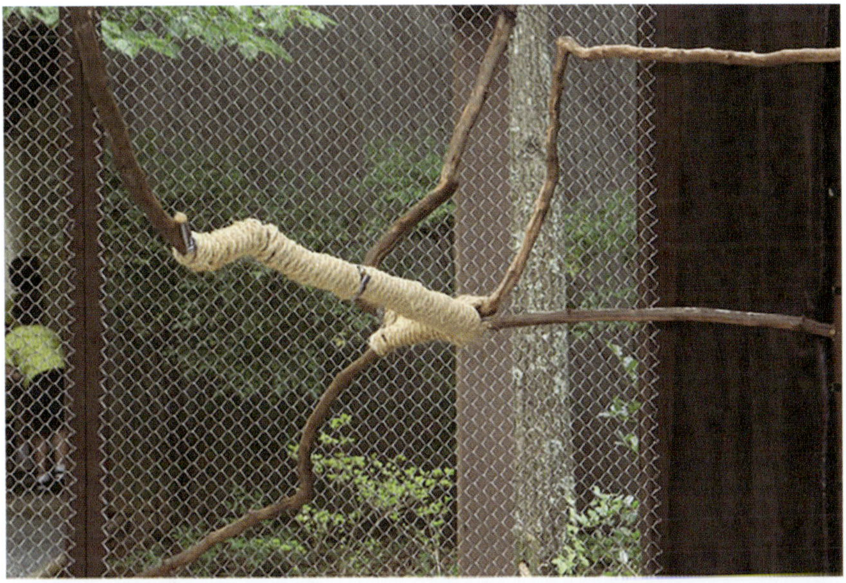

Fig. 15.6. Natural branches partially wrapped in rope make great perches.

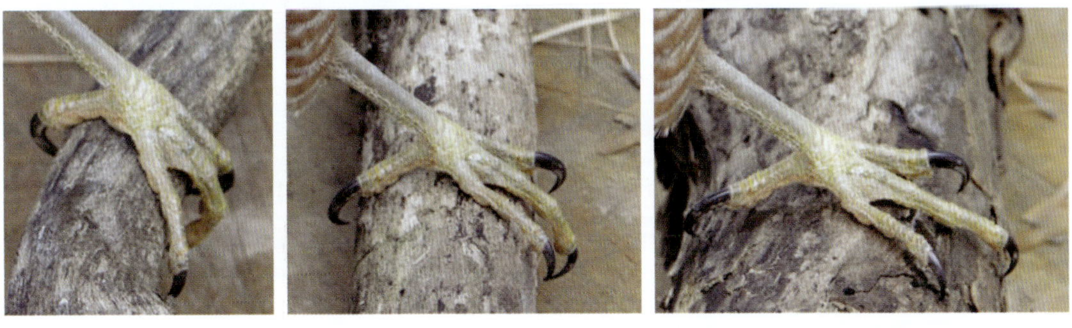

Fig. 15.7. An ideal perch diameter should share the load across the sole of the foot and the digits. The perch on the left is too small and the one on the right is too large. The one in the center is the correct diameter for this bird.

not intended for exercise can be smaller and do not need to be as tall.

An 8 × 16 × 8′ (2.5 × 5 × 2.5 m) cage is the standard non-flight cage at Carolina Raptor Center. This size cage can easily house two birds up to great-horned owl size.

Smaller 3 × 3 × 3′ (1 × 1 × 1 m) cubicles or "condos" which are completely protected from the weather are useful since they allow birds that have bandages to move outside quickly. These outdoor cages provide a quiet and less stressful environment for patients to relax and recuperate.

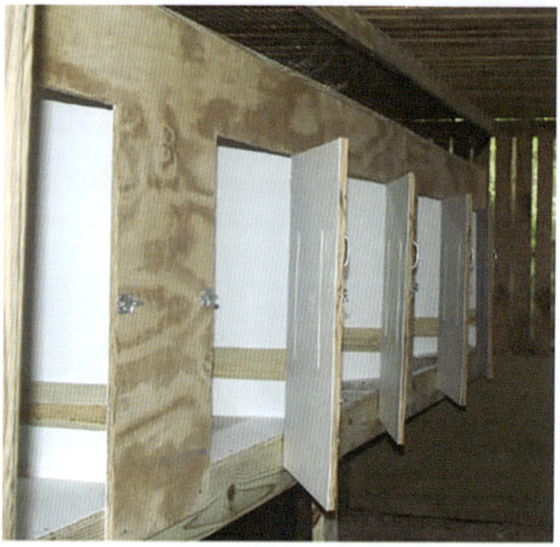

Fig. 15.8. A standard 8 × 16 × 8′ (2.5 × 5 × 2.5 m) cage has been converted into a five-unit condo.

Some species-specific housing concerns

- Accipiters (Cooper's hawk) hunt birds so they should be housed individually, especially when

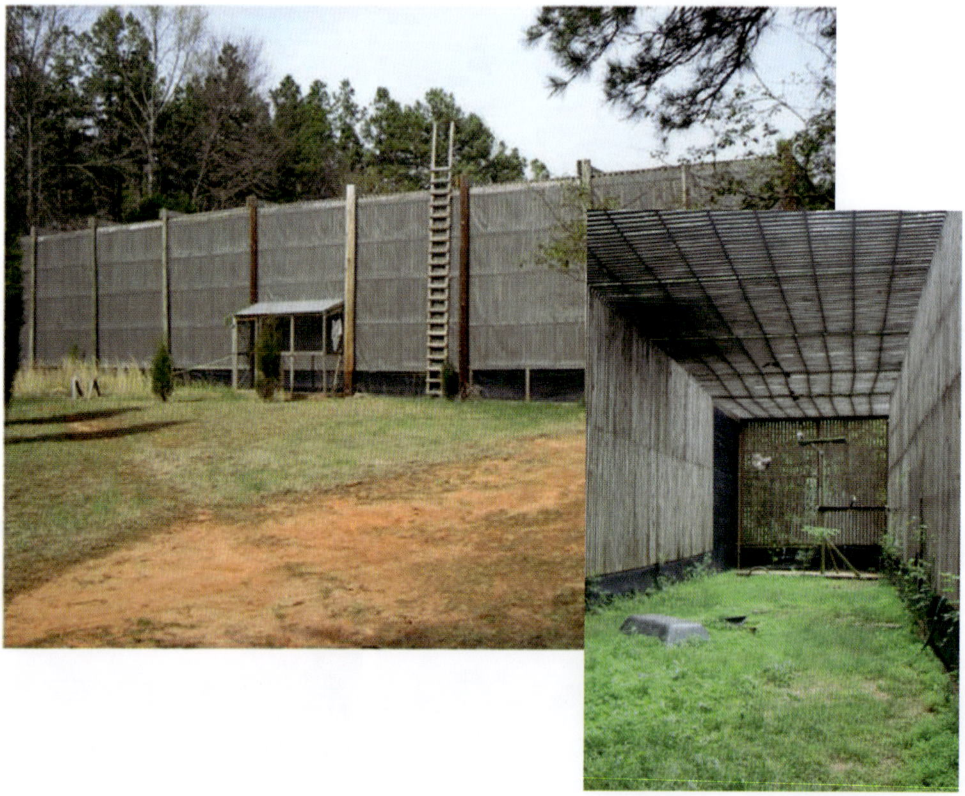

Fig. 15.9. A 100′ (30 m) flight cage is required for the larger species such as large hawks, vultures, and eagles.

Table 15.2. Flight cage sizes for various species.

Species	Cage size (L × W × H)
Kestrel, screech owl	30 × 10 × 8', 10 × 3 × 2.5 m
Red-shouldered hawk, barred owl	50 × 12 × 12', 15 × 4 × 4 m
Red-tailed hawk, great-horned owl	100 × 20 × 20', 30 × 6 × 6 m
Vulture	100 × 20 × 20', 30 × 6 × 6 m
Eagle	100 × 20 × 20', 30 × 6 × 6 m

considering birds of the opposite sex, since there is such a large disparity in body size.

- Screech owls are housed together with few problems, but cannibalism has been reported.
- Peregrine falcons require flat perches as well as traditional perches.
- All young birds are easily habituated so food hatches should always be used.
- Avoid housing different species of owls or hawks together. There are some combinations that work well but, in general, this practice should be avoided if possible.
- Large hawks seem to get along well with vultures and can be housed together.

Resident Bird Care

Resident birds and birds in a rehabilitation setting are managed very differently and have a different set of needs and requirements. There are many good references (Arent, 2007) on resident bird husbandry and this topic will not be discussed in depth here. This section is, however, a brief introduction to the more medically related aspects of resident bird care.

Quality of life

The quality of life (QoL) of any animal in long-term residence should be evaluated on a regular basis. There are many factors that affect the QoL and some become more important as an animal ages. Animals that do not have a satisfactory QoL should be humanely euthanized if their issues cannot be addressed. The QoL should also be evaluated carefully before an animal is accepted into your collection. Factors to consider fall into a few general categories, as follows.

- Existing injuries and problems:
  - Vision. All birds should be able to move about their enclosure safely and to find food. Many wild raptors coming from rehabilitation programs can have significant damage to one or both eyes, so a thorough ophthalmic exam is critical.
  - Mobility. All birds should be able to bear equal weight on both legs. If not, bumblefoot is likely to develop. Injuries such as fractures that affect a major joint can lead to degenerative joint disease (DJD), decreased ROM, and wing droops.
  - Plumage. All birds should have plumage sufficient to allow them to thermoregulate in all seasons throughout the year.
  - Beak. All birds should have a beak that is functional and allows them to feed and to preen. Beaks with misalignments may require repeated handling for coping.
  - Amputations of any part of a wing often lead to chronic stump wounds, repeatedly damaged blood feathers, and poor balance. These birds are generally not good candidates for long-term captivity.
- Chronic illness:
  - DJD is a common finding in older birds. This is a painful inflammatory condition that can degrade QoL. Some cases can be managed medically but these birds will need to be monitored with periodic physical examinations including radiographs.
  - Obesity is a common captivity problem. All birds should be provided with opportunities for exercise, they should receive a proper diet, and their weight and body condition score should be monitored carefully.
- Behavior:
  - All captive birds should have the appropriate personality and demeanor. Note that many/most wild birds received from rehabilitation programs are not good candidates for long-term captivity. It is

also generally accepted that adult birds do not make the transition to long-term captivity as well as younger birds and some species are generally much better candidates than others.
    - Self-mutilation is often a severe example of a maladjusted or stressed bird. The birds should be evaluated carefully. In some cases, there may be an underlying medical problem that can be addressed. However, in many there may not be an identifiable cause and these birds should be euthanized.
- Husbandry:
    - A bird should not be added to a collection if its basic husbandry needs cannot be met. This includes:
        - The natural history of this species should be very well understood. Are these birds social? When is their breeding season? Are males and females dimorphic? What type of nests do they build/utilize?
        - The appropriate housing/enclosure (Fig. 15.10) with proper perching (Figs 15.4–15.7) and ground substrate. Refer to Arent (2007) for required enclosure sizes.
        - Exposure to regular sunlight and the elements (i.e. rain).
        - The proper temperature range for the species.
        - The appropriate diet.
        - Enrichment.
        - Medical care (including periodic examinations).

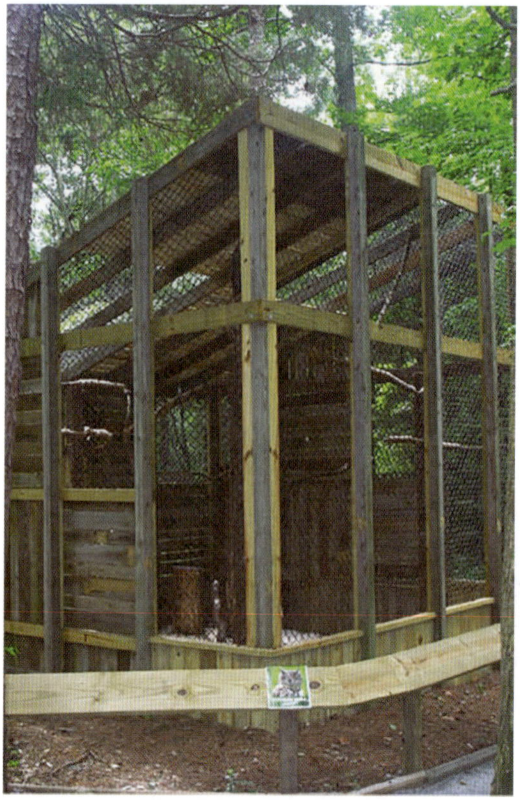

Fig. 15.10. Typical construction of a permanent resident enclosure.

Feeding

The Feeding Guide presented in Appendix A is for birds in a rehabilitation setting. These birds have an inherently higher caloric requirement than the typical resident bird in a static display. Because of this, the amounts fed to resident birds will be significantly lower than indicated in the Feeding Guide.

The appropriate amount of daily food will vary with the species, individual, level of activity, and season. It is critical that each bird's body condition score and weight are monitored carefully until a proper daily food amount is determined. Plan on increasing the daily food amount in the winter, especially for the smaller species.

Physical examination

Full health checks

Each bird should receive a full health check at least once a year. This consists of:

- Keel score and weight.
- Fat scores.
- Feet and talon check.
- Eye exam: anterior and posterior chambers.

- Feather check.
- Beak check and cope if necessary.
- Blood work: PCV/TP/CBC ± chemistry. This may seem like overkill, but it is very helpful to have previous bloodwork and trends to compare with if you suspect that a bird may be ill.
- Radiograph: should be done periodically if needed, especially in older birds, or to serve as a baseline for further reference.
- Deworm with fenbendazole and ivermectin.
- Apply Frontline® spray (Merial, Duluth, GA, USA) (not the top spot) for tick prevention if ticks are an issue in your area.

Mini health checks

These are done at 3- to 6-month intervals between the full health checks. These checks are quick and easy and typically consist of:

- Keel score and weight.
- Foot check.
- Beak check and cope if necessary.

For glove-trained birds, everything except beak coping can typically be done while on the glove.

Enrichment

It is important to provide enrichment opportunities for all birds in a permanent resident population. Some things to try:

- Vultures enjoy carcasses. Deer carcasses that have been mostly butchered for the meat are perfect for this purpose.
- Other birds seem to enjoy tearing up phone books, but any similar type of diversion is useful. Pine cones and Kong™ (The Kong Company, Boulder, CO, USA) dog toys filled with food can also be enjoyable.
- Providing real wild-type food (e.g. roadkill) provides variety. Squirrels are ideal. Radiograph all carcasses to ensure that they do not contain metal/lead fragments. At the Carolina Raptor Center, up to 30% of roadkill squirrels have metallic foreign bodies from previous gunshots.

Equipment maintenance

Resident birds trained to the glove typically require equipment to be placed around their tarsometatarsi. The equipment consists of a soft leather anklet (aylmeri) and a leather strip (jesse) that attaches to the aylmeri (Fig. 15.11).

It is important that the leather is well maintained to prevent chafing and sores from developing underneath. In addition, proper maintenance will prevent the leather from cracking or wearing out, which can result in an inadvertent escape. Glycerin-based saddle soap is useful for keeping leather aylmeri and jesses flexible and in good shape. In addition, the equipment should be checked regularly and replaced if there are any signs of cracking or wear.

Common issues

Obesity

Obesity is a serious concern in any resident bird population. This is particularly true for birds in static displays that do not get much exercise, or are not handled very much, and therefore do not get weighed often. It is very important to set an ideal weight for each individual bird and to check the weight periodically (at least four times per year). Glove-trained birds should be weighed weekly and this can be facilitated by training them to perch on a scale. The ideal weight may vary during the year and it may be wise to allow birds living in areas with cold winters to increase their weight a bit during the colder months.

Arthritis

It is not uncommon for older birds to develop DJD in the major joints. Radiographs should be a part of the yearly physical examination for geriatric birds to look for DJD, or to monitor the progression of existing conditions. Treatment with meloxicam and Cosequin® (Nutramax Laboratories, Lancaster, SC, USA) can be very beneficial, along with proper weight control and exercise. Intra-articular steroid injections may also be helpful, as can treatment with omega-3

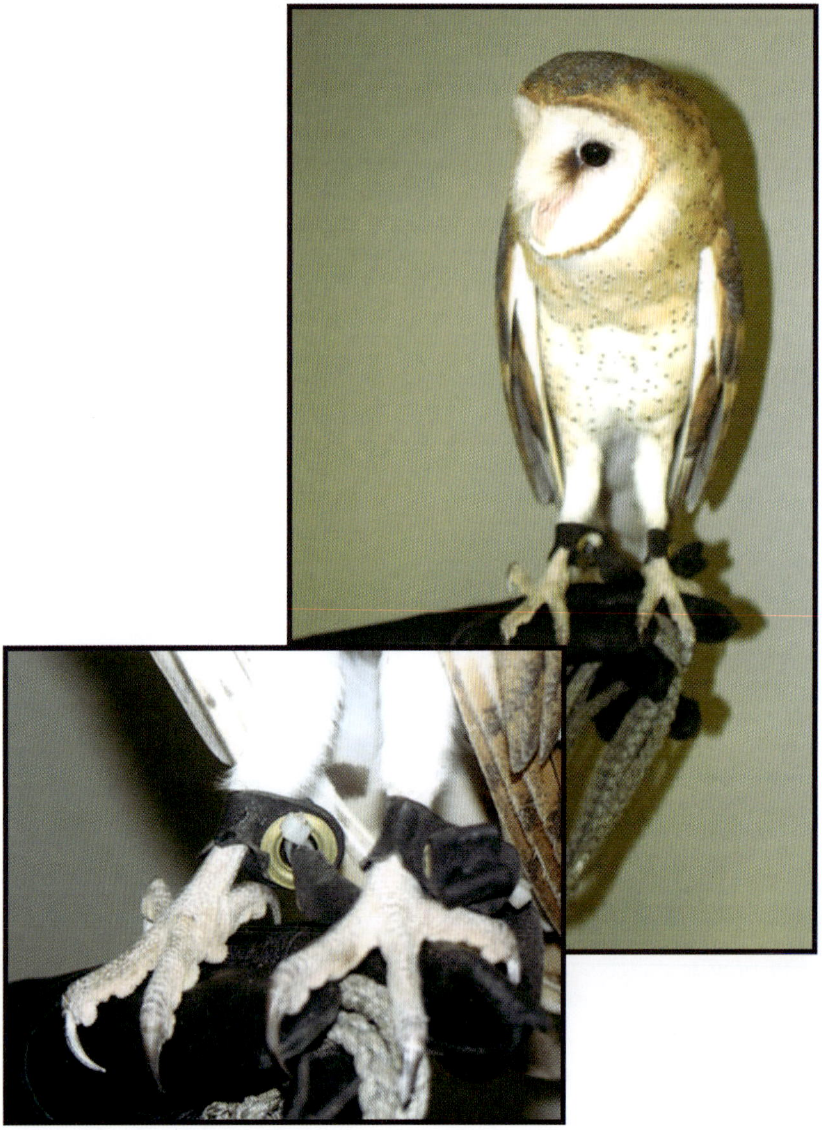

Fig. 15.11. Aylmeri and jesses on a barn owl.

fatty acids and various herbs such as white willow bark, devil's claw, meadowsweet, and turmeric (Bennett and Kelleher, 2008; Langhofer, 2010).

Bumblefoot

Bumblefoot (Chapter 7) is another common problem in resident birds. Since bumblefoot is often caused by obesity, proper weight control is the key to prevention. Other causes include inadequate perches or any non-weight-bearing lameness (including arthritis). Your standard procedure should include a quick visual examination of the feet whenever a bird is handled. Signs of redness, swelling, or lack of texture should be investigated immediately and the appropriate corrective measures taken. Although not truly bumblefoot, deep cracks in the plantar surface, particularly at the joints, can also occur from dryness and hyperkeratosis or thickening of the skin. Prevention and treatment can include the trimming of any excessively thickened skin and the application of Vitamin E mixed with a petroleum jelly product such as Bag Balm® (Vermont Original LLC, Lyndonville, VT, USA).

Overgrown beaks

The beak grows continuously. Wild birds generally maintain beak shape and length through normal use. Captive birds, however, do not always have the same opportunities and overgrown beaks are commonly encountered. Because of this, regular beak trimming or coping is required.

> **Terms**
>
> rhamphotheca—entire beak
> rhinotheca—upper beak
> gnathotheca—lower beak

Some signs of an overgrown beak are:

- The upper beak hook is long and may start to curve under. A healthy beak should form a 90° angle when lines are drawn along the edges to the tip. Fig. 15.12 shows a healthy beak.
- Non-falcons' beaks can overgrow and may develop an inappropriate tomial tooth (Fig. 15.13).
- Figs 15.14 and 15.15 show overgrown beaks with incorrect angles.
- The surface is cracked or flaky (Fig. 15.15).
- The edges of the lower beak can curve inwards and start to form a tube.
- The lower beak can grow long and prevent closure of the mouth.
- The defect in front of the overgrown falcon tooth in Fig. 15.15 can be caused by a bird clinging with its beak to chain link or some other form of mesh on the enclosure walls.

Hand-held grinding tools such as those made by Dremel® (Mount Prospect, IL, USA) and various nail trimmers are used to cope and shape beaks (Fig. 15.16). The head must be held securely with the fingers on the back of the head. The thumb is

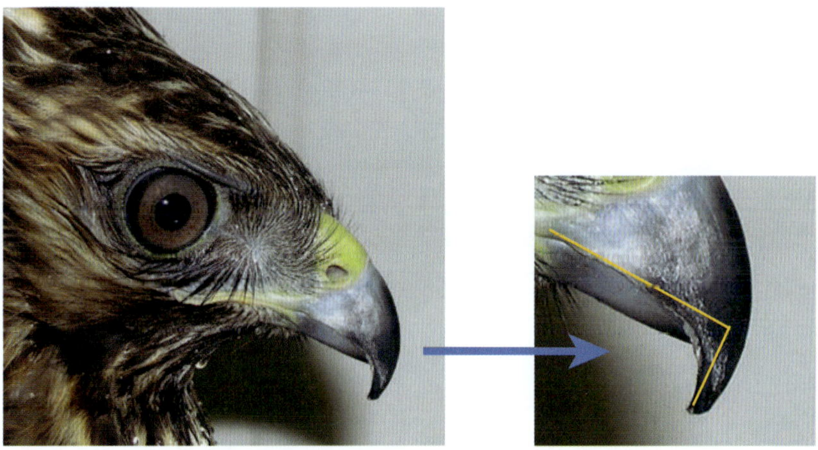

Fig. 15.12. A healthy beak has smooth sides, upper and lower edges that meet properly, and a hook of the proper length that forms a 90° angle (yellow lines).

pressed across the oral commissures to keep the beak open and to keep the tongue away from the grinding tool (Figs 15.17–15.21). Be careful to keep the bristle feathers around the mouth away from the spinning grinding tool. Also, a fine dust is created, so care must be taken to protect the bird's eyes. They may need to be flushed with saline when the procedure is complete. Note that some beaks in particularly bad condition may require multiple coping sessions to fix.

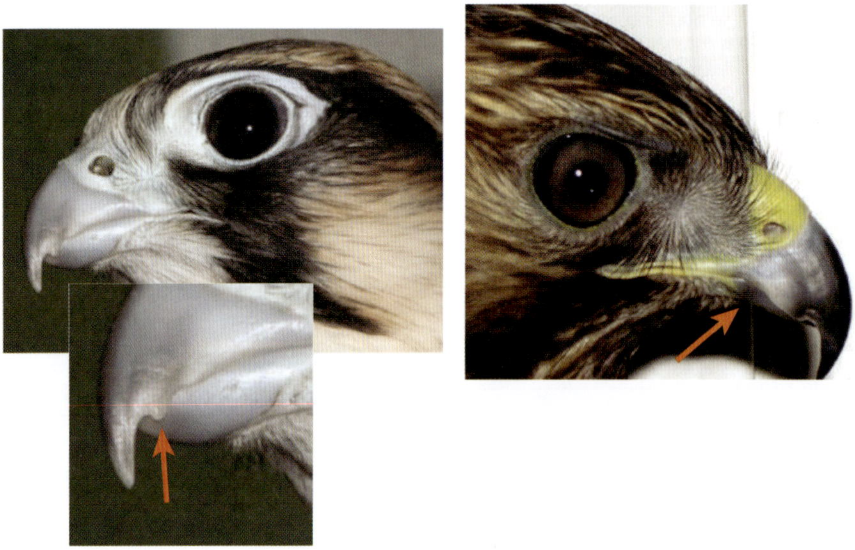

Fig. 15.13. The falcon's tooth or tomial tooth is normal in falcons (left) and should not be removed when coping. A similar structure will grow in other species (right) and this should be removed.

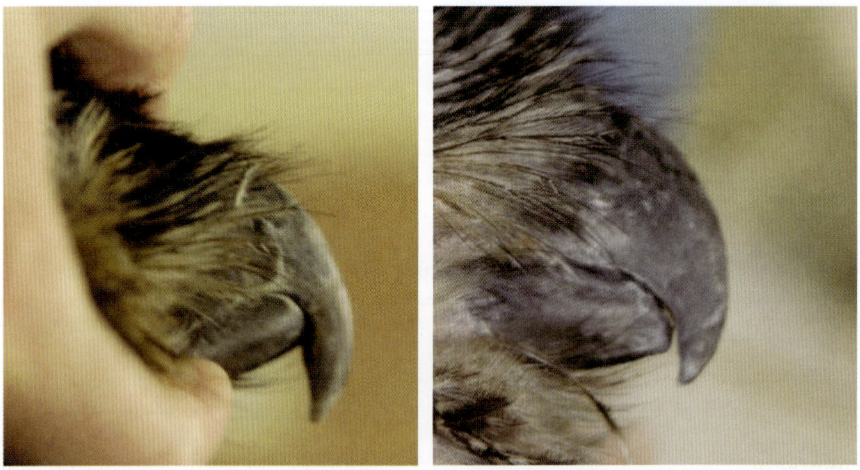

Fig. 15.14. A severely overgrown beak before (left) and after (right) it was coped.

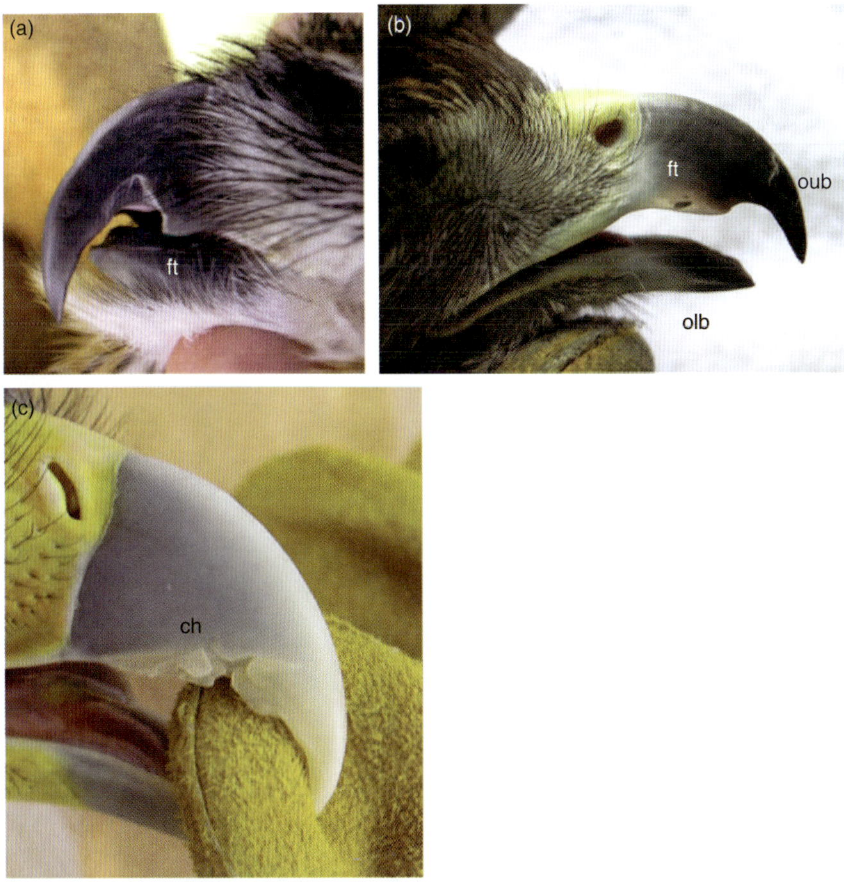

Fig. 15.15. Some beaks in need of coping. There are examples of falcon's teeth (ft), chips and cracks on the sides (ch), overgrown lower beak (olb), overgrown upper beak (oub).

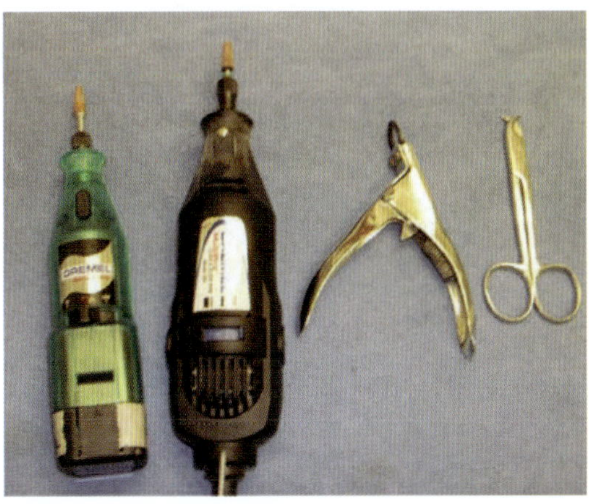

Fig. 15.16. Beak coping tools.

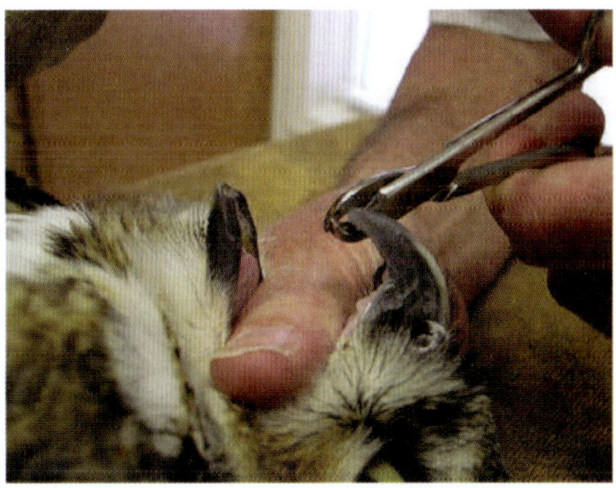

Fig. 15.17. Very long beaks can be shortened initially using a nail trimmer. However, do not take too much off at once since this can lead to bleeding and painful trauma to the underlying bone. Note how the thumb keeps the beak open.

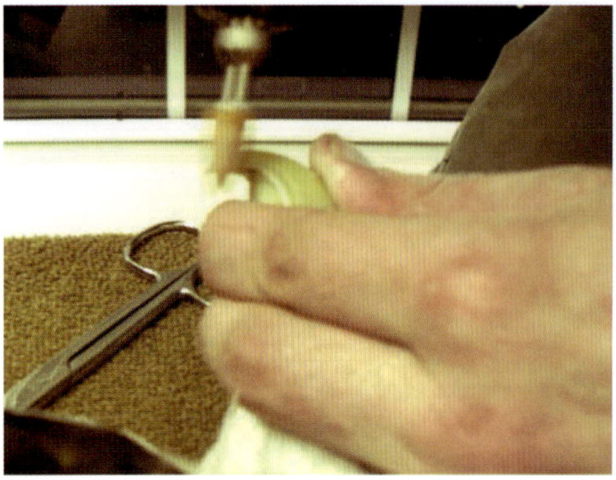

Fig. 15.18. The hook is then shaped and sharpened to a point.

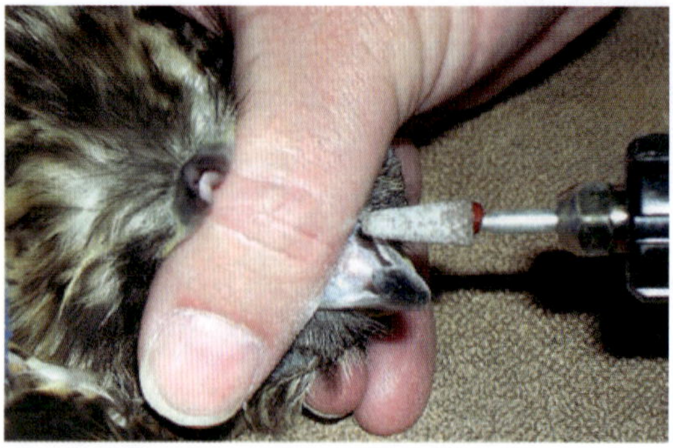

Fig. 15.19. The edges are ground and the "falcon tooth" is removed, if necessary. Note how the thumb protects the tongue from the grinding tool.

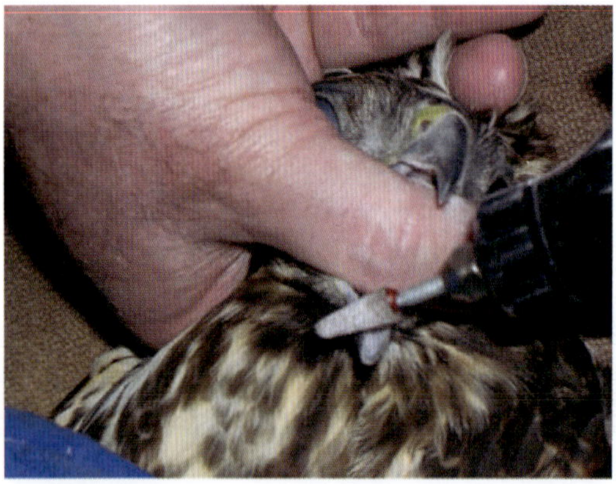

Fig. 15.20. The lower beak is shaped.

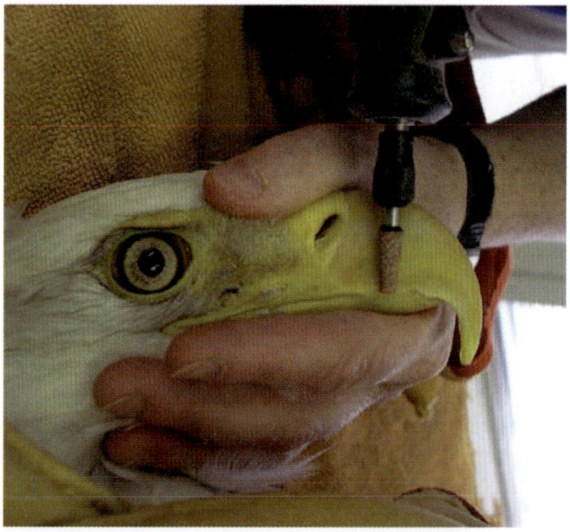

Fig. 15.21. The flakes are removed from the sides of the upper beak.

Bibliography

Arent, L. (2007) *Raptors in Captivity: Guidelines for Care and Management*. Hancock House Publishing, Surrey, BC, Canada.

Bennett, T. and Kelleher, D. (2008) Holistic treatment of osteoarthritis in psittacine birds. *Proceedings of the 29th Conference of the Association of Avian Veterinarians, Savannah, GA, USA*. Association of Avian Veterinarians, Teaneck, NJ, USA, pp. 49–52.

Langhofer (2010) Clinical therapeutic options for the treatment of osteoarthritis in avian patients with case reports. *Proceedings of the 31st Conference of the Association of Avian Veterinarians, San Diego, CA, USA*. Association of Avian Veterinarians, Teaneck, NJ, USA, pp. 85–89.

The Modern Apprentice. The modern apprentice. Falconry, ecology, education. Available at: www.themodernapprentice.com (accessed February 2016). [This website is an excellent reference for many falconry-related subjects.]

16 Capturing Trapped Birds

Learning Objectives

1. Problems to expect after birds have been trapped in a chimney.
2. Tricks to capture warehouse birds.

Birds Trapped in Chimneys

Owls may be trapped in chimneys during the nesting season when they are looking for a cavity to nest in. A bird may fall into the actual fireplace, but it is more common for it to be trapped above the flue. If the bird is located above the flue, the flue door may have to be removed in order to extract the bird. Wear goggles to protect your eyes from falling soot and debris. Use of a long flexible pole with a loop on the end can assist in snagging the bird and gently pulling it down.

Common problems to look for:

- Emaciation and dehydration.
- Blunt talons.
- Corneal ulcers.
- Wrist wounds.
- Soiled, sooty, or damaged feathers.
- Wounds on cere and supraorbital ridges.

Care must be tailored to the actual problems found. Time is also an important factor as many of these birds may have an active nest, so releasing them as soon as possible is critical.

Birds Trapped in Warehouses

Cooper's hawks or other accipiters can get trapped when chasing a songbird or pigeon. While most can find their way out, many will get trapped, especially if the entry/exit points are small. Before taking action, allow some time (up to 24 h, if possible) for the bird to free itself. Some helpful tips include:

- Opening all doors/windows and turning out lights.
- Turning off any ceiling fans.
- Trying to create an environment that is quiet and free of activity for at least a few hours.

If the bird is unable to free itself, attempting to capture with a live trap is the next step (Figs 16.1 and 16.2). Enlisting the help of a falconer is highly recommended. Capturing a raptor with a live-prey trap may not work until the bird is hungry, so you may need to wait a few days before making an attempt. If a bird does not come down to the trap within 30–45 min, you may need to try again the next day. The trap can be purchased at a falconry supply store or constructed out of metal mesh. It must have space for a live mouse to be able to move around. The trap must have a weight attached so that a bird cannot fly off with it, and it must have a series of leg snares attached to the top. The snares are made of monofilament fishing line and are very effective at tangling around a digit or ankle.

> **Raptor Tip**
>
> Never leave a trap unattended. A trapped bird can injure itself very severely in a matter of minutes!

Once the bird is caught in a snare, immediately remove it from the trap and examine its legs and toes for injury. Most trapped birds are healthy and can be released immediately. However, if it has been trapped for a longer period of time (i.e. 3 days or more), it may require treatment for emaciation and dehydration.

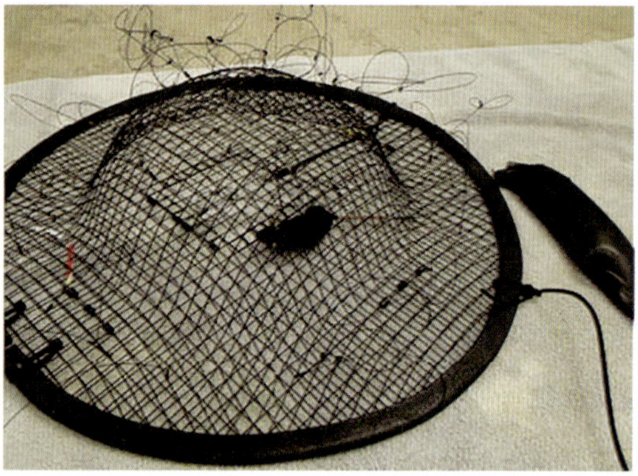

Fig. 16.1. A professional Bal Chatri falconry trap. It is dome-shaped with a trapdoor on the bottom to load a mouse. The weight is attached with a cord and you can see many fishing-line snares along the top.

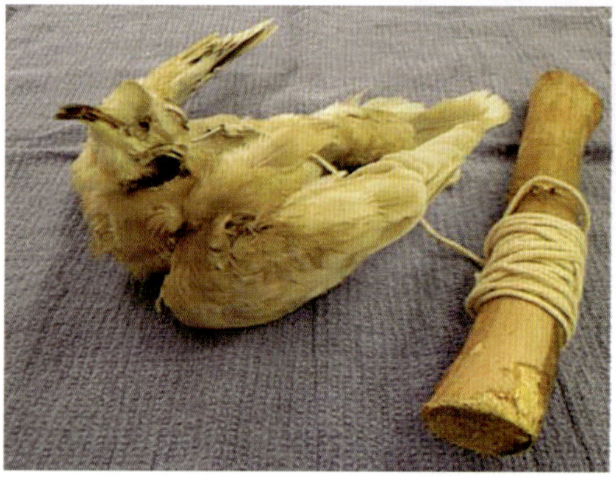

Fig. 16.2. Falconry lures can also be helpful.

Bibliography

International Association for Falconry and Conservation of Birds of Prey. Available at: https://iaf.org/ (accessed June 2020).

The Modern Apprentice. Available at: www.themodernapprentice.com (accessed February 2016). [This website is an excellent reference for many falconry-related subjects.]

North American Falconers Association. Available at: www.n-a-f-a.com (accessed July 2016).

Northwoods Falconry. Available at: https://northwoodsfalconry.com (accessed June 2020). [Supplier of all sorts of falconry equipment.]

17 Time for Release!

Learning Objectives

1. Determining if a bird is ready for release.
2. Common injuries that make a bird not releasable.
3. Release logistics: where, when, how.

There is nothing more rewarding than releasing a bird that was injured and in need of help. For many in this profession, this is what it is all about. Your patient has come a long way since admission, but there are a few final checks that are necessary before it is ready to be returned to the wild.

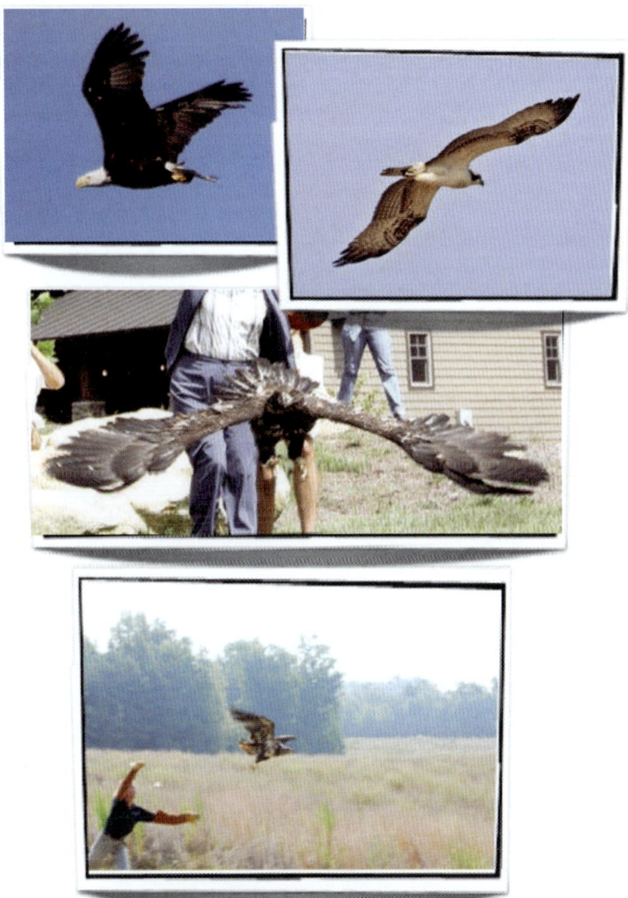

Pre-release Checks

Feather quality

The feathers must be in good condition with very little or no damage. They should be clean and waterproof and should repel water readily when sprayed or misted. Any significantly damaged feathers should be repaired if possible (Chapter 13) or the release must be postponed until a successful molt has occurred. There should be very little sound generated by the feathers in flight, and owls must be almost entirely silent in flight after the first one or two wing beats.

Flying ability

The bird must be physically fit and able to fly repeatedly without tiring. This is a subjective evaluation and heat/humidity can affect a bird's performance dramatically. Some details to look for:

- Open-mouthed or labored breathing after minimal exercise indicates a lack of conditioning, obesity, or illness. Check for excessive fat deposition and, if illness is suspected, the bird should be fully worked up.
- A bird's flight should appear effortless. If it is rough or if the bird is working exceptionally hard to fly, then there may be a problem or a lack of conditioning. This warrants further investigation.
- Inability to maintain level flight or reach a high perch indicates a lack of conditioning.
- Any asymmetry in wing extension or a tilt in the body during flight.
- Any wing droop before or after flying should be carefully scrutinized (see "Criteria for Nonreleasability" below).
- Unwillingness to fly. Most healthy birds will fly off when approached and usually require little or no provocation. Many cases are not always straightforward since some birds become accustomed to people after a prolonged stay in a rehabilitation facility and may not be so quick to fly off. Some species, such as great-horned owls, are particularly stubborn and may not fly even if prodded with a stick!

Although all release candidates should fly as close to perfectly as is possible, this is especially important in species that have long migrations such as broad-winged hawks. Any deviation from perfection should be assessed carefully.

Proper physical training and evaluation of flight ability requires appropriately sized cages (Chapter 15). One cannot expect a large hawk to soar in a 30′ (10 m) cage, for example. Additionally, flight patterns vary with species, and familiarity with each species is required before a proper evaluation can be made. For example:

- Vultures and red-tailed hawks soar and glide a great deal. In a 100′ (30 m) flight cage, these birds will soar 30′ (10 m) before landing.
- Accipiters are fast, maneuverable birds. They rarely glide but should be able to turn quickly.
- As stated above, owls should be silent in flight, even when maneuvering. Any noise in flight may be a result of feather damage or other problem that causes the bird to flap differently or less efficiently.
- Peregrine falcons stoop in a high-speed dive and cannot be effectively evaluated in a flight cage. They should be transferred to an experienced falconer for evaluation during free flight.

Vision

Any bird with evidence of eye trauma or damage should have its vision thoroughly tested. Evaluation of vision can include checking the pupillary light and menace responses, as well as use of an obstacle course (Chapter 5) and live-prey tests (Chapter 12).

Behavior

A bird's behavior must also be evaluated prior to release. This is especially important in young birds and orphans where the risk of habituation or improper imprinting can be significant. Things to look for:

- Food begging directed at people is a definite sign of mal-imprinting.
- Overly aggressive behavior towards humans. This determination can be subjective, since it

is not uncommon to have an especially nasty great-horned owl, for instance. However, this aggressive behavior can indicate a lack of the normal fear response and can be the result of imprinting.

- Normal evasive behavior around humans. A normal bird should try to flee. However, some adults will stand their ground and try to protect themselves with their talons, especially if they are guarding or protecting food.
- Normal behavior towards birds of the same species.
- Juveniles of the larger hawk species (such as red-shouldered and red-tailed hawks) will often lie on their keel when stressed or scared. This is normal behavior.
- All juvenile birds must have passed live-prey testing to ensure that they can recognize, catch, and eat appropriate prey (see Chapter 12).

Body condition and overall health

A quick physical exam should always be performed prior to release. This should include:

- Feather evaluation.
- Weight and keel score. Ideally, all birds should be released with a keel score of 3.5–4.0. This gives them a little "buffer" since it may take some time to be re-acclimated into the wild. In addition, birds released in the winter months should have a nice store of fat.
- PCV/TS, if possible.

Release Site, Season, and Time of Day

It is critical that the appropriate site be chosen for release. Ideally, the bird would be taken back to where it was found. Obvious exceptions to this are sites that pose a danger, such as a high-traffic area or if the original injury was due to human activity such as gunshot. Refer to Chapter 3 for the appropriate habitat types for the various species.

It is often difficult to find transport back to the original site for every bird. Therefore, it is critical that new and constantly varying release sites be used. If this is not done, very high local concentrations of birds may result, and this could potentially lead to excessive competition and decreased longevity. Release sites should be recorded and mapped out to avoid overcrowding (Fig. 17.1).

Realize that there is a predator–prey relationship between owls. Therefore, do not release smaller owl species where larger owl species are known to be present in large numbers.

The season can also play an important role in the release. Does this species normally occur in this area at this time of year? This is especially important for highly migratory birds (broad-winged hawks) or those that are sensitive to cold (barn owls, osprey). In these cases, these birds may need to be transported long distances before release or held over winter for release during the next spring.

The time of day is also critical. Owls should always be released at dusk and diurnal birds released during the day. Note that it is not uncommon for released birds to be mobbed by small birds such as crows. Releasing owls at the appropriate time of day can help avoid this problem.

Some other helpful guidelines include:

- Do not release within 200′ (60 m) of barbed wire or electric fences.
- Do not release near busy roads or other high-traffic areas.
- Owls should not be released earlier than 1 h before dusk.
- One bird per location for most species. Vultures are the exception and can be released in groups.
- Avoid releases during major storms and heavy rain. Consider the weather forecast for the next 24 h when releasing small species and slim-bodied species (screech owl, American kestrel, barn owl).
- The safest technique for release is to simply set the carrier/box on the ground and open the top. Grabbing the bird from the box and then releasing makes for a better photo opportunity but represents an increased and unnecessary risk of injury or broken feathers.
- All participants should step away from the box at least 20′ (6 m) and create an open

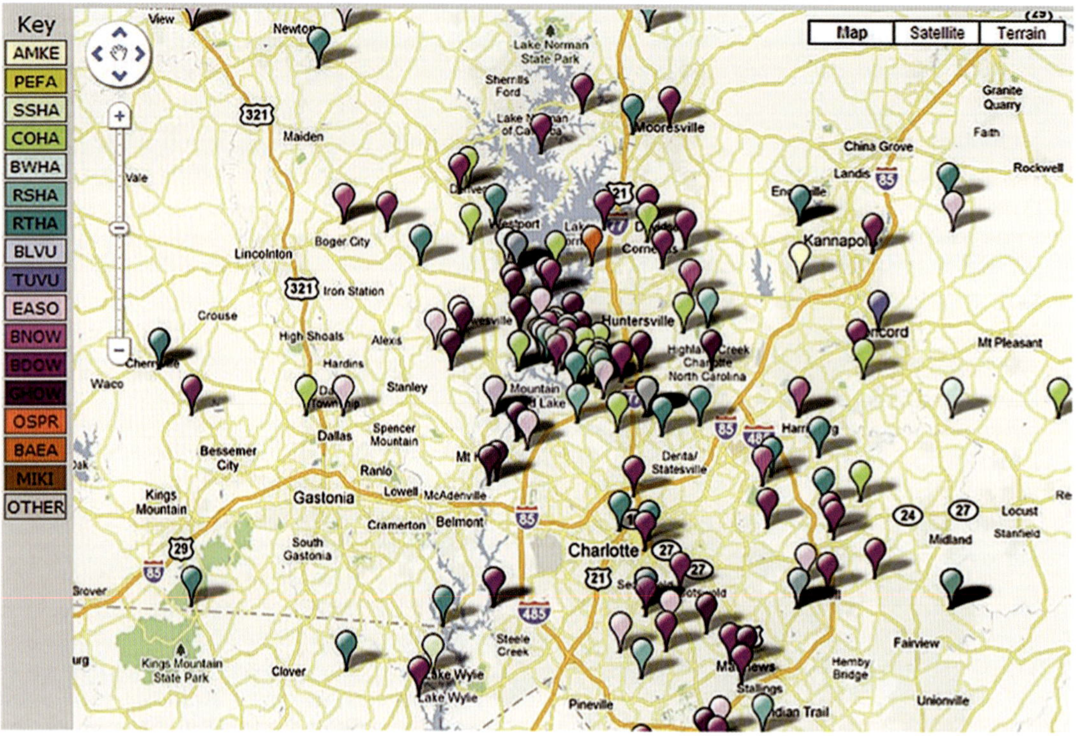

Fig. 17.1. Releases plotted on a Google map. These data were exported from the RaptorMed™ medical records software. Map data © 2015 Google.

lane for the bird to take off into (although the direction of the first flight can be very unpredictable).

Releases Requiring Special Attention

Most birds can simply be transported to a release site in a kennel or cardboard box and let go by opening the door or flaps. There are a few instances, however, where this is not the case.

Juvenile bald eagles and ospreys

These birds are ideally released from a hack tower (an elevated platform in a suitable habitat) (Fig. 17.2). This is very important because it is difficult or impossible to effectively live-prey test the fish-eating species otherwise. The tower provides protection and seclusion for the young bird and allows it to imprint on an appropriate environment. In addition, the tower provides a safe haven for the bird to return to for food while it is learning to hunt. The tower must be designed with food hatches so that people can deliver food without being seen by the bird. The following guidelines are helpful when hacking a bird out:

- Move the bird out to the tower at around 4–6 weeks of age. This is after it is self-feeding but before it is fully feathered and attempting to fly.
- Keep the tower doors closed for 2 weeks while the bird acclimates. Provide fresh food daily and take all appropriate measures to avoid imprinting (see Chapter 12).
- After about 2 weeks, open the doors to allow the bird to start exercising and exploring. Continue to provide fresh food daily until it is clear the bird is no longer returning to eat.

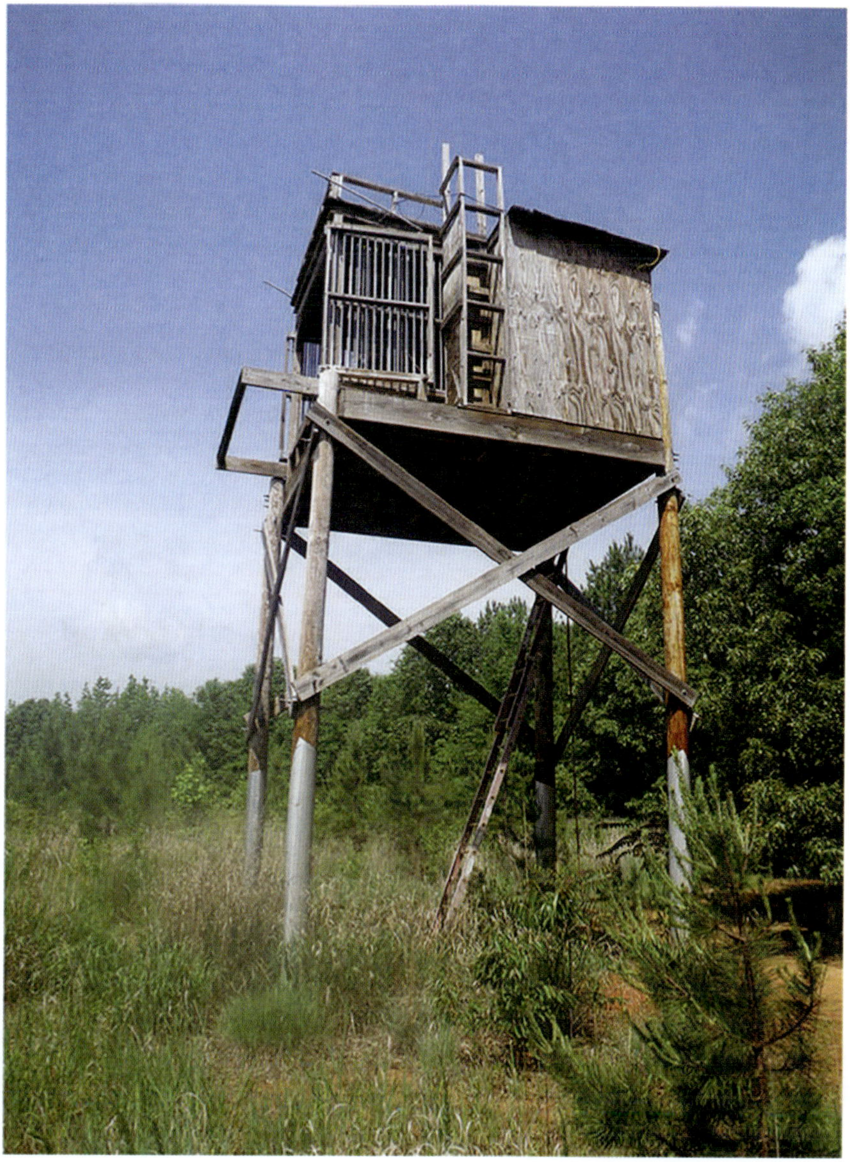

Fig. 17.2. A hack tower with a perch out front. Notice that the front doors are open.

The bird will usually continue to return to the tower for the first 1–2 weeks.

Falcons

Falcons also require special treatment to release and this is due to the way that they hunt in a high-speed stoop. Clearly, it would be impossible to test this hunting behavior in a flight cage or on a creance line. Because of this, any large falcon (such as a peregrine falcon) that has sustained an injury which could affect its flight ability should be transferred to an experienced falconer for proper free-flight evaluation. A falconer can train the bird to a glove and then evaluate its flight and hunting ability. The bird can then be released and will quickly lose any habituation or dependence that may have developed in the process.

Criteria for Non-releasability

There are several types of injuries which rule out release. The most obvious issue is the inability to fly to an acceptable standard. Clearly there is some subjectivity in this criterion, but each bird should be as near-perfect as possible before release can be considered. One rule of thumb: if you can tell the bird has been in rehab from its appearance or flight patterns, then you may need to re-evaluate it before releasing. Some other problems that can make release impossible are given below.

Vision loss

As discussed in Chapter 5, release of one-eyed birds is a judgement call and a matter of great debate. Remember that hawks rely heavily on stereoscopic vision, so loss of vision in an eye is very serious and generally prohibits release. Owls, on the other hand, rely on their sense of hearing as well as vision, so they tolerate the loss of vision in one eye better (Scott, 2013).

Feather condition

Feather damage can easily result when a bird is very jumpy and stressed in captivity. In cases that are otherwise ready for release, the best option is to repair/imp (see Chapter 13) as many feathers as possible and release the bird immediately before further damage is done. Remember that flight ability and sound level (especially in owls) must be carefully evaluated.

Beak issues

Malocclusion of the beak can result from old fractures or trauma to the jaw or the beak itself. If the upper and lower beak do not mesh properly, they will not wear well. Over time, the beak will overgrow, and this will cause serious problems with the ability to feed. Many of these cases are not releasable.

Inability to bear full weight on both feet

This condition will inevitably result in bumblefoot which is invariably a painful and debilitating condition. These birds are not fit for release and are extremely poor candidates for permanent placement. These birds should be euthanized.

Toe/talon loss

Digits 1 and 2 are the most important, and damage to or loss of either makes release impossible (vultures are an exception to this rule). Birds adapt to damage or loss of digits 3 and 4 quite well and release of these birds is generally not a problem. In fact, it is common to admit birds with old, traumatic amputations of digits, so there does seem to be a bit of flexibility when it comes to digit injuries.

Wing droops

There will be the occasional bird that flies well but has a nagging wing droop that just will not go away no matter how long you wait or how much you exercise it. In these cases, it may be acceptable to release these birds if the droop is minor. If the wing droop is severe enough that it drags on the perch or may be stepped on, then release is clearly out of the question since the feathers will eventually become damaged.

Identification Bands

Ideally, all birds are banded prior to release since this can provide very valuable information if and when the bands are eventually recovered. At the Carolina Raptor Center, approximately 20 band reports are received each year. Although the numbers are small and likely statistically insignificant, it can be very informative to receive a band return on a bird with a specific injury that received a specific treatment.

Note that, in the USA, a special banding permit must be obtained from the US Geological Survey (USGS) Bird Banding Lab in order to permanently band birds of prey (Fig. 17.3). Different rules may apply depending on your locale.

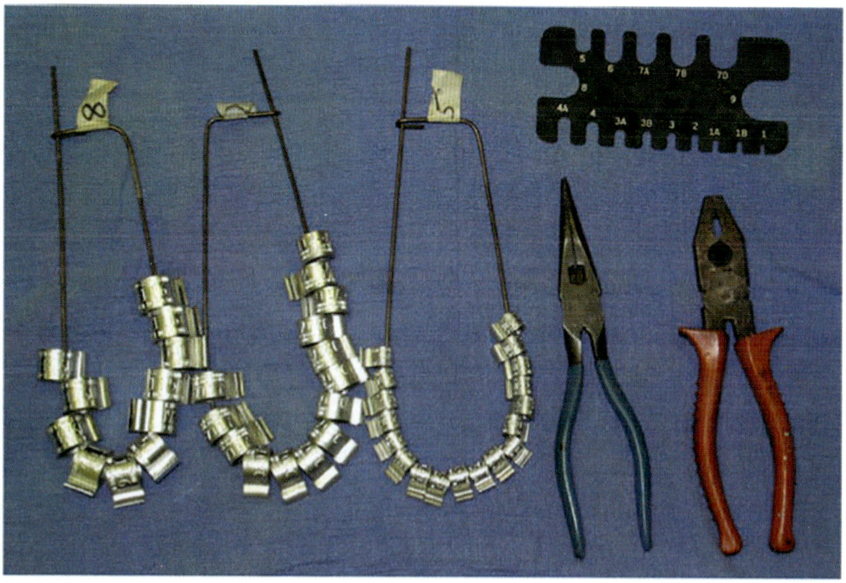

Fig. 17.3. Official USGS permanent bands.

Bibliography

Scott, D. (2013) A retrospective look at the survival of birds of prey released from a rehabilitation center in North Carolina. *Proceedings of the 2013 Association of Avian Veterinarians Annual Conference, Jacksonville, FL, USA*. Association of Avian Veterinarians, Teaneck, NJ, USA, p. 359.

Appendix A: Feeding Guide

The feeding guide in Table A.1 should be used as a starting point for determining how much to feed. It is based on species but realize that there are many factors that will affect what should be considered a proper diet for a specific individual. These factors include:

- Activity level.
- Individual metabolism.
- Individual size. Red-tailed hawks, for example, can range from 800 g in a small male to over 1500 g in a large female. Obviously, they will require a different amount of food.
- Breeding status and sex.
- Time of year/average temperature.
- Injuries and molt status.

It is critically important that the bird's weight be monitored closely and that leftovers are collected and weighed. The amount fed can then be adjusted as needed.

Notes:

1. The amounts listed are for adult birds in a rehabilitation setting. Permanent resident birds will require substantially (20–25%) less, especially if sedentary.
2. All values are in grams except chicks, which are in the number of whole day-old chicks. A typical weight for a chick is approximately 45 g.
3. Quail may be substituted for chicks but can vary widely in weight.
4. Nestlings/orphans should receive 2–3 times the above amounts. Refer to Chapter 12 for more information.

Table A.1. Feeding guide: total daily amount (g).

Species	Rat	Mouse	Day-old chick	Fish
American kestrel		20–30	1	
Bald eagle	350–375			350–375
Barn owl	80–90	80–90	3	
Barred owl	60–70	60–70	2	
Black vulture	150–180	–		
Broad-winged hawk		40–50	2	
Cooper's hawk	Male: 80–90 Female: 100–110	Male: 80–90 Female: 100–110	3	
Eastern screech owl		20–30	1	
Great-horned owl	90–100	90–100	3	
Osprey				200–275
Red-tailed hawk	90–100	90–100	3	
Red-shouldered hawk	60–65	60–65	2	
Sharp-shinned hawk	50–60	50–60	2	
Turkey vulture	200–225	–		

5. Exercising birds should receive amounts at the high end of the ranges.
6. Venison should not be fed more than once a week and should be supplemented with vitamins and calcium.
7. Fish should be supplemented with vitamins such as VitaHawk (DB Scientific, Oakley, CA, USA) to correct for potentially low levels of thiamine.
8. Diurnal birds are fed in the morning or afternoon and nocturnal birds are fed at dusk.

Raptor Tip

Live prey can be used to stimulate anorectic patients to start eating. This is especially useful with red-tailed hawks.

Roadkill

Roadkill can be an excellent source of natural prey food, and squirrels are especially useful. However, it is critical that all roadkill food items be radiographed to look for metallic foreign bodies from previous gunshot, as these may contain lead (Fig. A.1). At Carolina Raptor Center, approximately 30% of the roadkill squirrels received contain previous gunshot fragments and must be discarded.

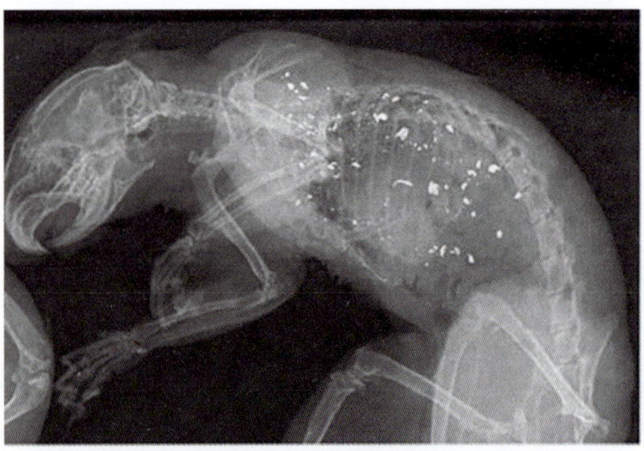

Fig. A.1. A typical roadkill squirrel loaded with metallic foreign bodies resulting from previous gunshot.

Energy Requirement Calculations

The feed amounts in Table A.1 were derived from many years of treating and feeding actual birds and can be used as a starting point when determining your bird's food requirements.

The theoretical amounts can also be calculated by estimating the basal metabolic rate (BMR):

$$\boxed{\mathrm{BMR} = k \times \mathrm{BW}^{0.75}}$$

where BW is in kilograms and $k = 78$ for non-passerines.

The maintenance energy requirement (MER) is the amount of energy required for normal physical activity. It is generally assumed to be:

$$\mathrm{MER} = 1.5 \times \mathrm{BMR}$$

The actual energy requirement for a particular patient depends on the circumstances/injury and is a multiple of the MER (Table A.2). For reference, a typical mouse contains 55–65 kcal of energy.

Table A.2. Energy requirements. (Data from Samour, 2008, p. 179.)

Energy requirement	Multiple of MER
Starvation	0.6
Mild trauma	1.1
Severe trauma	1.5–2.0
Growth	2.5
Sepsis	1.5
Burns	2.0

Example A.1

A 700 g barred owl is admitted with head trauma:

$$BMR = 78 \times 0.7^{0.75} = 60\,kcal/day.$$

$$MER = 1.5 \times 60 = 90\,kcal/day.$$

Assume severe trauma.

$$Energy\ required = 1.5 \times 90 = 135\,kcal/day.$$

$$135/60\,kcal\ per\ mouse = 2.25\ mice\ per\ day.$$

Calcium:Phosphorus Ratio

The Ca:P ratio should be approximately 1.5:1. Some commonly used prey items are low in calcium so supplementation with bonemeal powder is recommended. Raw beef/venison have a particularly poor Ca:P ratio and should never be used as a significant portion of the diet. Mouse and rat "pinkies" are also very poorly balanced and should never be part of a raptor's diet. Skinning a mouse actually improves its ratio, and quail are almost perfectly balanced with respect to Ca and P if eaten whole. Ca:P ratios of commonly available types of food are summarized in Table A.3.

Table A.3. Ca:P ratio. (Data from Chitty, 2008, p. 196.)

Diet	Ratio
Beef	0.05
Rat	1.2
Eviscerated rat	1.33
Mouse	1.38
Day-old chick	1.4
Skinned mouse	1.5
Quail	1.54

Bibliography

Arent, L. (2007) *Raptors in Captivity: Guidelines for Care and Management*. Hancock House Publishing, Surrey, BC, Canada.

Chitty, L. (2008) *BSAVA Manual of Raptors, Pigeons and Passerine Birds*. BSAVA, Gloucester, UK.

Samour, J. (2008) *Avian Medicine*, 2nd edn. Mosby-Elsevier, Philadelphia, PA, USA.

Appendix B: Formulary

Drug dosages were derived from several sources, including those listed in the Bibliography. Many have been used by the author at the Carolina Raptor Center.

Drug	Dosage
Acid citrate dextrose (ACD)	0.15 ml/ml blood for transfusions
Activated charcoal	10–20 ml/kg PO
Adequan	5 mg/kg IM q7d × 4, then monthly as needed
Albon (sulfadimethoxine 12.5%)	25–50 mg/kg PO SID × 3–5 days
Alfaxalone	15 mg/kg IM for sedation (Escalante *et al.*, 2018)
Allopurinol	For hyperuricemia/gout: 10 mg/kg PO BID Toxic in red-tailed hawks at 50 mg/kg
Aminophylline	4 mg/kg PO BID/QID. Prepare suspension with a compounding syrup 10 mg/kg IV/IM TID May have diuretic effects but may not be an effective bronchodilator in birds
Amoxicillin	150 mg/kg PO BID
Amoxicillin with clavulinic acid	125–150 mg/kg PO BID Not metabolized by liver. Good for anaerobes and penetrates lungs well
Amphotericin B	1.5 mg/kg IV TID × 3–5 days. Dilute in largest bolus of D5W possible 1 mg/kg IT TID Not absorbed orally Nebulize 1 mg/mg saline for 15 min BID
Ampicillin	150 mg/kg IM QID
Atropine (0.54 mg/ml)	For organophosphate toxicity: 1.0 mg/kg IM q3–4h In fowl: a dose of **50** mg/kg (yes, fifty!) was effective (Shlosberg *et al.*, 1997) Bradycardia: 0.04–1.0 mg/kg IV/IO. Double dose if IT. Triple dose if IM
Azithromycin	50 mg/kg SID PO × 5 days for *Chlamydophila*
Barium sulfate	25–50 ml/kg via crop gavage. Do not use if perforation is suspected. Take radiographs at 0, ½, 1, 2, and 4 h 20 ml/kg of 60% w/v suspension (Liquid E-Z-Paque®, E-Z-EM Inc., Westbury, NY, USA) Transit time (minutes, for a hawk): crop, 0; ventriculus, 10–15; intestines, 15–120; cloaca, 90–360
Bupivicaine	<2 mg/kg local, can dilute in saline

Continued

Continued.

Drug	Dosage
Buprenorphine	0.1–0.6 mg/kg IM BID, TID (American kestrel: Ceulemans *et al.*, 2014) 0.6 mg/kg IM TID – lasts 6 hours but can cause severe sedation
Butorphanol	1–4 mg/kg IM, IV BID–QID. Not effective PO, SQ
CaEDTA—calcium disodium versenate	35–50 mg/kg SQ SID, BID, 5 days on, 2 days off. Continue for 4 weeks or until blood lead level returns to normal. Can also be given IM but this can be irritating. Tends to chelate from bone predominantly. Can be given in combination with DMSA
Ca glubionate	25 mg/kg PO SID for osteopenia 100 mg/kg PO
Ca gluconate 10% (100 mg/ml)	50–100 mg/kg IV slowly (0.1–1.0 ml/kg) Can also give SQ or IM, if diluted
Ca gluconate 23% (230 mg/ml)	For hypocalcemic seizures, egg binding 5–10 mg/kg IM, SQ BID 50–100 mg/kg slowly IV 1 ml/30 ml H_2O
Carnidazole (Spartrix)	100 mg/kg PO once. May need to repeat dose in falcons (Samour, 2008) 30 mg/kg PO SID × 3 days
Carprofen (Rimadyl)	2–10 mg/kg IV/IM/SQ SID as needed
Cefadroxil	100 mg/kg PO BID × 7 days
Cefatoxime Na	100 mg/kg IM, IV BID
Cefazolin	50–100 mg/kg IM, IV BID, TID
Ceftiofur (Naxcel)	10 mg/kg IM, SQ BID
Ceftriaxone	75–100 mg/kg IM, IV TID, QID
Cephalexin	50 mg/kg PO BID–QID
Cephalothin	30 mg/kg TID 50–100 mg/kg TID
Chloroquine	Erythrocytic forms of malaria For clinical malaria: 15 mg/kg once then 10 mg/kg at 6, 18, 24 h 0.5 ml/kg (25 mg chloroquine + 1.3 mg primaquine) PO q7d × 2
Clindamycin	100 mg/kg PO BID Very good bone penetration. Use for osteomyelitis
Clomipramine	4 mg/kg PO for mutilation/behavior disorder in an ibis
Clotrimazole	Nebulize 10 mg/ml for 30–60 min BID. Mix 1:10 with NaCl Inject 10 mg/kg into air sacs. Can dilute in propylene glycol to 2.5 mg/ml and dose into 4 different air sacs 2 mg/kg IT SID × 5 days (under anesthesia) (10 mg/ml flush)
Colchicine	Anti-fibrotic for chronic liver disease 0.04 mg/kg PO BID Can also be used for hyperuricemia
Deslorelin acetate (Suprelorin)	4.7 mg implant placed SQ between the shoulder blades

Continued

Continued.

Drug	Dosage
Dexamethasone Dox SP	1–4 mg/kg IM once Single dose 2–4 mg/kg IM for eye trauma
Dextrose 50%	50–100 mg/kg IV slowly (0.1–0.2 ml/kg) 1.0 ml/kg IV slowly for sepsis or hypoglycemia
Diazepam	For seizures: 0.5–1.0 mg/kg IV, IO, IM/cloacally × 3 Painful and unpredictable IM. Midazolam is better
Dimercaptosuccinic acid (DMSA)	25–35 mg/kg PO BID Can be given in combination with CaEDTA. Tends to chelate from soft tissues predominantly
Diphenhydramine	1–4 mg/kg PO, IO, IV, IM BID, TID
Doxapram	5–10 mg/kg IV, IM, SQ for apnea
Doxycycline	25–50 mg/kg IV, PO SID (not IM) 25 mg/kg PO BID For *Hemoproteus/Leukocytozoon*: 12 mg/kg BID for 2 weeks For *Chlamydophila*: 50–75 mg/kg PO BID × 45 days 35 mg/kg PO SID × 21 days (Guzman *et al.*, 2010)
Enrofloxacin	15 mg/kg BID, 25 mg/kg SID PO or SQ into fluid pocket. Do not use IM Do not use in young, developing birds
Epinephrine	0.5 mg/kg IV, IO, IT, IC For 1:1000: 0.5 ml/kg Topical: 0.1–0.2 mg/kg of 1:10,000
F10	Nebulize or apply topically at dilution of 1:250 in saline
Fenbendazole	25 mg/kg either once or SID for 3–5 days Ascarids: 2× q10d *Capillaria*, flukes: 25 mg/kg PO SID × 5 days *Syngamus*: 20 mg/kg PO SID × 14 days Possible toxicity in vultures? Possible feather damage in young birds? Can cause bone marrow suppression (leukopenia)
Fipronil (Frontline)	Use spray, not top spot Max. 3 ml/kg Apply to featherless areas (keel, abdomen, axillas, leg web, between scapulas) and behind the ears
Fluconazole	10 mg/kg load then 5 mg/kg In cockatiels: 5 mg/kg PO q24h or 10 mg/kg PO q48h. Compound with deionized water and Ora-Plus® (Perrigo, Dublin, Republic of Ireland) then vortex mix. Stable in refrigerator for 14 days (Ratzlaff *et al.*, 2011)
Flumazenil	0.05 mg/kg to antagonize midazolam
Flunixin/Banamine	1.5 mg/kg IM 5 mg/kg Do not use in ducks
Furosemide	102 mg/kg SID to QID as needed
Gabapentin	10 mg/kg BID PO

Continued

Continued.

Drug	Dosage
Glucosamine	35 mg/kg SID then 2–3 times weekly for maintenance 100 mg/kg PO SID × 6 weeks, then 50 mg/kg PO SID Cosequin Feline contains 125 mg glucosamine
Haloperidol	Feather picking: 0.4 mg/kg SID for 7 months
Heparin (1:1000)	For flush: 1.75 ml to 250 ml NaCl Draw into a 3 ml syringe to coat the inner surface. Then push it all out and refill syringe with NaCl
Hetastarch	5 ml/kg + LRS 15 ml/kg IV
Hyaluranidase	75–150 units/l LRS SQ to aid in absorption
Iohexol	20 ml/kg PO
Iron Dextran	10 mg/kg IM q7–10d
Isoxsuprine	5–10 mg/kg/day
Itraconazole	10 mg/kg PO BID 10 mg/kg PO SID, BID prophylactic × 21 days 10–15 mg/kg BID therapeutic
Ivermectin	0.2–0.4 mg/kg PO, IM, SQ once or q7d, undiluted Dilute as follows for smaller birds: 0.1 ml 1% + 0.9 ml propylene glycol = 1 mg/ml 1 mg/kg SQ single dose for *Capillaria* 2–3 mg/kg IM/SQ for *Syngamus/Serratospiculum* **CAUTION**: 3 mg/kg is toxic in falcons (temporary blindness, vomiting, ataxia). 1 mg/kg is ok
Ketamine/Medetomidine	3 mg/kg ketamine + 0.06 mg/kg medetomidine IM for premedication/ induction prior to isoflurane Reverse with atipamezole: 0.15 mg/kg IM. May substitute dexmedetomidine if medetomidine is unavailable
Ketoconazole	10–30 mg/kg PO BID *Candida*: 15 mg/kg BID for 7–14 days, then recheck (cytology, culture)
Lactulose	200 mg/kg PO BID 0.2–0.5 ml/kg PO BID
Leuprolide acetate (Leupron)	750 µg/kg IM. Twice at 2-week intervals to suppress ovarian activity and follicular maturation. Can also use Suprelorin (deslorelin acetate) implant
Levothyroxine	To stimulate molt: 25 µg/kg SID × 7 days 50 µg/kg SID × 7 days 75 µg/kg SID × 7 days 50 µg/kg SID × 7 days 25 µg/kg SID × 7 days Or can use whole bovine thyroid gland: 15 g/kg SID for 3–5 days 0.02 mg/kg PO SID, BID
Lidocaine	<2.5 mg/kg local, can dilute in saline For 2%: 0.1 ml/kg For local block: 5 mg/kg + 0.3 ml NaCl. Lasts 2–4 h (shorter than bupivicaine) but has quicker onset (5 min versus 15 min)

Continued

Continued.

Drug	Dosage
Magnesium sulfate (Epsom salts)	0.5–1 g/kg SID for 1–3 days. Acts as a cathartic and helps precipitate lead
Mannitol	500 mg/kg slow (over 20 min) IV q8h × 3. Followed by crystalloids for diuresis. Only effective in first 24 h Intermittent boluses are better than a constant rate infusion. Crystallizes at room temperature. Store in a warmer or incubator
Mefloquine (Larium)	30 mg/kg PO BID × 1 day, then SID × 2 days, then q7d for 6 months 50 mg/kg PO SID × 7 days
Meloxicam (Metacam)	0.5–1.0 mg/kg PO, IM BID 2 mg/kg PO BID safe and effective in pigeons. 0.5 mg/kg was not effective (Desmarchelier *et al.*, 2012) Use higher doses (1–2 mg/kg BID) for WNV
Methylprednisone acetate (Depo Medrol 40 mg/ml)	5 mg/kg. For joint injections
Metoclopramide	0.5–2.0 mg/kg IM, IV SID–TID
Metronidazole	50 mg/kg PO SID, BID for 5–30 days. Use carnidazole for *Trichomonas* infections
Midazolam	0.5–1.0 mg/kg IM, IV q8–12h 0.5–1.25 mg/kg IM for pre-anesthetic 2 mg/kg intranasally for sedation (Mans *et al.*, 2012) 0.6 mg/kg intranasally
Milk thistle	Liver protective: 30–50 mg/kg PO TID
Mineral oil	6–10 ml/kg PO BID, TID via tube as a laxative to aid in the removal of GI foreign bodies
Nalbuphine	12.5 mg/kg IM q4h. Effects can last up to 3 h
Nitenpyram (Capstar)	Can use topically in maggot-infested wounds. Dilute a 57 mg tablet with 60 ml water and apply liberally with spray bottle. Can also give ½ tablet orally for 1 kg bird
Nystatin 100,000 IU/ml	300,000 IU/kg PO 2–3 ml/kg BID for 7 days Not absorbed orally
Orbifloxacin	15–20 mg/kg PO SID
Oxyglobin	5–15 ml/kg IV/IO PRN slow bolus (over 20 min) usually preceded by LRS 15 ml/kg
Peanut oil	For catharsis: 1 ml/100 g (metallic foreign bodies)
Pentoxyfilline	For peripheral vasodilation: 5 mg/kg PO BID
Permethrin spray	Insecticide that is safe for birds. Use for environmental control
Piperazine	100 mg/kg
Pipericillin	100 mg/kg IM BID, TID
Ponazuril (Marquis)	20 mg/kg PO SID for *Sarcocystis* Also effective against other Coccidias
Pralidoxime, 2-PAM	For organophosphorus toxicosis: 100 mg/kg IM. Must be given within 24 h of exposure May be toxic in raptors?

Continued

Continued.

Drug	Dosage
Praziquantal	10–20 mg/kg IM, PO, SQ q7–10d × 2
Prednisone	2 mg/kg PO BID
Primaquine	Tissue forms of malaria 0.03 mg/kg PO SID × 3 days Redig: 0.75–1.0 mg/kg
Psyllium	Hydrophobic fiber solution. Used to lavage/evacuate the stomach to remove foreign bodies
Pyrantel	4.5 mg/kg PO q10d × 2 20 mg/kg PO once
Pyrethrin	0.15% topical spray
Selamectin	For mange: 23 mg/kg topically q30d × 2 (Sadar *et al.*, 2015)
Sertaline	1.5 mg/kg PO SID for feather picking
Sucralfate	25 mg/kg PO TID, post-op × 7 days
Sulfamethazine	For coccidia: not effective any more 50–65 mg per pigeon PO × 3 days. Repeat in 3 days or treat for 5 days
Terbinafine	10–15 mg/kg PO BID, can combine with itraconazole. Can be dissolved in water 15 mg/kg PO SID in penguins (Bechert *et al.*, 2010a) 22 mg/kg PO SID in red-tailed hawks (Bechert *et al.*, 2010b)
Terbutaline	Effective bronchodilator in birds 0.1 mg/kg PO SID, BID 0.01 mg/kg IM BID–QID
Thyroid gland (fresh beef gland)	Molt induced in penguins. 10 g/kg PO SID. Molt complete in 18–26 days (Webster *et al.*, 2016)
Toltazuril (Baycox 2.5%)	For coccidiosis: 25 mg/kg PO weekly × 3 Mix with soda to neutralize high pH and reduce vomiting
Tramadol	5 mg/kg PO BID (bald eagle; Souza *et al.*, 2009) 30 mg/kg PO BID/TID/QID (parrot; Sanchez-Migallon Guzman *et al.*, 2012; Souza *et al.*, 2013) 5 mg/kg IV/IM Can make a suspension by crushing the tablets, mixing with glycerin to make a paste, and diluting to the required concentration with water Dosage is very species-specific and effectiveness is variable
Trimethoprim/Sulfadiazine (Tribrissen, DiTrim)	50 mg/kg PO BID Coccidia: 60 mg/kg combined BID PO; 3 days on, 2 off, 3 on
Trimethoprim/Sulfamthox-azole	50 mg/kg PO BID Penetrates lungs and bone well
Ursodeoxycholic acid	Can help decrease liver damage (antioxidant?)
Vitamins A, D, E	Vitamin A: 30,000 IU/kg IM Vitamin D: 3000 IU/kg IM Vitamin E: 3000 IU/kg IM Vitamins A, D, E (Injacom 100, Hoffman-La Roche, Nutley, NY, USA): 0.5 ml/kg q7d Vitamins A, D: 0.06 ml/kg Can also use oral β-carotene

Drug	Dosage
Vitamin B_1 (thiamine) 12.5 mg/ml in B-complex 200 mg/ml thiamine only	1–3 mg/kg (0.1–0.3 ml/kg) SQ, IV, IM q7d For neurologic cases: 25 mg/kg IM SID for 3–5 days. Use more concentrated formulation
Vitamin C	100–150 mg/kg
Vitamin-B complex	0.06 mg/kg SQ/IM
Vitamin D	For egg binding see Vitamins A, D, E
Vitamin K_1	2.5 mg/kg SQ, IM BID for 3–4 days, then PO SID for 4 weeks 2.5 mg/kg IM SID until stable, then q7d (Carpenter *et al.*, 2001) 5 mg/kg IM BID for second-generation rodenticides In general, treat at high dose for 1 week for warfarin and at least 2 weeks for brodifacoum
Voriconazole	12.5 mg/kg PO BID × 21 days

Bibliography

Altman, R.B., Clubb, S.L., Dorrestein, G.M. and Quesenberry, K. (1997) *Avian Medicine and Surgery*. W.B. Saunders Company, Philadelphia, PA, USA.

Bechert, U., Christensen, J.M., Poppenga, R., Le, H., Wyatt, J. and Schmitt, T. (2010a) Pharmacokinetics of orally administered terbinafine in African penguins (*Spheniscus demersus*) for potential treatment of aspergillosis. *Journal of Zoo and Wildlife Medicine* 41(2), 263–274.

Bechert, U., Christensen, J.M., Poppenga, R., Fahmy, S.A. and Redig, P. (2010b) Pharmacokinetics of terbinafine after single oral dose administration in red-tailed hawks (*Buteo jamaicensis*). *Journal of Avian Medicine and Surgery* 24(2), 122–130.

Carpenter, J., Mashima, T. and Rupiper, D. (2001) *Exotic Animal Formulary*, 2nd edn. W.B. Saunders Company, Philadelphia, PA, USA.

Carpenter, J.W. (2012) *Exotic Animal Formulary*, 4th edn. W.B. Saunders Company, Philadelphia, PA, USA.

Ceulemans, S.M., Guzman, D.S., Olsen, G.H., Beaufrère, H. and Paul-Murphy, J.R. (2014) Evaluation of thermal antinociceptive effects after intramuscular administration of buprenorphine hydrochloride to American kestrels (*Falco sparverius*). *American Journal of Veterinary Research* 75(8), 705–710.

Chitty, L. (2008) *BSAVA Manual of Raptors, Pigeons and Passerine Birds*. BSAVA, Gloucester, UK.

Desmarchelier, M., Troncy, E., Fitzgerald, G. and Lair, S. (2012) Analgesic effects of meloxicam administration on postoperative orthopedic pain in domestic pigeons (*Columba livia*). *American Journal of Veterinary Research* 73(3), 361–367.

Escalante, G.C., Balko, J.A. and Chinnadurai, S.K. (2018) Comparison of the sedative effects of alfaxalone and butorphanol-midazolam administered intramuscularly in budgerigars (*Melopsittacus undulatus*). *Journal of Avian Medicine and Surgery* 32(4), 279–285.

Guzman, D.S., Diaz-Figueroa, O., Tully, T. Jr, Ciembor, P., Morgan, T., Walden, M., *et al.* (2010) Evaluating 21-day doxycycline and azithromycin treatments for experimental *Chlamydophila psittaci* infection in cockatiels (*Nymphicus hollandicus*). *Journal of Avian Medicine and Surgery* 24(1), 35–45.

Mans, C., Guzman, D.S., Lahner, L.L., Paul-Murphy, J. and Sladky, K.K. (2012) Sedation and physiologic response to manual restraint after intranasal administration of midazolam in Hispaniolan Amazon parrots (*Amazona ventralis*). *Journal of Avian Medicine and Surgery* 26(3), 130–139.

Ratzlaff, K., Papich, M.G. and Flammer, K. (2011) Plasma concentrations of fluconazole after a single oral dose and administration in drinking water in cockatiels (*Nymphicus hollandicus*). *Journal of Avian Medicine and Surgery* 25(1), 23–31.

Ritchie, B.W., Harrison, G.J. and Harrison, L.R. (1994) *Avian Medicine: Principles and Application*. Wingers Publishing, Inc., Lake Worth, FL, USA.

Sadar, M.J., Sanchez-Migallon Guzman, D., Mete, A., Foley, J., Stephenson, N., Rogers, K.H., *et al.* (2015) Mange caused by a novel *Micnemidocoptes* mite in a golden eagle (*Aquila chyrsaetos*). *Journal of Avian Medicine and Surgery* 29(3), 231–237.

Samour, J. (2008) *Avian Medicine*, 2nd edn. Mosby-Elsevier, Maryland Heights, MO, USA.

Sanchez-Migallon Guzman, D., Souza, M.J., Braun, J.M., Cox, S.K., Keuler, N.S. and Paul-Murphy, J.R. (2012) Antinociceptive effects after oral administration of tramadol hydrochloride in Hispaniolan Amazon parrots (*Amazona ventralis*). *American Journal of Veterinary Research* 73(8), 1148–112.

Shlosberg, A., Bellaiche, M., Hanji, V. and Ershov, E. (1997) New treatment regimens in organophosphate (diazinon) and carbamate (methomyl) insecticide-induced toxicosis in fowl. *Veterinary and Human Toxicology* 39(6), 347–350.

Souza, M.J., Martin-Jimenez, T., Jones, M.P. and Cox, S.K. (2009) Pharmacokinetics of oral and intravenous tramadol in bald eagles. *Journal of Avian Medicine and Surgery* 23(4), 247–252.

Souza, M.J., Gerhardt, L. and Cox, S. (2013) Pharmacokinetics of repeated oral administration of tramadol hydrochloride in Hispaniolan Amazon parrots (*Amazona ventralis*). *American Journal of Veterinary Research* 74(7), 957–962.

Webster, R.K.E., Aguilar, R.F., Argandona-Gonzalez, A.-K., Conayne, P., De Sousa, D., Sriram, A., *et al.* (2016) Forced molt in four juvenile yellow-eyed penguins (*Megadyptes antipodes*). *Journal of Wildlife Diseases* 52(4), 809–816.

Appendix C: Anesthetic Record

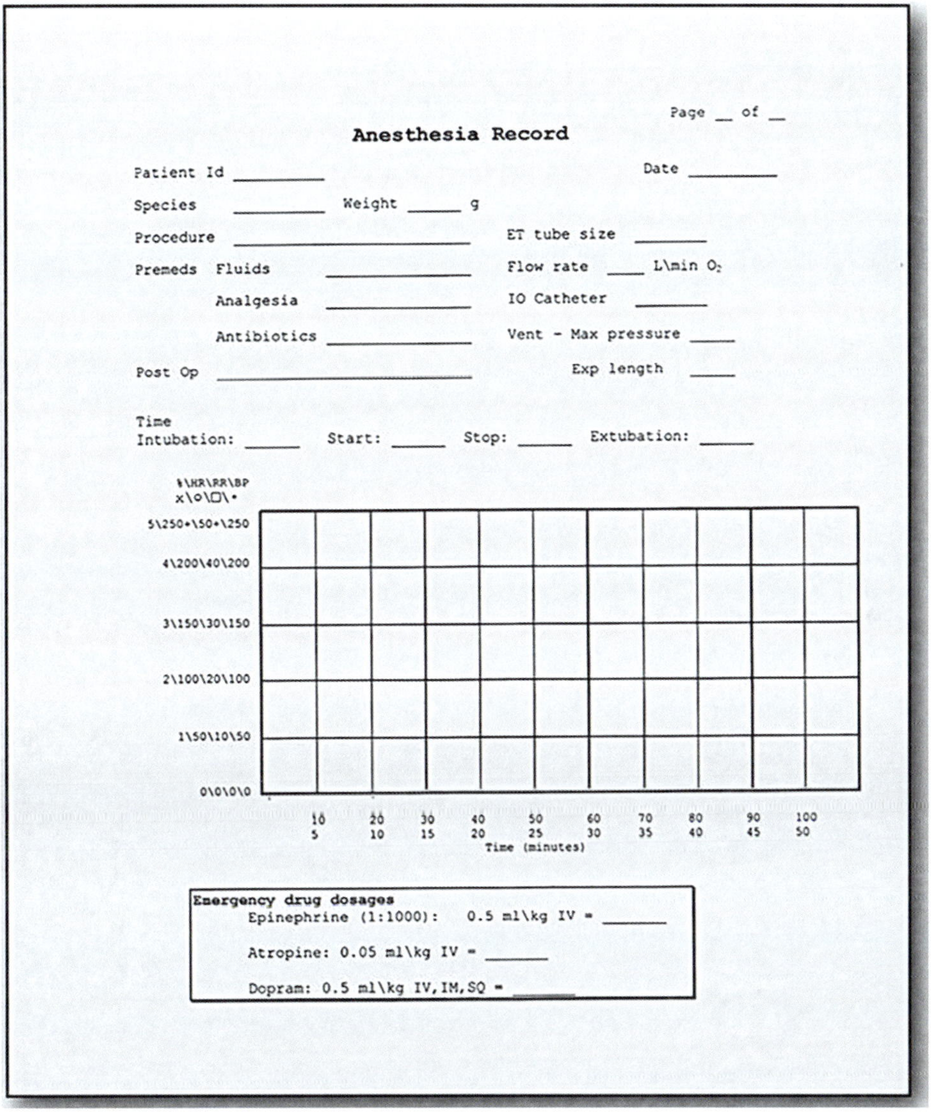

Page __ of __

Anesthesia Record

Patient Id ________ Date ________

Species ________ Weight _____ g

Procedure ______________________ ET tube size ______

Premeds Fluids ____________ Flow rate ___ L\min O_2

Analgesia ____________ IO Catheter ______

Antibiotics ____________ Vent - Max pressure ___

Post Op ______________________ Exp length ____

Time
Intubation: _____ Start: _____ Stop: _____ Extubation: _____

Emergency drug dosages
Epinephrine (1:1000): 0.5 ml\kg IV = ______
Atropine: 0.05 ml\kg IV = ______
Dopram: 0.5 ml\kg IV,IM,SQ = ______

Appendix D: Wrapper Patterns

Velcro® (Velcro® USA Inc., Manchester, NH, USA) wrappers are very useful for restraint since the wings are effectively immobilized in a comfortable position after the bird is slid into the wrapper and the Velcro® is secured. There are three types of wrappers:

- Open-ended body wrappers. These are useful for eye examinations and for force-feeding, or when carrying and weighing larger birds such as vultures or eagles.
- Closed-ended body wrappers. These do not allow for good air flow so should only be used for very short periods (i.e. 10–15 s) but are very useful when weighing birds. The bird is slid into the wrapper, the Velcro® is secured, and the bird is placed on its back on the scale (Fig. D.1).
- Wing wrappers. These are great as a replacement for the traditional elastic wrap figure-8 bandage and are especially useful when there are feathers in blood, since these wraps allow the feathers to continue to grow and slide underneath. They are reusable, can be applied and removed quickly, and save on the use of bandage material. They can also be placed over a normal figure-8 bandage to help protect it from the bird picking at it. Duct tape should be placed over the Velcro® to prevent the bird from removing the wrapper. See Figs 4.13, 4.14, and 8.3.

Materials

- Light- to medium-weight canvas, pre-washed.
- Binding/piping (to attach to all cut edges to prevent unraveling).
- Velcro® strips.

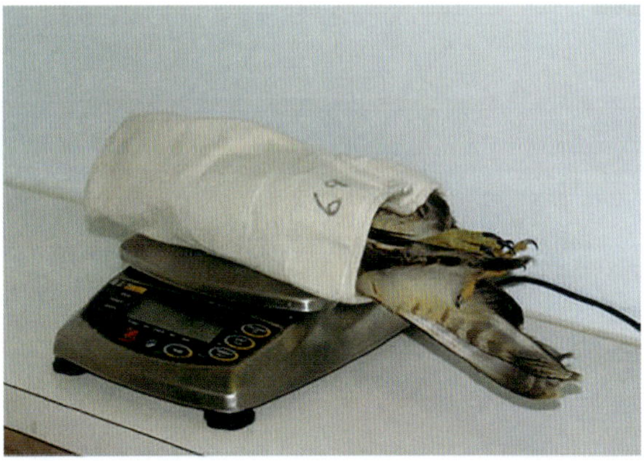

Fig. D.1. A closed-ended wrapper being used when weighing a red-shouldered hawk.

Patterns and Dimensions

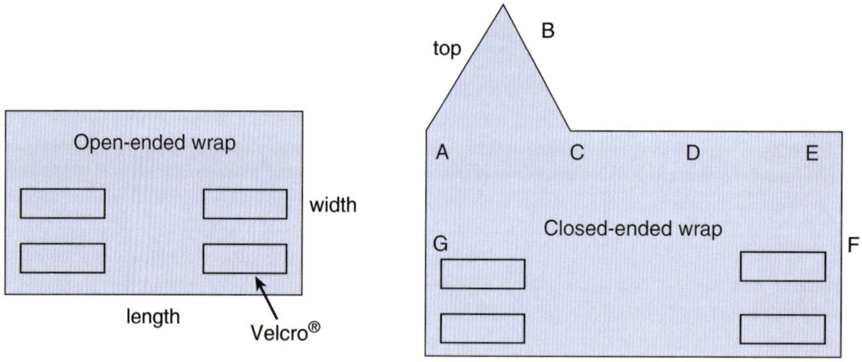

Fig. D.2. Body wrapper patterns. For the closed wrap, fold so that B meets D, A meets E, and F meets G. Sew together along edges from C to B/D to A/E to G/F.

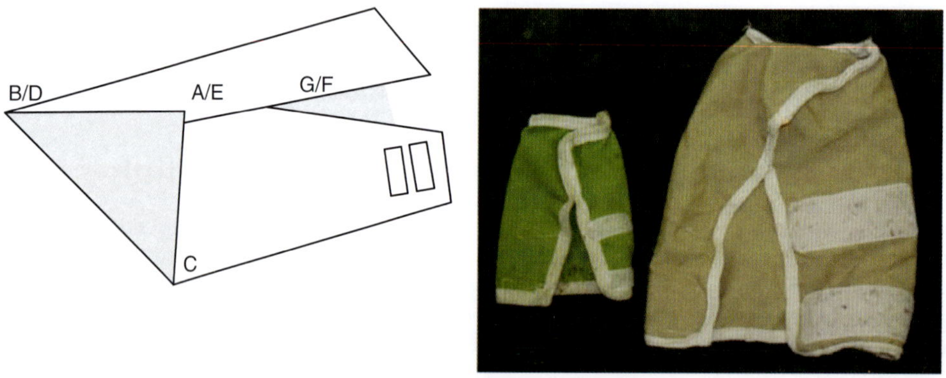

Fig. D.3. Completed closed-end wrappers.

Table D.1. Dimensions in inches (centimeters) for open and closed-end body wrappers.

Wrapper size	Species	Width, " (cm)	Length, " (cm)	Top, " (cm)	Velcro® pieces, " (cm)
Small	American kestrel, eastern screech owl	7 (18)	10.5 (27)	3.5 (9)	1 × 2 (2.5 × 5)
Medium	Cooper's hawk, barn owl, broad-winged hawk	8 (20)	14 (36)	4.5 (11)	2 × 2 (5 × 5)
Large	Barred owl, red-shouldered hawk, red-tailed hawk	12 (30)	19.5 (50)	6.5 (16)	2 × 4 (5 × 10)
XL	Great-horned owl, red-tailed hawk	14 (36)	24 (61)	8 (20)	2 × 5 (5 × 12)
XXL	Vultures, eagles	19 (48)	30 (76)	10 (25)	2 × 6 (5 ×16)

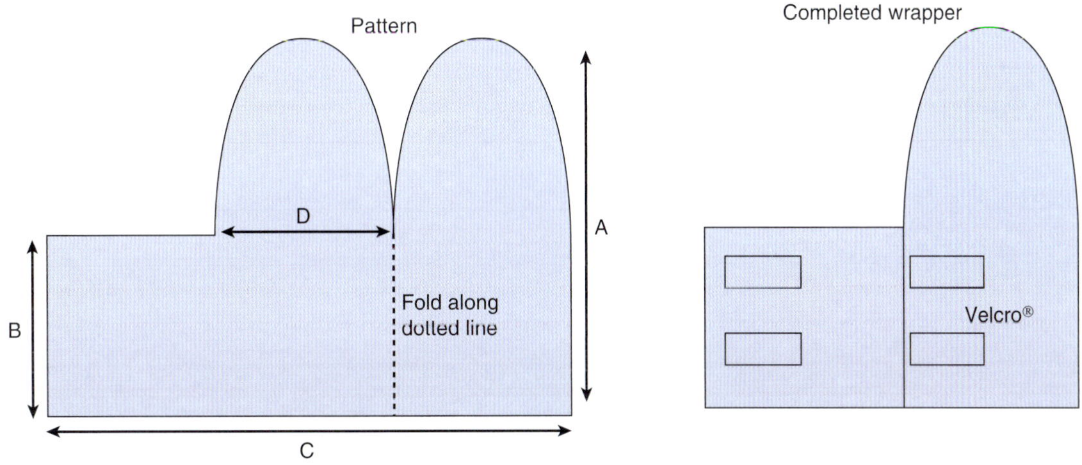

Fig. D.4. Wing wrapper pattern.

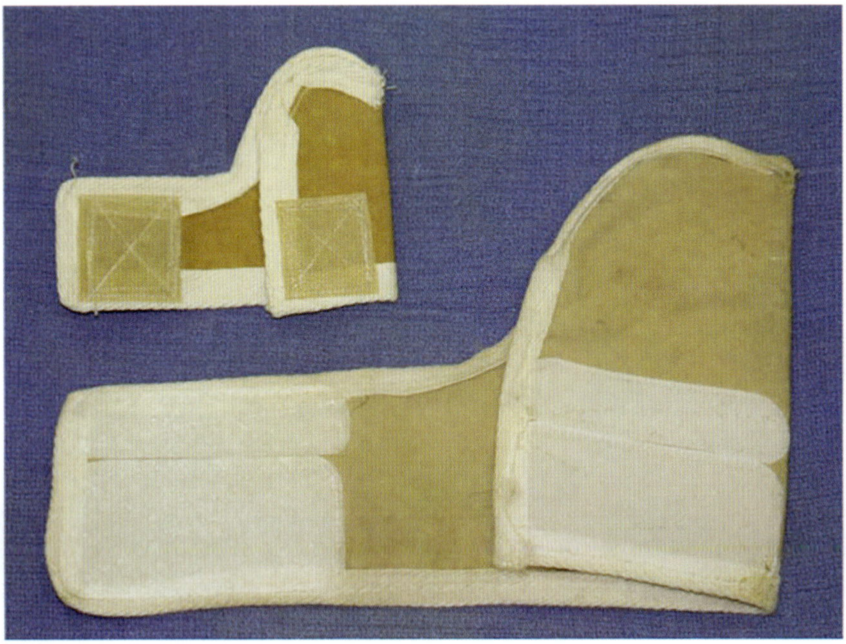

Fig. D.5. Completed wing wrappers.

Table D.2. Dimensions in inches (centimeters) for wing wrappers.

Wrapper size	A, " (cm)	B, " (cm)	C, " (cm)	D, " (cm)
Small	3.5–4 (9–10)	1.5–2 (4–5)	4.5–5 (11–12)	2 (5)
Medium	5 (12)	2.5–3 (6–7)	7.5 (19)	3 (6)
Large	7 (18)	3–3.5 (7–9)	11 (28)	4 (10)

Appendix E: Laws and Regulations

The following laws and treaties are relevant to the process of rehabilitation and for obtaining a permit. Each country may have similar laws and regulations so it is important to familiarize yourself with the local laws.

USA

In the USA, federal and state laws require individuals to be licensed in order to rehabilitate wildlife. Federal permits are granted by the US Fish and Wildlife Service (USFWS) and each state also has a Department of Natural Resources that performs a similar function.

In general, it is illegal to attempt to rehabilitate a wild animal without the proper permits. However, veterinarians are allowed to treat injured wildlife legally as long as they transfer the animal to a licensed rehabilitator as soon as it is stable enough for transfer.

A USFWS web page[1] has information about obtaining a rehabilitation permit, and the National Wildlife Rehabilitators Association (NWRA) website[2] has additional information that may be useful.

Migratory Bird Treaty Act (MBTA)

Established in 1918 and expanded over the years in cooperation with other nations. The law makes it illegal for people to "take" migratory birds, their eggs, feathers, or nests. In effect, it is illegal to possess any part of a live or dead migratory bird without a permit. All birds of prey are protected under this law.

Bald and Golden Eagle Protection Act

This law provides additional protections for eagles.

UK

In the UK, the following pieces of legislation and organizations are important:

- The Animals Act of 1971 provides for civil liability for damage done to animals.
- The Wildlife and Countryside Act of 1981 provides various protections for species of special concern.
- The Animal Welfare Act of 2006 provides minimum guidelines for the proper care and overall welfare of any captive animal.
- British Wildlife Rehabilitation Council[3] (BWRC) provides resources to promote the welfare of injured wildlife.

International

- The International Wildlife Rehabilitation Council[4] (IWRC).

[1] https://www.fws.gov/permits/#MBTA (accessed June 2020).
[2] www.nwrawildlife.org (accessed June 2020).
[3] www.bwrc.org.uk (accessed June 2020).
[4] www.theiwrc.org (accessed June 2020).

- International Association for Falconry and Conservation of Birds of Prey[5] (IAF).
- Convention on International Trade in Endangered Species of Wildlife and Flora[6] (CITES) is an international agreement between governments. Its aim is to ensure that international trade in specimens of wild animals and plants does not threaten their survival.

[5]https://iaf.org/ (accessed June 2020).
[6]www.cites.org (accessed June 2020).

Appendix F: Body Weights during Development

Species	Hatch	Weeks								3 months
		1	2	3	4	5	6	7	8	
Barn owl	15–20	25–30	90–100	250–300	450–500	550–600	650–700	600+	600+	500+
Barred owl	30–40	100–150	250–300	400–450	525–575	550–600	575–650	600+	600+	600+
Black vulture	75–85	100–200	275–375	600–800	950–1200	1300–1500	1600–1800	1900+	2000+	2100+
Eastern screech owl	UNK	25–30	50–70	100–110	110–120	130–140	140+	140+	140+	140+
Red-shouldered hawk	30–40	30–40	30–70	175–275	350–450	400–600	450+	450+	450+	450+
Turkey vulture	UNK	100–150	300–400	750–850	1100–1200	1500+	1500+	1500+	1500+	1500+

All data collected from the RaptorMed™ database at Carolina Raptor Center and compiled by Carly Smith.
All weights are in grams.
UNK, unknown.

Appendix G: Building a Nest

Artificial nests can be made from many materials, but nests woven from actual foliage are ideal as they look natural and the parents may be more likely to return to a more natural-looking nest. In addition, a landowner may be more likely to allow a natural-looking nest to be placed in a tree on his or her property. Finally, since they are all natural, they will eventually degrade and come down without a future visit.

1. The ideal plant for nest weaving has long, straight, slender shoots or branches (Fig. G.1). In the southeast United States, an invasive bush called the autumn olive (*Elaeagnus umbellate*) or the Russian olive (*Elaeagnus angustifolia*), or even Kudzu vines work well.

2. Tools and materials (Fig. G.2):

- **a.** 80 to 120 thin shoots or branches.
- **b.** Three thicker branches 3–5′ (1–1.5 m) in length and about ½″ (1 cm) in diameter. These will form the main ribs of the nest.
- **c.** Pruning shears.
- **d.** Twine.

3. Cut the three ribs to the same length and gently bend one end about ⅓ from the end. The bend will not stay but your goal is to weaken the end so it can be bent easily later.

4. Bind the three ribs with twine and fan them out so they are equally spaced in a star pattern (Fig. G.3).

5. The three ribs are now bent up to form a bowl shape. Opposite branches are bound together with twine to maintain the bowl (Fig. G.4).

6. Weave the floor of the nest with the thinner shoots (Fig. G.5a). The weave should be dense enough so there are no larger holes that a bird could slip through. It may be helpful to turn the nest upside-down when weaving (Fig. G.5b). Be sure to remove any thorns or sharp points.

7. Bind the weave with twine, especially the shoots and branches near the rim (Fig. G.6).

8. Keep the twine that is binding the larger branches into the bowl shape in place for 3–5 days. Then you can remove the twine and the nest should retain its shape (Fig. G.7). When installing in a tree, use biodegradable rope and make sure the rope passes through and around the three ribs. A carefully placed nail and bailing wire can also be useful. Each installation is unique so you may need to improvise a bit.

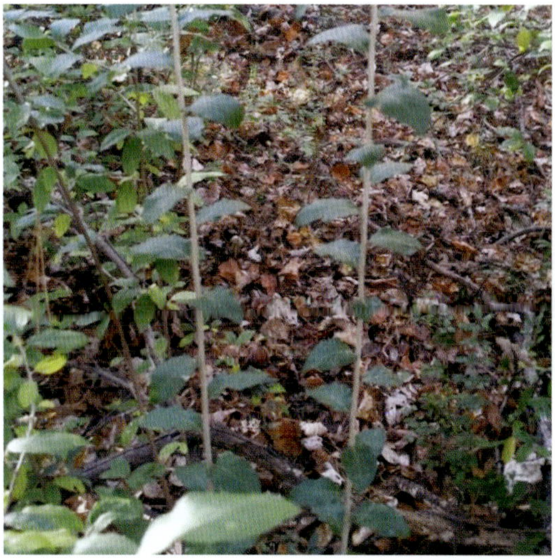

Fig. G.1. Slender, straight shoots or branches are great for nest weaving.

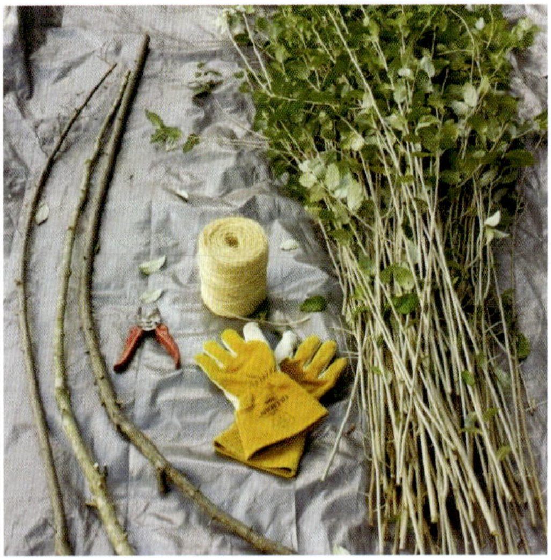

Fig. G.2. Materials for nest building.

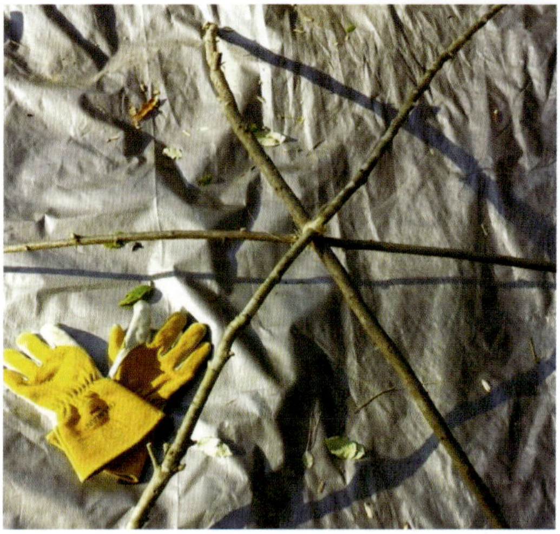

Fig. G.3. Bind the three ribs together.

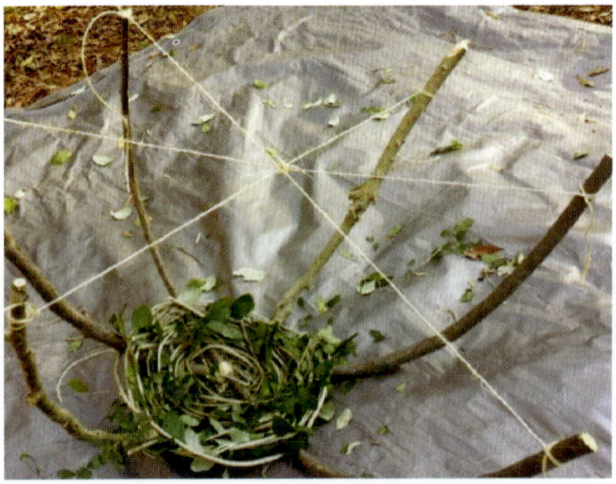

Fig. G.4. The three ribs are bent into a bowl shape.

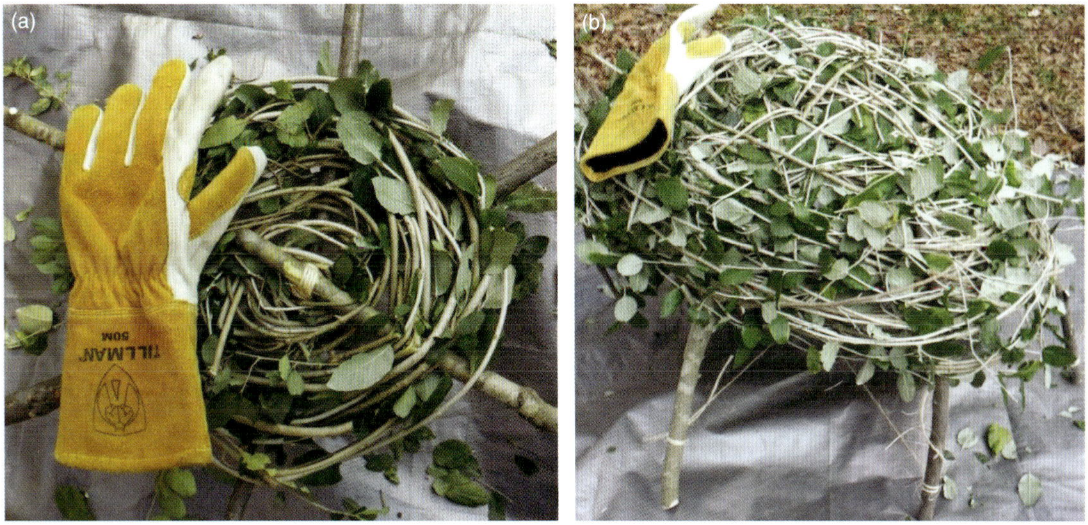

Fig. G.5. Weave the shoots between the three main ribs (a). Weaving can be easier with the nest upside-down (b).

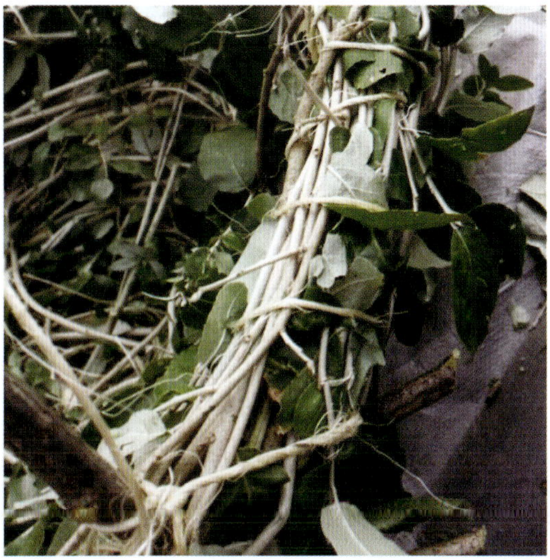

Fig. G.6. Bind the weave with twine.

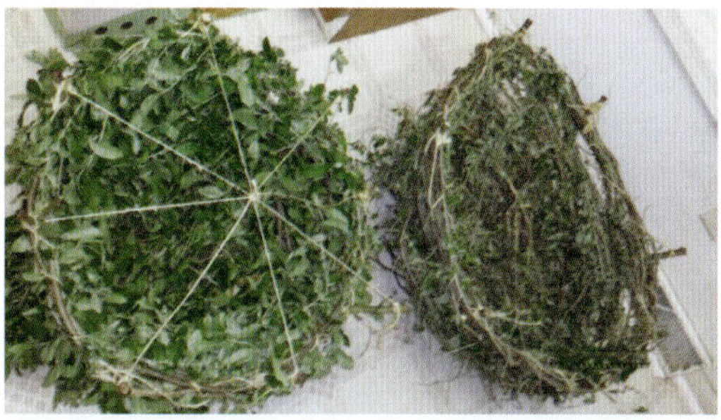

Fig. G.7. The finished product. The nest on the left was just finished and needs to sit for a few days before the twine can be removed.

Appendix H: Feeding Puppets

Feeding puppets are very helpful when caring for nestlings. At this age, they are usually fed by their parents and this exposes them to important sensory cues that allows for normal development. Failure to receive the proper cues can lead to mal-imprinting and a non-releasable bird. Using puppets is recommended whenever you must have contact with a young bird, whether they are being fed or not. Acquiring species-specific puppets is crucial but you may need to obtain special permits in order to create and own these puppets.

Puppets are created from fresh cadavers. The cadaver is skinned from around the mid-abdomen up towards the head. The entire thorax, abdomen, and legs are discarded. The harvested section is then wrapped around an appropriate-sized plastic beverage bottle. The bottle acts as a form to maintain the puppet's shape, and also provides an easy way to hold and manipulate the puppet when in use (Fig. H.1).

Some tips for creating your puppets:

- Try to remove the entire harvested part in one piece.
- Use corn meal to help desiccate the inside surface of the skin.
- Use borax to preserve the tissue.
- Remove the wings at the shoulders before removing the skin. Remove and discard the humerii. Preserve the distal wing sections with borax and allow them to dry in a natural folded position. They can be re-attached to the sides of the puppet using fishing line, wire, or twine.
- In general, remove as much soft tissue and muscle as possible. Remove the eyes, and as much tissue as you can from the oral cavity, neck, and inside the skull. Pack the skull cavity with cotton balls after preserving with borax.
- Remove the bottom half of the plastic bottle. Use a small length of PVC pipe or a wooden dowel rod to create a handle inside the plastic bottle. The handle can be secured to the bottle's screw-on cap which will end up inside the puppet's neck near the base of the skull.
- Once the skinned section is preserved with borax and wrapped around the plastic bottle, let the puppet dry for 2 weeks. It should naturally adhere to the plastic bottle.
- Glue on the eyes. Eyes with the appropriate appearance/iris color can be found online from multiple sources.
- Canned spray foam can be used in small amounts if applied under the skin over the neck and up inside the skull. The foam is quite rigid when it dries, and it will help stiffen the neck and keep it from loosening and/or breaking after use.

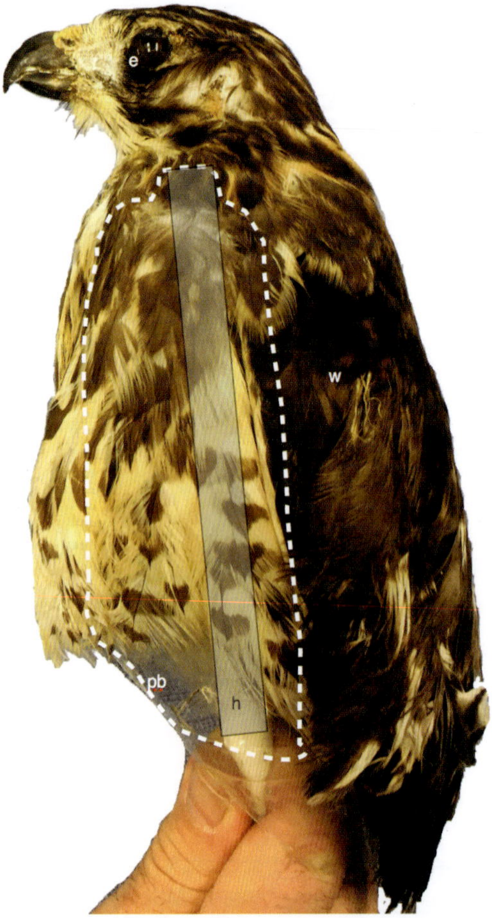

Fig. H.1. A typical feeding puppet: artificial eyes glued into place (e), the wings (w) are secured to the sides of the puppet, the plastic bottle (pb) is outlined. Note that the bottom has been removed. The handle (h) runs up to the neck of the bottle.

Appendix I: Resources

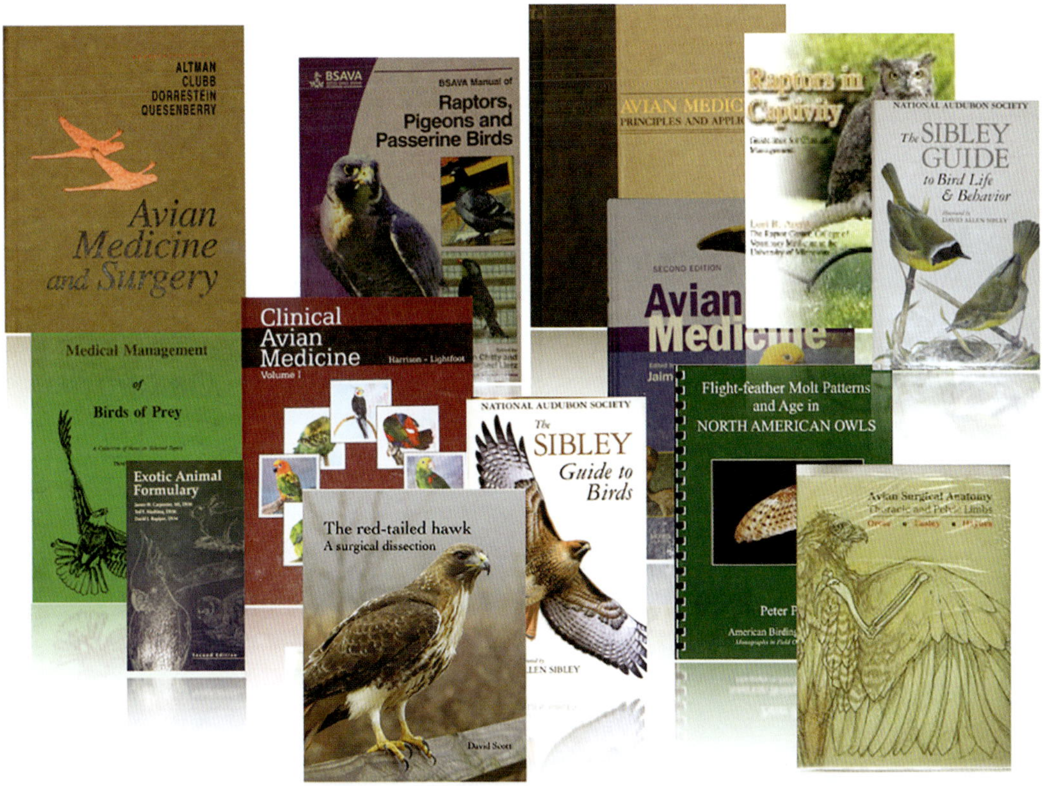

Books

- Altman, R.B., Clubb, S.L., Dorrestein, G.M. and Quesenberry, K. (1997) *Avian Medicine and Surgery*. W.B. Saunders Company, Philadelphia, PA, USA.
- Arent, L. (2007) *Raptors in Captivity: Guidelines for Care and Management*. Hancock House Publishing, Surrey, BC, Canada.
- Campbell, T.W. and Ellis, C.K. (2007) *Avian and Exotic Animal Hematology and Cytology*. Blackwell Publishing, Ames, IA, USA.
- Carpenter, J., Mashima, T. and Rupiper, D. (2001) *Exotic Animal Formulary*, 2nd edn. W.B. Saunders Company, Philadelphia, PA, USA.
- Chitty, L. (2008) *BSAVA Manual of Raptors, Pigeons and Passerine Birds*. BSAVA, Gloucester, UK.

- Harrison, G.J. and Lightfoot, T. (2006) *Clinical Avian Medicine*. Vols I & II. Spix Publishing, Palm Beach, FL, USA.
- Orosz, S.E., Ensley, P.K. and Haynes, C.J. (1992) *Avian Surgical Anatomy: Thoracic and Pelvic Limbs*. W.B. Saunders, Philadelphia, PA, USA.
- Pyle, P. (1997) *Flight-Feather Molt Patterns and Age in North American Owls*. American Birding Association, Colorado Springs, CO, USA.
- Pyle, P. (1997) *Identification Guide to North American Birds. Parts 1 & 2*. Slate Creek Press, Point Reyes, CA, USA.
- Redig, P. (1993) *Medical Management of Birds of Prey*, 3rd edn. The Raptor Center, St. Paul, MN, USA.
- Samour, J. (2008) *Avian Medicine*, 2nd edn. Mosby-Elsevier, Philadelphia, PA, USA.
- Scott, D. (2018) *The Red-tailed Hawk: A Surgical Dissection. Blurb*. Available at: www.blurb.com (accessed June 2020).
- Sibley, D.A. (2000) *The Sibley Guide to Birds*. Alfred A. Knopf, Inc., New York, NY, USA.
- Sibley, D.A. (2001) *The Sibley Guide to Bird Life & Behavior*. Alfred A. Knopf, Inc., New York, NY, USA.

Web Links

- International Association for Falconry and Conservation of Birds of Prey. Available at: https://iaf.org/ (accessed June 2020).
- International Wildlife Rehabilitation Council (IWRC). Available at: www.theiwrc.org (accessed June 2020). This group is very helpful in placing and finding non-releasable animals for permanent placement.
- The Modern Apprentice. Available at: www.themodernapprentice.com (accessed June 2020). This website has an excellent glossary of falconry terminology.
- North American Falconers Association. Available at: www.n-a-f-a.com (accessed June 2020).
- US Fish & Wildlife Service (USFWS). Available at: www.fws.gov (accessed June 2020).
- US Geological Service (USGS) Bird Banding Lab. Available at: https://www.usgs.gov/centers/pwrc/science/bird-banding-laboratory (accessed June 2020). This site distributes the Bandit software.

Suppliers and Products

- Abaxis. Available at: www.abaxis.com (accessed June 2020). VetScan chemistry analyzer.
- Allard USA. Available at: www.allardusa.com (accessed June 2020). X-Lite® Classic cast VTP material.
- Compounded Solutions. Available at: www.compoundedsolutions.com (accessed June 2020). Compounded drugs such as CaEDTA and DMSA.
- IMEX. Available at: www.imexvet.com (accessed June 2020). Orthopedic supplies.
- MiceDirect. Available at: https://micedirect.com/ (accessed June 2020).
- Millbrook. Available at: www.millbrookcrickets.com (accessed June 2020). Crickets and superworms.
- Nanric Inc. Available at: www.nanric.com (accessed June 2020). Advanced Cushion Support™.
- National Band and Tag Company. Available at: https://nationalband.com/ (accessed June 2020). Temporary ID bands.
- Northwoods Falconry. Available at: https://northwoodsfalconry.com (accessed June 2020). All sorts of falconry supplies (gloves, Vitahawk, etc.).
- Prescription Specialties. Available at: www.rxspecialties.com (accessed June 2020). Compounding pharmacy.
- RaptorMed™ software. Available at: www.raptormed.com (accessed June 2020).
- Vitahawk. Available at: www.vitahawk.com (accessed June 2020).
- Zoogen. Available at: www.antechdiagnostics.com (accessed June 2020). DNA sexing.

Index

Note: Page numbers in **bold** type refer to **figures**; page numbers in *italic* type refer to *tables*; page numbers followed by 'a' refer to appendices; page numbers followed by 'n' refer to notes.